HEALTH ADMINISTRATION AND MEDICAL CITIES IN MIDDLE EAST COUNTRIES

Health Tourism and Cultural Issues

HEALTH ADMINISTRATION AND MEDICAL CITIES IN MIDDLE EAST COUNTRIES

Health Tourism and Cultural Issues

DR. R. KUMAR

MBBS, MS, Ex. PGI, Eye Specialist

Author of Books on Health Care, Hospitals, Women Empowerment, NGOs, Social Sciences, Health, Fiction, Biography, etc.

Columnist on Health Education, Medical Tourism and Management.

REGAL

REGAL PUBLICATIONS

New Delhi

HEALTH ADMINISTRATION AND MEDICAL CITIES IN MIDDLE EAST COUNTRIES
Health Tourism and Cultural Issues

ISBN 978-81-8484-240-1

Typeset by
S.S. COMPOSERS
3190, Mohindra Park, Shakur Basti,
Delhi-110034.

Printed in India at
MAYUR ENTERPRISES
WZ Plot No. 3, Gu[illegible] Market, Tihar Village,
New Delhi-110018.

Published by
REGAL PUBLICATIONS
F-159, Rajouri Garden, New Delhi-110027.
Phone: +91-11-45546396, 25435369
E-mail: regalbookspub@yahoo.com, regaldeepbooks@yahoo.com

Contents

Contents

Preface

Modern technologies and outlook, have transformed the globe's vast population into a boundary-less "Global Village Community." From a 'consumer' point of view, it is now possible to take advantage of both cheap airfares and often higher standards or more affordable medical treatment in foreign countries, than those available in their own countries. From a patient perspective, the benefits of global health care are numerous. The Arab nations are facing an unprecedented surge in demand for health care products and services and the same is going to increase in the next few years. Socio-economic development, characterized by increasing income and access to modern amenities and services, has led to changes in the population's nutritional and lifestyle habits, increasing the prevalence of lifestyle-related medical conditions such as obesity, heart disease and diabetes. The expectations of better care, together with growing populations and better-informed patients, are driving investment in hospitals and medical facilities, and pushing up demand for health care services, innovative drugs and the latest medical technologies. With the tightening of immigration rules and security checks, the US has seen a decline in the number of foreign patient visits. More patients, especially those from the Middle-East, are moving towards alternatives like Thailand, Singapore and India.

Medical Cities in the Middle East

Many countries in the Desert are setting up medical cities for providing the very best health care service not only for the growing local population but also for expat workers and patients from across the region. The notable examples are Dubai Health Care City (DHCC), Sheikh Khalifa Medical city (SKMC) Abu Dhabi, King Abdulaziz Medical City (KAMC), Saudi Arabia, Jordan Hospital and several others. However several other countries in the Middle East are struggling with over-burdened government-run health care systems, and are turning to the private sector for much-needed investment and expertise. Given the current economic situation, there does not appear to be any reduction in the appetite for, nor supply of, capital for health care-related projects in the region. It seems that investors are willing to bet that the demographic, economic and social forces driving demand for high quality health care in the Middle East are forthcoming. In fact Middle East has taken giant strides in setting up

Medical cities in their countries and have set-up an example for the rest of the world that medical city model of health care can deliver well for the natives as well as for health tourists from other countries.

Why should the Medical Tourist come to Middle East?

In the past 30 years or so, the costs of health care have soared in developed countries, especially the United States. Americans and, to some extent, the British, Canadians, Australians began to look for ways to reduce these expenses. Certain services and procedures in American hospitals are now being contracted out to Third World countries, from transcriptions of medical records to the reading of X-rays. Medical tourism presents an opportunity for hospitals to fuel economic growth by tapping the potential of the international patient market. To attract foreign patients, health care providers may consider leveraging on both business and clinical considerations. Though cost is the over-riding factor, the wait for surgeries in some developed nations can also be annoying. USA, Canada and Great Britain have reported a surge in the number of people traveling outside the country to avoid long queues in the National Health Service, which can often be for a year or more for some surgical procedures. The South East Asian countries such as Thailand, Malaysia, Singapore, Korea and Philippines are the popular destinations for medical treatment. India is also positioning itself as the primary destination for advanced medical procedures in the world. Some of Indian hospitals are also competing with their Asian peers to get a slice of the cake in the booming health tourism market for international patients. But the Medical cities in the desert have a potential for the people of the region as well as from the East and West, because of huge 'Oil money' being ploughed for improving health care. They have better discipline in various fields and they can employ the best of talent from all over the world.

Oases of Health Care: Lessons from the Desert

As we talk about desert states, it conjure-up the images of traditional backward civilization of warring people with lack of education and health care. Being associated with Chandigarh Medi-city project we traveled to Dubai and Abu Dhabi to have first hand study of health care in UAE in general and the medical cities model in particular. We were simply delighted to see their all round socio-economic development and by the progress made in dispensing health care. While it is difficult to find poor and unemployed people in the desert, we also missed absenteeism, indiscipline, unethical approach, brawls, traffic chaos on the roads and queues of patients in public hospitals. We visited Dubai Health Care City (DHCC) and Abu Dhabi's Sheikh Khalifa Medical City (SKMC). We also learnt about the excellence of King Fahad Medical city in Saudi. Dr. Neerod Jha, a leading cardio-thoracic surgeon in UAE (formerly from PGI Chandigarh) facilitated our visit and study.

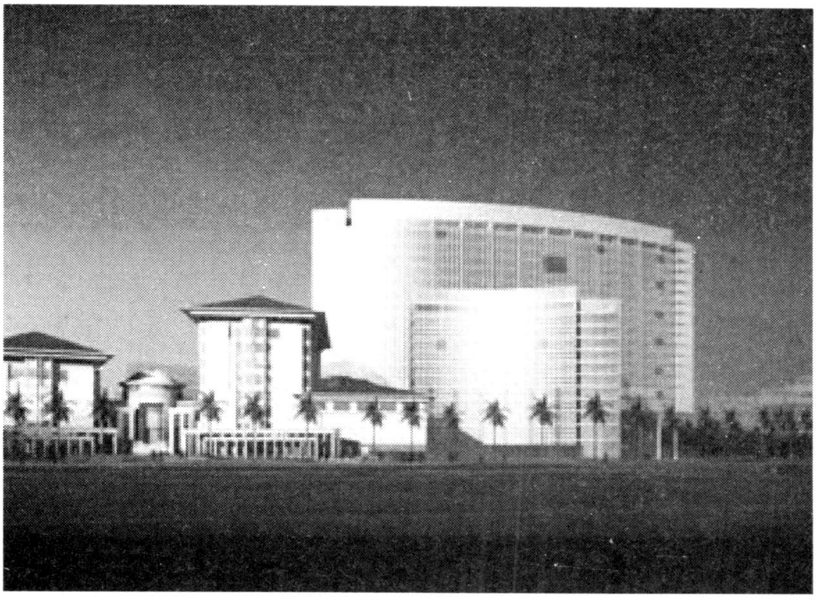

Dubai Health Care City

DHCC is the first medical free zone in the world. It means it is tax free, foreign ownership, no restrictions on capital, no trade barriers or red-tape or pricing control. The DHCC has been planned to provide world class facilities to patients coming from 32 countries of the region, including India. DHCC boasts of two complementary communities, namely, the Medical Community and the Wellness Community. The Medical Community, which focuses on acute care services, occupies 4.1 million square feet. The Wellness Community covers 19 million square feet and completes DHCC`s

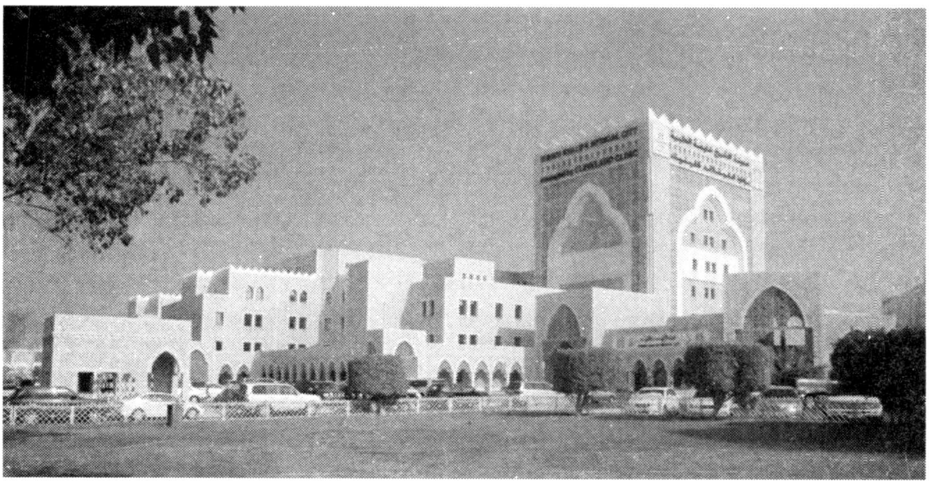

Sheikh Khalifa Medical City (SKMC)

health care continuum by housing hospitals, outpatient clinics, luxury spa resorts and the entire spectrum of wellness services. The Medical Community is also home to medical, dental, nursing and allied health schools. These schools offer Continuous Medical Education courses and postgraduate education. The key members of this community are the Harvard Medical School Dubai Centre and Boston Dental University. Harvard Medical International and DHCC have jointly established the Centre for Health care Planning and Quality (CPQ) as a regulatory body implementing rigorous high quality clinical standards to ensure safe quality patient care. CPQ also plays a major role in planning to ensure an appropriate balance between clinical services within DHCC to meet patient needs, demands and expectations.

Sheikh Khalifa Medical City (SKMC)

Abu Dhabi health authority owns and operates 12 hospital facilities, 2,644 licensed beds, and more than 40 ambulatory and primary health care clinics with more than 16,500 doctors, nurses and other clinical and administrative staff, making it one of the largest employers in the Middle East. SKMC encompasses several 'Centres of Excellence' in Abu Dhabi. It serves as the flagship institution for Abu Dhabi's public health system and is managed by Cleveland Clinic, which is heralded as one of the top hospitals in the USA. It is committed to providing health care that meets international standards through accessibility, affordability, choice, superior physician care, advanced technology and patient satisfaction. It ensures not only optimal levels of patient care and satisfaction but is also promoting general health and well-being through education and awareness. While the best of physicians and surgeons are recruited from all over the world, there is no constraint on their salaries or state of the art equipment. The world class care is absolutely free for the local citizens. The serious or catastrophic ailments do not leave behind any one homeless or orphan.

This book on "Health Tourism and Cultural Issues" focuses on Islamic socio-religious behaviour as well. It has been designed to help doctors, nurses, midwives, health administrators and planners to better comprehend the needs and preferences of the modern day patients/clients living or visiting Gulf countries. The need for specific cultural information on different ethnic groups and people of differing linguistic and religious backgrounds is increasingly important for health care providers and other care givers. The health care professionals in other countries where migrants from the Middle East reside/visit would also find this book useful in meeting with their aspirations.

We have dealt with various issues in the following chapters:

1. Health Care and Cultural Issues in the Middle East.
2. Health Tourism in Middle East: Understanding Ethos of the Locals.

3. Health Care and Health Cities in Qatar and other Gulf Cooperation Council (GCC) Countries.
4. Dubai Health Care City (DHCC): Oases for Health Tourism.
5. Sheikh Khalifa Medical City (SKMC), Abu Dhabi.
6. King Abdulaziz Medical City (KAMC), Saudi Arabia.
7. Medical Cities in Jordan.

Chandigarh DR. R. KUMAR

1

Health Care and Cultural Issues in the Middle East

The Arab nations will face an unprecedented surge in demand for health care products and services in the next few years. Socio-economic development, characterized by increasing income and access to modern amenities and services, has led to changes in the population's nutritional and lifestyle habits, increasing the prevalence of lifestyle-related medical conditions such as obesity, heart disease and diabetes. The expectations of better care, together with growing populations and better-informed patients, are driving investment in hospitals and medical facilities, and pushing up demand for health care services, innovative drugs and the latest medical technologies. Many countries in the region are setting up medical cities for providing the very best health care service not only for the growing local population but also for expatriate workers and patients from across the region. Other countries are struggling with over-burdened government-run health care systems, and are turning to the private sector for much-needed investment and expertise. Given the current economic situation, there does not appear to be any reduction in the appetite for, nor supply of, capital for health care-related projects in the region. It seems that investors are willing to bet that the demographic, economic and social forces driving demand for high quality health care in the Middle East are forthcoming. Reduced public investment at home and a hostile environment of health care cost containment is making the Middle East more attractive to Western health care companies. Zakat, the Islamic principle of charity, is the underlying driving force. As a result, the public and private sectors need to cooperate. Governments are keen to supervise and regulate the health care system to make sure private health care players fully understand and embrace this unique concept and preserve the culture that exists.

The issues

Public sector health care facilities in the region are finding it increasingly difficult to keep up with the growing demands of their people. In Kuwait, the Ministry of Health admitted that nearly 1.6 million patients had switched from public hospitals to private hospitals in 2007 because of the poor quality at government-run hospitals. Unsatisfactory health care has resulted in residents seeking medical treatment abroad. According to Dubai Health Care City officials, Arabian Gulf citizens spend an estimated US $25 billion a year receiving treatment elsewhere. Meanwhile, patients from the region are the life-blood of medical tourism markets such as Singapore. With governments struggling to cope with the changing demographics and onset of chronic diseases, it is clear the public sector now needs to take action.

WHO Ranking of World Health Systems—190 Countries (2000)

Country	*Ranking*
France	1
Oman	8
Saudi Arabia	26
UAE	27
USA	37
Bahrain	42
Qatar	44
Kuwait	45
Malaysia	49
Egypt	63
Jordan	83
Libya	87
Lebanon	91
Iran	93
Iraq	103
Syria	108
India	112
Yemen	120

Source: © World Health Organization.

Poor allocation

Low levels of provision of national wealth to health care is at least partly responsible for the poor quality of health care in the Middle East. Although in some countries, notably Jordan and Lebanon, the proportion of gross domestic product. (GDP) spent on health care is as high as, or higher than, that in more developed economies, in much of the region the figure is very low. Many relatively rich countries such as Saudi Arabia, the UAE

Life Expectancy in Different Countries (F v/s M)

Country	*Female*	*Male*
Bahrain	75	73
Egypt	68	66
France	81	79
India	63	61
Iran	71	68
Iraq	56	67
Jordan	71	70
Kuwait	78	76
Lebanon	70	69
Libya	72	72
Malaysia	72	71
Oman	74	73
Qatar	77	76
Saudi Arabia	70	70
Syria	72	71
UAE	78	76
USA	78	77
Yemen	61	60

Source: © World Health Organization (WHO).

and Kuwait spend a surprisingly small proportion of GDP on health care. Perhaps even more surprisingly, while this proportion rose in most countries between 2000 and 2006, from 2.3 per cent to 4.3 per cent in Qatar for instance, and 5.6 per cent to 6.3 per cent in Egypt, most of the countries that spend the lowest on health care actually saw this proportion fall. Kuwait, for example, spent just 2.2 per cent of GDP on health care in 2006, down from 3.1 per cent in 2000. In absolute terms there is no reductions in health care investment. Health care spending has in fact risen in nominal and per capita terms in nearly all the countries of the region. In many countries, however, this increase was combined with high rates of economic growth. For instance in Kuwait, per capita health spending actually increased by 52 per cent between 2000 and 2006, from US $523 to US $796, but in the same period fell by 29 per cent as a proportion of GDP.

Government led privatization programmes are now being used to address these issues. For instance, Oman has one of the most efficient health systems in the world, with a government that advises and strongly supports the private sector.

There is a severe shortage of trained medical workers in the region. This shortage has become particularly acute in the Gulf Cooperation Council (GCC) countries, as the investment in health care cities and other new health care facilities increases the demand for medical workers.

Historically, the GCC states have responded by recruiting foreign medical staff, mainly from the West, but increasingly from the Indian sub-continent and the Philippines. In some places, it is virtually impossible to find a local medical practitioner—for instance in Qassim province, north of Riyadh, just 2 per cent of practicing physicians are Saudi nationals. Bahrain on the other hand has a long history of medical training and employs a comparatively high proportion of nationals in health care. Bahrain has set-up its own medical education infrastructure, including a medical school owned and operated by the Royal College of Surgeons in Ireland. Other Gulf governments are following suit, investing in the development of medical education and training programmes for nationals, and recruiting the services of internationally recognized health care brands. Dubai has attracted Harvard Medical School to Dubai Health Care City (DHCC), while Qatar is building a specialty teaching hospital run in association with Weill Cornell Medical College in its US $2.3 billion Sidra Medical and Research Centre in Doha.

In Saudi Arabia, the government announced plans to recruit 13,000 family doctors by the end of 2010, partly through sending nationals abroad for training while it builds more teaching hospitals, with the help of private investment. It has also announced its intention to increase capacity in the five established medical schools, increase the opportunities for scholarships in various health specialties, and enlarge the base of medical postgraduate studies in the country. Countries such as Saudi Arabia have a large base of citizens to train and compete with their foreign counterparts. But in other GCC countries, and in particular the UAE, there is an insufficient local population willing and able to undertake the training required to generate the extra health care professionals. These countries will continue to rely on expatriate workers to staff their medical facilities. But expats are extremely mobile, and high global demand for health care workers raises the risk of them leaving for better opportunities elsewhere. To make a success of the investment being poured into the health care cities and elsewhere, governments will need to find ways to retain experienced personnel and reduce staff turnover.

Private expenditure high

As per The WHO statistics on private expenditure on health, private sector accounted for the highest proportion of overall health care expenditure in Egypt, where it produced 59 per cent of spend in 2006. The vast majority of this (95 per cent) was out-of-pocket spending, indicating the low provision of health insurance in Egypt. Lebanon also had a large private health sector in 2006 although Lebanon's share shrank from 70 per cent of the market in 2000 to 53 per cent in 2006. In Qatar, the government has encouraged the private sector to play a greater role in providing health care, with the opening of the first private hospital in 1999. However, in recent years the government has been investing its oil wealth in publicly funded and operated health care facilities, causing private sector involvement to fall from 31 per cent in 2000 to just 27 per cent in 2006. Meanwhile, in Saudi Arabia and Kuwait, the influence of the private sector remained stable from, while in the UAE it grew from 21 per cent of spending in 2000 to 27 per cent in 2006.

GCC member-states, in particular, have been looking to the private sector to take a more active role in the financing and provision of health care in the public sector, thus blurring the lines between public and private provision. The governments of these countries are using sovereign wealth funds such as Dubai Holding or Abu Dhabi's Mubadala Development Company to build the much-needed health care infrastructure. For example, the new Dubai Health Care City, a US $3 billion development by Tatweer, a subsidiary of Dubai Holding, is expected to add 17 hospitals, with 2,325 new beds, at the same time as welcoming medical tourists.

Saudi Arabia is also committed to increasing the role of the private sector. In January 2006, expatriate health insurance became mandatory for all firms employing more than 500 foreigners, and in 2008 was extended to all expatriate workers. The scheme is intended to be expanded to encompass all Saudi nationals, but this has proved controversial. From January 2009 affordable health insurance was made available to all Dubai residents. Bahrain is also planning on introducing compulsory health insurance for expatriates, and therefore shift some treatments to the private sector. In the past, countries which have part or fully-privatized their health care systems have experienced many difficulties. In Malaysia, for instance, the main thrust of health care reform since 1980 has encouraged greater private sector involvement, and this has resulted in an increase in the number and variety of private hospitals and clinics. The Malaysian government has for several decades been contemplating the introduction of a national health insurance scheme to replace tax revenue and out-of-pocket spending as the main source of financing for the health care system, but has so far failed to make any progress.

Arab culture, ethos and health care

Arab World has 21 different countries, numerous sub-cultures, and religious and ethnic minorities. A great danger lies in the misuse of a little knowledge without critical thought. Diversity exists in every group of humans. Each individual needs to be assessed along a scale of acculturation. We must avoid jumping to assumptions. Just because a person wears traditional ethnic dress may not mean that they lack English language skills or if a women wears traditional clothing that she does not work outside the home. And the converse may be true of someone wearing typical western clothing. No one wants to admit that we may suffer from cultural insensitivity, cultural blindness, or in the worse case, harbor negative stereotypes and prejudice.

Ethos and cultural mores conceive of sickness in terms of the perceptions and experiences of patients. As individuals grow up in society, they are taught how to label their sickness experiences; they learn the cultural explanations of these conditions, the standard treatments, and the appropriate responses to others with the same conditions. It is the patient's experiences that define the distinction of normal and abnormal function. Modern health care practice needs study of Arab ethos and culture, to make the delivery and accessibility more effective. The myths, stereotyping, and ignorance about Islamic culture stand in the way of providing quality health care to Arab patients.

Health and Healing in the Middle East

The sciences of health and healing among the Arabs is a tradition with roots in the earliest of recorded history. In the 7th century AD, Islamic civilization emerged from the Arabian Peninsula, expanding east and west and ultimately extending from Morocco and Spain (Andalusia) across the spice route to China.

This emerging civilization synthesized wide ranging ancient Greek, Turkish, Indian, Persian, and indigenous Arab traditions within an Islamic framework, producing a comprehensive, analytic and scientific system of healing. Arab medical texts were among the foundations of the Western modern medical tradition; the canon of Ibn Sina formed half of the medical curriculum of European medical schools until the mid-17th century (*Ibid.*: 196-97). Microbial diseases were identified in a basic fashion (named madah) within Arabic medicine, and were described in terms of mode of infection and particular pathological effects on organs and tissue. Numerous internal and external etiologies were identified. Islamic medicine followed the system of humoral pathology developed by Hippocrates.

Fire, air, water, and earth : basis of health and disease

This healing system envisions the body in terms of humors—blood, phlegm, yellow bile, and black bile, corresponding to the elements of the natural world—fire, air, water, and earth. Each bodily humor possesses two natures. For example, blood is considered hot and moist, phlegm cold and moist, yellow bile hot and dry, and black bile cold and dry. The body brings together these four elements, and when this mixture is in equilibrium the human body is in a state of health.

Traditional cures were generally aimed at countering an excess or deficiency in one of the humors. For example, a particular problem might be described as an excess of cold and moisture that has invaded a particular humor or organ system. Pharmaceutical extractions might be prescribed and particular foods, spices, and teas might be taken to heat this system and to rebalance the humoral disunity. Beliefs about hot and cold effects on the bodily humors are maintained to varying degrees among Arabs as part of the transmitted cultural folk wisdom. (See Appendix attached to this chapter, to know more about the concept of disease in middle east).

Early history of wellness in Islam

A fountainhead of medical wisdom during the Islamic era, al-Razi, was a fine teacher and a compassionate physician, who brought rations to the poor and provided nursing for them. He was also a man devoted to common sense. al-Kindi, the first Muslim philosopher to use Aristotelian logic to support Islamic dogma, also wrote on logic, philosophy, geometry, calculation, arithmetic, music, and astronomy, Cause of Vertigo, etc. Ibn al-Haytham, wrote, 'The Book of Optics', in which he gives a detailed treatment of the anatomy of the eye, correctly deducing that the eye receives light from the object perceived and laying the foundation for modern photography. Agricultural advances are also part of the Muslim legacy. Important books were written on soil analysis, water, and what kinds of crops were suited to what soil. Because there was considerable interest in new varieties—for nutritive and medicinal purposes. The 'Abbasids, were forced to develop extensive trade to obtain food, e.g. Baghdad had to import wheat from Syria and Egypt, rice from the Fayyum in Egypt, southern Morocco, and Spain, and olive oil from Tunisia. To obtain scarce metals the 'Abbasids had to turn elsewhere. They imported the technologically advanced "ondanique" steel from India, and then processed it at such famous centres of weapons manufacture as Damascus and Toledo, both of which cities won fame for their blades. The 'Abbasids also imported iron from Europe, tin from the British Isles and Malaya, and silver from northern Iran, Afghanistan, and the Caucuses. For these necessities the 'Abbasid traders exchanged a wide variety of products: pearls, livestock, paper, sugar, and luxurious cloth. The cloth trade produced a number of auxiliary exports: gold and silver thread for embroidery, gum from the Sudan for glazing, and needles, looms, and dyestuffs. Closely connected with the trade in dyestuffs was the trade in medicines, an offshoot of 'Abbasid advances in medicine and the spread of hospitals in all major Islamic cities. As scientific research and translation of medical texts from India and possibly even China expanded the earlier pharmacopoeia, ingredients for medicines were brought from all over the known world.

The first hospital in the Islamic world

It was established as early as the 7th century in Damascus to help lepers, the blind, and disabled (Hamarneh, 1983:178). This hospital utilized sophisticated methods of admission, discharge, record keeping, and administration. The hospitals attracted gifted students and were generously endowed by rich patrons (*Ibid.*: 179). Hospitals also served as schools of medicine to teach interns and residents. Through this system, an impressive method of testing and licensing doctors with rules and regulations for standards of practice was developed. Medical treatment relied primarily on exercise, baths, and diet and its modification. By the 13th century Ibnal-Bitar had recorded over 1300 drugs that were derived from plants, animals, or minerals. Surgical techniques were known and utilized. Techniques were employed for fractures, treatment of trauma, and obstetrics. A number of

Arab physicians compiled textbooks and case histories compendiums in the process of their professional duties. The golden age of Islamic medicine extended from the 9-12th centuries. Islamic medicine did not disappear at the end of the Middle Ages with the unseating of the Arabic empire. It continued in the form of traditional healers following the Unani or Greco-Islamic system.

The traditional health system of Arabs is still present to varying degrees throughout the Middle East, though today, the number of adept practitioners (hakim) of the traditional Islamic medical system are few. The traditional medical system is more pervasive in rural regions, while in the cities, Western technological medicine is now almost exclusively utilized. In other nations with significantly strong Islamic medical traditions, India and Pakistan state regulations have allowed practitioners to be licensed after completion of special four year courses, where the curriculum includes the Canon of Avinciena.

Health and evil spirits

Some health disorders are attributed to unseen forces, most commonly jinn, or evil spirits. Mental disorders in particular are often attributed to the disruptive influence of these spirits. The traditional view understands the human consciousness within this realm as a non- local entity, subject to influencing and being influenced by the thoughts and intentions of other individuals (human and jinn). There is a widespread belief that bad intentions toward a person can cause illness. The evil eye is said to affect a person when another individual is envious toward them, either knowingly or unknowingly. People are particularly aware of the evil eye around children. Turquoise pendants or verses from holy books are commonly worn. When a person complements a child, care is taken to mention God in the compliment so as to exclude jealousy that might make the child ill. These beliefs are ubiquitous in the Middle East and should be understood as an important part of the traditional world view to which disease causality is often attributed. It must be understood that the assumptions about health and illness held by Arabs is embedded in this time-held traditional system.

Health Context of the Modern Middle East

It is important for health practitioners to understand the Middle Eastern medical context in their Arab patients' countries of origin. Throughout the Arab World today, the Western allopathic system of medicine is widely available, often through a socialized government system. Public health and health education tend to be limited in the Arab nations. The idea of preventive care is an unknown luxury. Moreover, health education is highly limited. The general level of public awareness about health issues tends to be low.

Traditional Sector

Alongside the Western medical services are a number of traditional practitioners for particular health needs. These practitioners are not officially established and certified by state, but tend to exist in many areas as individual practitioners who have apprenticed and learned their skill from other expert lay practitioners. For example, traditional bone-setters are still considered effective healers for broken bones and some people even view their services as superior to the Western method of bone-setting. Similarly, mid-wives in the Levant continue to be skilled attendants for birth. Birth in the hospital, however, is considered more prestigious.

Service Sector Structure

In general, there are two distinct types of health providers in the Arab world: the government and the private providers. The government system is the largest of the sectors. These services are funded by general taxes and are established on the basis of a social insurance system. Government services are usually open for everybody, but the quality, efficiency, and effectiveness of this system is markedly inferior to private services.

Private services are perceived to be of better quality and impart higher social status. Health ministries in the Middle East, in general, have a strong urban bias in their priority distribution of medical and health services geographically. Practically all comprehensive secondary and tertiary care is provided in the city. Doctors tend to think that city practice is more prestigious and a greater experience than is rural practice. Residents from rural areas generally visit the rural primary care centres for most conditions, and only travel to the city for care when they are very sick.

Among the basic pillars of the religion that a health professional would be most likely to encounter is the Islamic prayer and fasting. Prayer is required in Islam five times a day (before sunrise, noon, mid-day, sundown, and night-time), and must be preceded by a ritual ablution. This ablution is called wudu' and Islam stipulates that the performance of this washing include intention to purify one's bad acts and the washing of the mouth, nose, face, ears, back of the neck, hands, arms up to the elbows, and feet to the ankles. Prayer includes the recitation of certain Qur'anic verses and series of prostrations to God in the direction of Mecca (East). Sick patients who are unable to pray with full prostrations are allowed to pray sitting up in a chair or bed, and if that is not possible, then allowed to pray in the position from which they cannot move. Obligations are removed when health is threatened. Keeping this in mind health care professionals should be aware and respectful of these needs for prayer should a Muslim patient want to exercise his or her religious obligations. Clinical staff should not be taken aback if a patient asks them, "which way is east?", and staff may even volunteer this information if they know the patient is religious.

Fast for health

An additional pillar encountered by health professionals is the fast. Muslims observe a month long period of fasting from any sexual activity, food, or drink from dawn until dusk daily, as stipulated by the Qu'ran during the lunar month of Ramadan. Fasting is considered a method of both physical and spiritual purification and as a means to annually re-acquaint the observer with the physical sensation of hunger to foster empathy toward the poor. Because Muslims follow a lunar calendar year, the time of year that this month occurs by the solar calendar each year varies. Muslims are exempt from the fast if they are traveling or if their health is jeopardized. Women are not required to fast during menstruation or forty days postpartum. Fasting is dictated by medical considerations while women are pregnant or nursing. Despite their illness, the Muslim patient may attempt to fast during this month. This fasting would involve the refusal of any food, drink or other substance (including pharmaceuticals) from before sunrise to after sunset. This would involve the refusal of I.V.s, tablets and enemas. If this appears to be a life threatening situation, health care practitioners may talk with an elder in the patient's family or an Imam from the community Mosque who may persuade the patient that in his or her current state fasting is not appropriate. For the Muslim patient observing the fast, a light meal (suhour) before dawn should be provided. At the time of sunset, a larger meal is taken (iftar) and this meal is often eaten with a group of other Muslims.

Public Health in the Arab World

Public health is notably under-developed in many Arab countries. Epidemiological data is difficult to obtain due to the lack of consistent medical charting and absence of health information collection at the state level. There is little widespread public discourse about health (e.g. cancer prevention or early detection screening, cholesterol, high-fat diet) putting the entire health sector at a disadvantage. Mental illness is a condition that is highly shunned in the Middle East. While Islamic norms dictate kindness and care be given to the mentally ill, Arab social norms tend to approach mental illness with fear and social avoidance. It might be said of the ill person that he is touched by demons (jinn) or that God is punishing him.

Both chronic diseases, and mental illness are viewed as a matter of shame with this Context. An example was an Arabic woman who refused further diagnostic work-up after having mammogram suggestive of malignancy. Her refusal was based in her belief that if it is known that she is going to the clinic for evaluation of breast cancer her daughter would be undesirable to other families in the community as a marital partner. Sick individual would often prefer to hide than to seek care and face open disclosure of the 'defect'.

The age of marriage for women is low and many Arab women have married during their teenage years. Marriage is often arranged to secure wealth within a family. Thus, while marriage between two first cousins may be considered incestuous in the modern context, it will be socially acceptable in Arabic contexts. The most common form of familial marriage is between paternal first cousins. The average rate for inter-marriages for most Arabic countries is about 40%. This practice may predispose some groups to genetic disorders including certain hemoglobinopathies (Teebi, 1997).

Polygyny not frequently practiced

While Polygyny is allowed in the words of Qu'ran, it is not frequently practiced. Less than 5% of Muslim men had more than one wife (Deeb and Sayegh, 1997). Divorce is very rare among Arabs, especially in rural areas since marriage is viewed as a relationship between two hammulas rather than two individuals. The man is required to pay for food, clothing, and shelter for his wife and children, and failure to do so is grounds for dissolution of the marriage contract. Some scholars, even recognize sexual dissatisfaction as fair grounds for acceptance of a woman's divorce petition, thus alleviating the possibility that the woman will seek satisfaction outside of the marriage and create a serious social ill. The Prophet was reported to have said "with Allah, the most detestable of all things permitted is divorce". Non-religious factors also discourage divorce. Important among these is the economic loss involved in a divorce case. Divorce is also considered a shameful act among the Arabs, and individuals worry that once they divorce, it will be difficult to remarry. This is reflected in an attitude that "if she was worthwhile, her husband would not have divorced her". A reciprocal, though not as prominent, attitude looks down on the divorced man.

Pregnancy is celebrated

The pregnant mother is given a lot of attention from members of the family and community. A woman is often seen to be truly mature by other women only after bearing a child. Infertility within the context of marriage is viewed as a mark of shame rather than a medical condition. It can ultimately be the cause of marital separation due to the level of pressure applied by the couple's extended families. Family pressure, similarly, tends to create strong incentive for large numbers of children. The birth and care of children, especially males (who act as future means of security for the parents) play a very important role in Arab culture. As a general principle, all children born in wedlock are regarded as legitimate and viewed as gifts from God. A well-developed system of etiquette is present within the Arab family for relationships between parent and child. In general, children are highly obedient to their parents and view this obedience as a lifelong commitment that supersedes all other social commitments, including marital allegiance. Discipline of the child tends to be punishment-oriented rather than reward-oriented. In Arab norms, light physical discipline and strong verbal reprimands of the child or even screaming at the child is considered proper parenting and is viewed as correcting the child's etiquette (adib al-walad) rather than being seen as violence.

As-salaamu alaykum: wa-alaykum as-salaam

In general, the well-being of the child is of concern and the fulfilment of educational and economic needs of the child is considered of great importance. Once the child is about age seven, it is the father who becomes the most important disciplinarian in the child's life. The child is expected to rise and offer his/her seat to an older person, to talk in a respectful manner, and to kiss the hand of the elder when introduced to him. Generosity is an important behavioural norm transmitted to children. Emphasis is also placed on bravery for male children. Children are expected to courteously greet everyone that they meet regardless of whether the person is known. The phrase used in this respect is "as-salaamu alaykum" (peace be upon you) which is answered with "wa alaykum as-salaam wa rahmatu Allah wa barakatuh" (and upon you peace and God's mercy and blessings). The growing child has to learn to subordinate his wishes to his family.

Sex outside marriage is considered a social evil

The sex impulse in both men and women is strictly suppressed before marriage. Sexual relations outside of marriage are considered a great social ill and a behaviour that is divisive and undermines societal stability. As such, premarital and extra-marital sexual relations are considered highly shameful and blameworthy. Girls are expected to be virgins (physically intact) at their marriage. If either a man or woman is found to be unchaste, harm and shame comes to that individual and his/her family. On one occasion a pediatrician asked his adolescent patient, a 14 year-old, Arab girl, if she had sex. The mother, upon hearing this question became irate at her daughter thinking that because the doctor asked this question he must believe that she had intercourse. It took several days to calm the family and the girl was still obviously upset. Polygamy is the exception, not the rule in the Arab community.

The social dimension of health care

Many of the region's most prestigious hospitals and health centres owe their existence to such charitable organizations, predating the establishment of health ministries and other state-level institutions. A large number of health facilities, ranging from outpatient clinics to hospitals, are still run by charitable groups, and many more are being built. Egypt's Cairo Children's Cancer Hospital, which opened to patients in 2007, is an example of a medical project funded entirely by charitable donations.

The health care sector is uniquely positioned at the heart of business, social and community life, and as such should be an example of responsible business. A good example is the Saudi-German Hospital Group, which as well as several hospitals in place or in development throughout the region, operates several not-for-profit entities in health care, including the Jeddah Chairy Blood Bank and the Health Management Research Institute, a collaboration with the Indian Institute of Health Management

Research. By helping to build physical and human resources, private players can support disease prevention, diagnosis, treatment and care, and support community-based efforts to train and educate health care professionals.

Egypt

Egypt's health care system is run by many different public and private providers, with private sector facilities concentrated in Cairo and in other large cities. Unlike some of its neighbours, Egypt does not suffer from medical staff shortages. Half the population is covered by basic government health insurance, with the rest being either enrolled in private insurance schemes or uninsured. Although basic primary health care services are offered free of charge and hospital services in public hospitals are free for the uninsured, the geographical coverage and the quality of care received is not consistent. So, citizens increasingly seek outpatient care in expensive private facilities, which are perceived as providing better services. However, this would not be the case, if a reasonably-priced universal insurance was available. Economic growth rates together with an aging and growing population, which is expected to reach 83 million by 2013, are driving health care reforms. A change of attitude by the public is also needed towards paying for health services (which will come if services are improved). Privatization could help deliver high quality facilities and run services, and this would be paid for by social insurance.

United Arab Emirates

The rapid population growth being experienced by the UAE, driven mainly by the influx of expatriate workers, has placed huge pressure on its health care infrastructure. There are now some 65 hospitals in the UAE, up from just seven in the 1970s. This phenomenal growth was originally driven by the public sector. In recent years, the private sector has taken up the running with around half the hospitals in the UAE, including the dozen or so hospitals in DHCC (a number that is due to grow to 17 by 2010). According to a report the number of hospital beds in Dubai is expected to nearly double from 2,934 in 2007 to 5,415 in 2010, with most of this increase in capacity being provided by the private sector.

UAE nationals enjoy free health care under the thiqa health insurance scheme, enrolment is free of charge for Abu Dhabi citizens. DAMAN has already led to increased demand for health services and products. The partnership with Munich Re is typical of the approach being adopted in the UAE. This approach is exemplified by Dubai Health Care City (DHCC) and Du-Biotech, which have been established as 'free zones', actively encouraging international companies to introduce the latest approaches to the delivery of health services, as well as making investments in medical education and research and development (R&D).

DHCC has attracted many international health care brands, including Harvard Medical School, the Mayo Clinic and Great Ormond Street

Hospital, as well as leading pharmaceutical and medical technology suppliers such as Johnson and Johnson, Novartis and Novo Nordisk. As part of their vision, DOHMS has initiated laws making it mandatory for all health care facilities in Dubai to attain international accreditation by 2010 or face closure.

Companies locating in the Du-Biotech Park receive 100 per cent exemption on corporate and personal tax guaranteed for 50 years, 100 per cent ownership of their business, 100 per cent repatriation of capital and profits, no currency restrictions, support services, simplified incorporation, and a fast-track visa-application process. Du-Biotech has already attracted over 40 companies active in R&D, scientific discovery, clinical testing, manufacturing, sales and distribution, as well as business support and legal services, and venture capital firms, among others.

Saudi Arabia

Saudi Arabia is by far the largest health care market in the Middle East, with a total health care spend valued at over US $15 billion per annum. Some three quarters of this currently comes from government spending, a proportion that is generally recognized as being unsustainable, with demand growing and government revenues constrained by falling oil revenues. This will mean a much greater role for the private sector in health care, which has been identified as one of the key sectors to be targeted in the government's privatization programme.

Under the plan, which was first unveiled in 2002, the hospitals would either be sold outright or leased out under a management contract. A further 2,000 hospitals and clinics that are planned or under construction will be established under a fund to be set-up and monitored, but not controlled by the Ministry of Health, as part of a gradual shift by the Ministry to become a regulator rather than provider.

This will provide opportunities for private providers. Saudi Arabia is another participant in the vogue for 'health care cities' in the Gulf region. The Kingdom has already established the 1400-bed King Fahd Medical City (KFMC), which it claims is the largest medical complex in the Middle East, in Riyadh. The King Abdullah Medical City (KAMC) will house three 500-bed hospitals, with the first due to open to patients in the second half of 2009. No big international names are involved, and no plans to promote the developments for medical tourism.

Saudi Arabia does already have a unique medical tourism offering, being the gateway to the holy sites of Mecca and Medina. During the Hajj, many pilgrims combine the trip with treatment in the clinics of Jeddah, and over this period the city's dental, medical and cosmetic surgery clinics experience a huge surge. Demand for health care services will be driven by the rapidly expanding and aging local population, which is predicted to grow from just under 25 million today to nearly 29 million in 2013, with the number of over-60s increasing from about a million today to 2.5 million in 2020. And as the population grows bigger, it will become more susceptible to chronic lifestyle diseases. Already some 20 per cent of Saudi nationals over the age of 20 suffer from type-2 diabetes, due to poor diet and sedentary lifestyles. According to the WHO there will be 2.5 million diabetes sufferers in Saudi Arabia by 2030, a much greater absolute number than anywhere else in the region.

By 2025 the need for hospital beds will more than double to about 165,000, and "treatment demand" will rise 240 per cent, predicts McKinsey. Health care costs will rise five-fold to US $60 bn. In fact, a potent combination of high population growth, rapid economic growth and openness to global capital, expertise and innovation will make the Middle East a major growth centre for the health care market over the next few years. The UAE will continue to be the main focus for foreign investment in hospitals and medical facilities, insurance and consultancy services, as PPPs are formed to deliver leading health care services demanded by locals and expatriate workers alike.

There may also be the opportunity to work in other GCC countries, such as Bahrain, Qatar and Kuwait. Some of the biggest opportunities are likely to be found in health care infrastructure projects, which have already attracted companies such as General Electric (GE) and Siemens, both of which have large infrastructure businesses as well as being major suppliers of health care IT and diagnostic imaging technologies. GE has already opened their new headquarters in Dubai Internet City, as well as a production facility in Saudi Arabia, manufacturing diagnostic imaging systems.

Leading international biotech companies, including Amgen and Genzyme, have already set-up operations in Du-Biotech, and smaller players seem certain to join them. Whether this will be enough to create 'critical mass' and establish a cluster to rival those around Boston, Massachusetts, or Research Triangle Park in North Carolina, remains to be seen—there is a lot of global competition for biotech talent and funds. Nevertheless, the ambition and drive to succeed is certainly there, and Dubai has an admirably positive 'build it and they will come' attitude, which has already worked in other sectors.

The lack of government experience in running large and complex health insurance schemes will provide openings for international insurance players, either by partnering with governments to create and run a scheme from the start, or by providing services on an outsourced basis. Certain key functions such as claims processing and management will be able to tap into a strong international outsourcing industry of specialist companies, but others will have to be provided on the ground, often for regulatory reasons.

In addition to the market for health care products and health care-related services, there will be a growing market for regulatory consultancy services as the region's governments struggle to adapt international best practices to local organizational, legislative and legal frameworks.

The ministry of health is responsible for the supervision of health care and hospitals in both the public and private sectors. The system offers universal health care coverage. The health care system has two tiers. One is a network of primary health care centres and clinics that provide preventive, prenatal, emergency, and basic services, as well as mobile clinics for remote rural areas. The second tier is represented by the hospitals and specialized treatment facilities located in urban areas.

Gross Domestic Product: Current Prices

(US $ billion)

Location	2008	2009	2010	2011	2012
Bahrain	21.2	18.1	19.9	21.6	23.4
Egypt	162.2	188.1	203.8	227.8	254.3
France	2,865.7	2,499.2	2,527.6	2,811.7	2,716.9
India	1,209.7	1,185.7	1,234.0	1,323.2	1,441.1
Iran	344.8	343.0	374.2	401.5	425.0
Iraq	90.9	68.6	80.5	91.9	102.8
Jordan	20.0	21.7	23.3	25.0	26.8
Kuwait	158.9	106.2	121.2	133.5	143.5
Lebanon	28.9	31.3	33.2	35.6	37.9
Libya	100.1	62.9	74.0	84.9	96.6
Malaysia	222.2	212.5	220.7	235.4	254.5
Oman	52.6	43.1	49.0	54.6	59.9
Qatar	102.3	99.7	133.3	157.0	170.8
Saudi Arabia	481.6	374.0	423.8	468.7	512.5
Syria	54.8	52.8	58.5	64.5	70.6
UAE	260.1	215.2	235.5	256.9	280.8
USA	14,264.6	14,002.7	14,050.8	14,633.1	15,390.0
Yemen	27.2	28.7	35.0	40.8	46.9

Population *(Million)*

Location	2008	2009	2010	2011	2012
Bahrain	0.8	0.85	0.8	0.8	0.8
Egypt	75.0	76.5	78.1	79.6	81.2
France	62.3	62.6	62.9	63.2	63.5
India	1,190.5	1,207.5	1,224.4	1,241.2	1,257.8
Iran	72.9	74.1	75.4	76.6	77.9
Iraq	30.4	31.2	32.0	32.8	33.6
Jordan	5.9	6.0	6.1	6.3	6.4
Kuwait	3.4	3.5	3.6	3.7	3.8
Lebanon	3.8	3.8	3.9	4.0	4.0
Libya	6.2	6.3	6.5	6.6	6.7
Malaysia	27.3	27.8	28.2	28.7	29.2
Oman	2.8	2.8	2.8	2.9	2.9
Qatar	1.1	1.2	1.4	1.5	1.7
Saudi Arabia	24.9	25.5	26.2	26.8	27.6
Syria	19.9	20.4	20.9	21.4	21.9
UAE	4.8	4.9	5.1	5.2	5.4
USA	304.4	307.4	310.5	313.6	316.7
Yemen	23.0	23.7	24.4	25.1	25.9

Source: IMF Economic Outlook Database (estimated), April 2009.

In 1970, the first of the government's five-year plans to promote development in a variety of areas, including health care, was instituted. In health care, the plan only meant establishing the necessary infrastructure of hospitals, clinics, pharmacies, laboratories, and research facilities, but hiring expatriate staff to work in the facilities and encouraging Saudis to pursue careers in the health care field. In 1970, there were 74 hospitals with 9,039 beds; by 2005, there were 350 hospitals with nearly 48,000 beds. The Ministry of Health operates 62% of the hospitals and 53% of the clinics and centres; the remaining facilities are operated by government agencies, including the Ministry of Defense, the National Guard, the Ministry of the Interior, and several other ministries, as well as by private entities.

Total Expenditure on Health as Percentage of Gross Domestic Product (%)

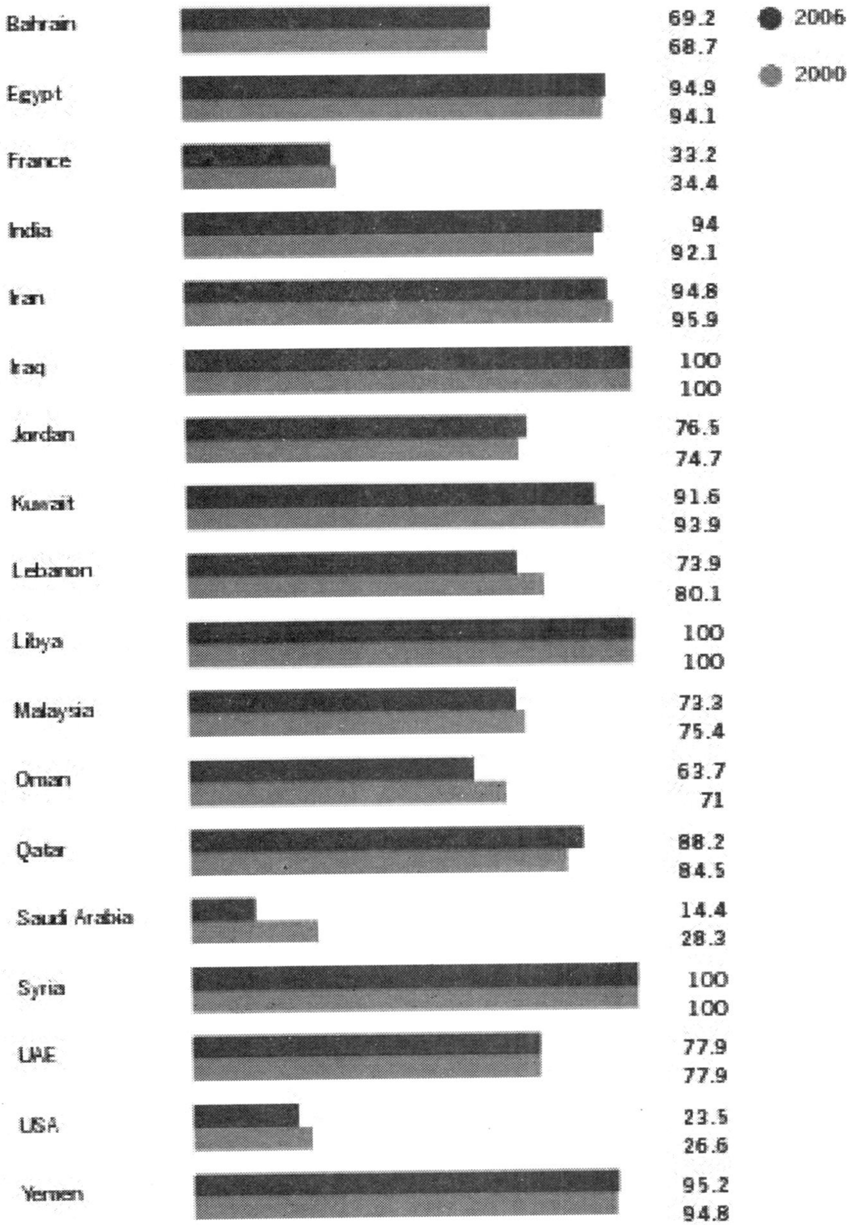

Source: þ World Health Organisation (WHO).

Private Prepaid Pland as Percentage of Private Expenditure on Health (%)

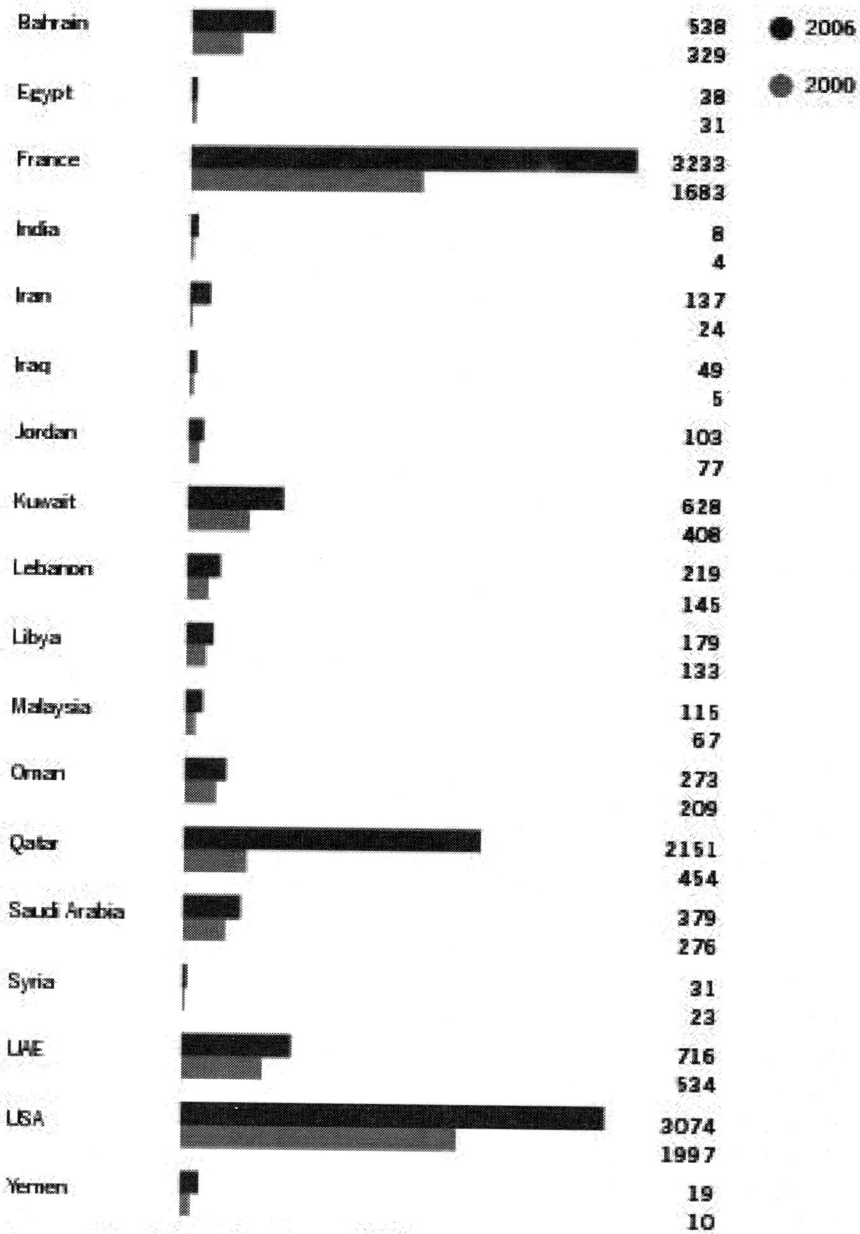

Source: þ World Health Organisation (WHO).

Out-of-pocket Expenditure as Percentage of Private Expenditure on Health (%)

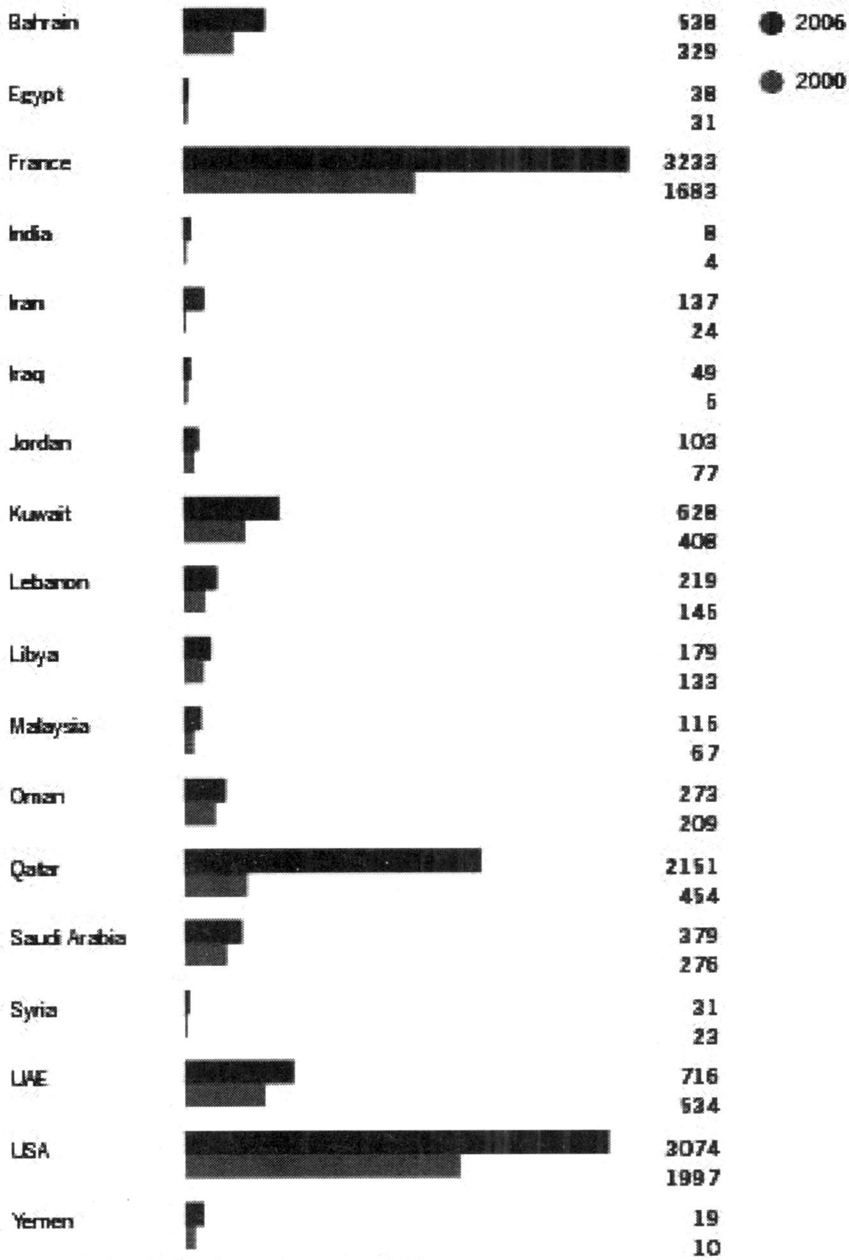

Source: World Health Organisation (WHO).

Per Capita Government Expenditure on Health at Average Exchange Rate (US $)

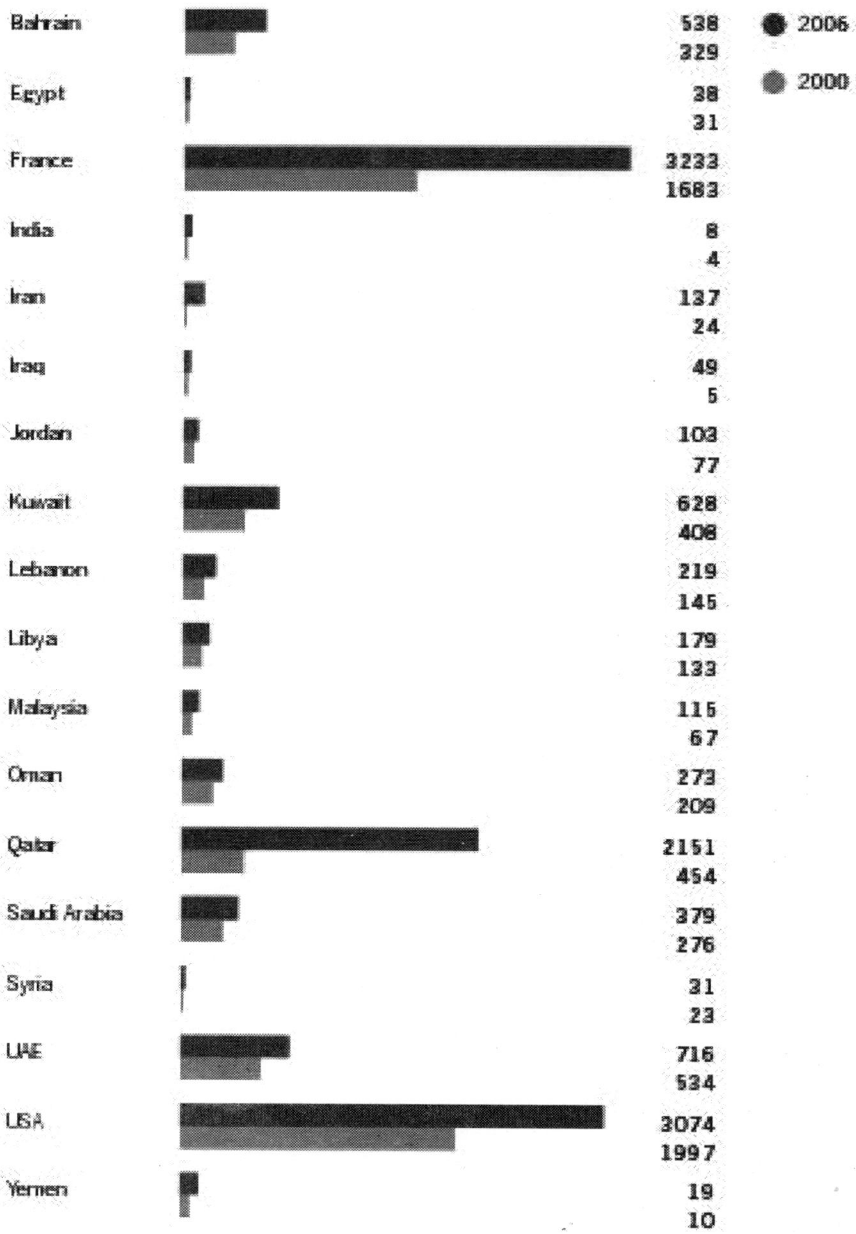

Source: þ World Health Organisation (WHO).

Total Expenditure on Health at Average Exchange Rate (US $)

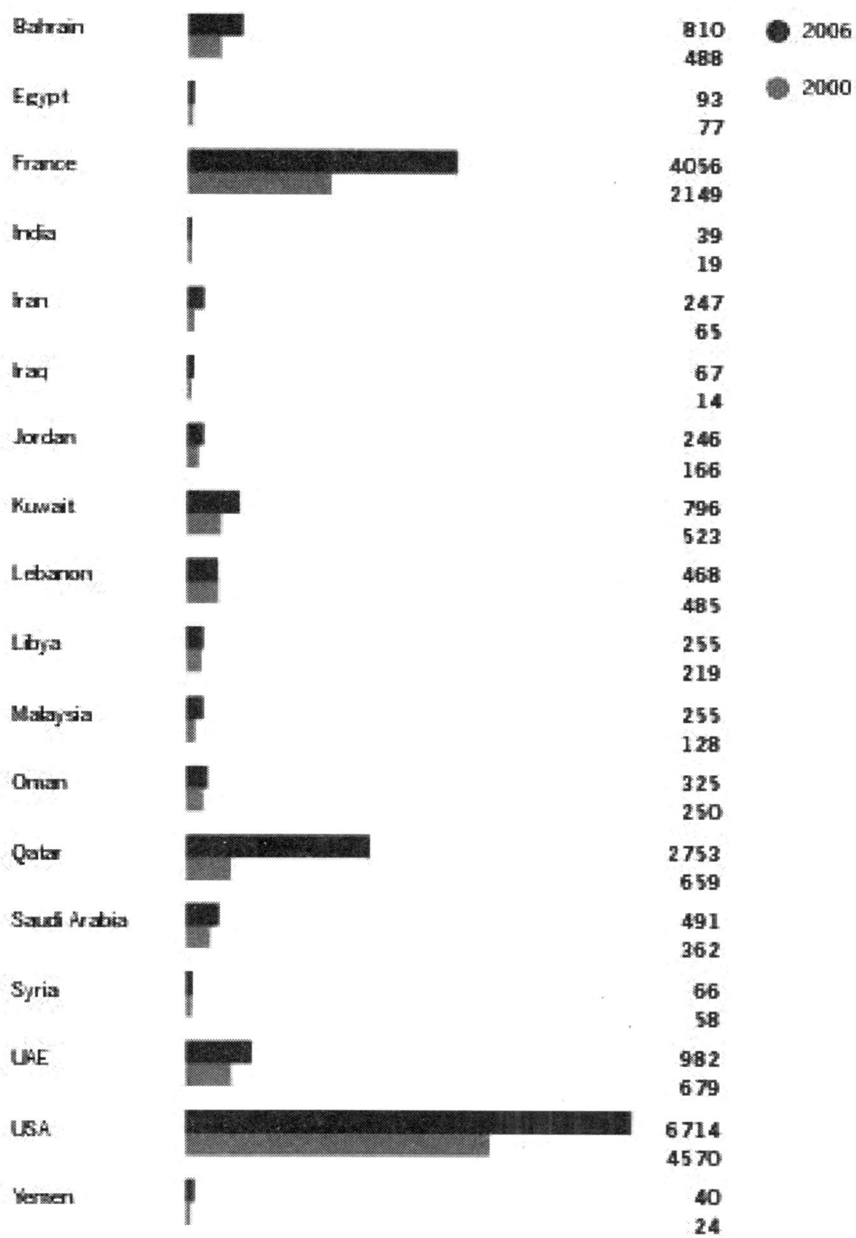

Source: b World Health Organisation (WHO).

Private Expenditure on Health as Percentage of Total Expenditure on Health (%)

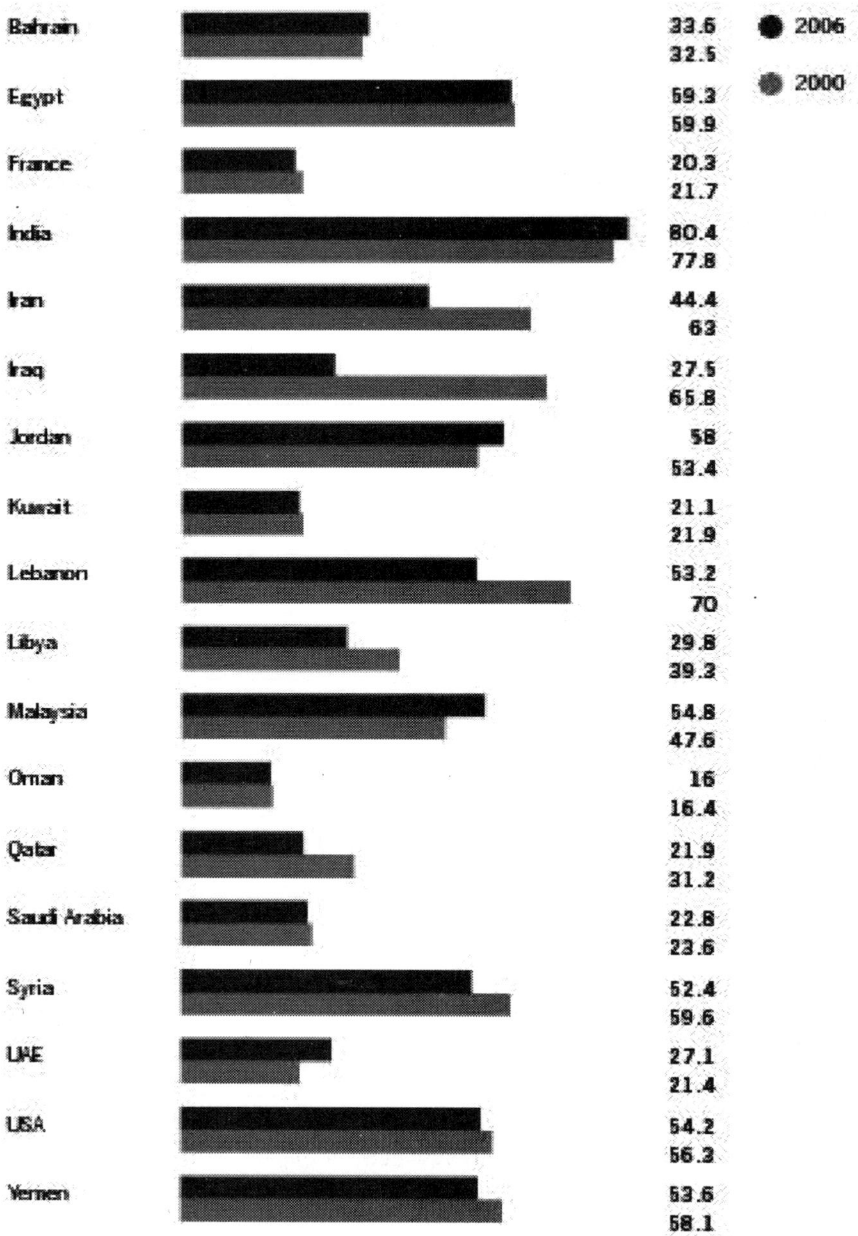

Source: þ World Health Organisation (WHO).

Total Expenditure on Health at Percentage of Gross Domestic Product (%)

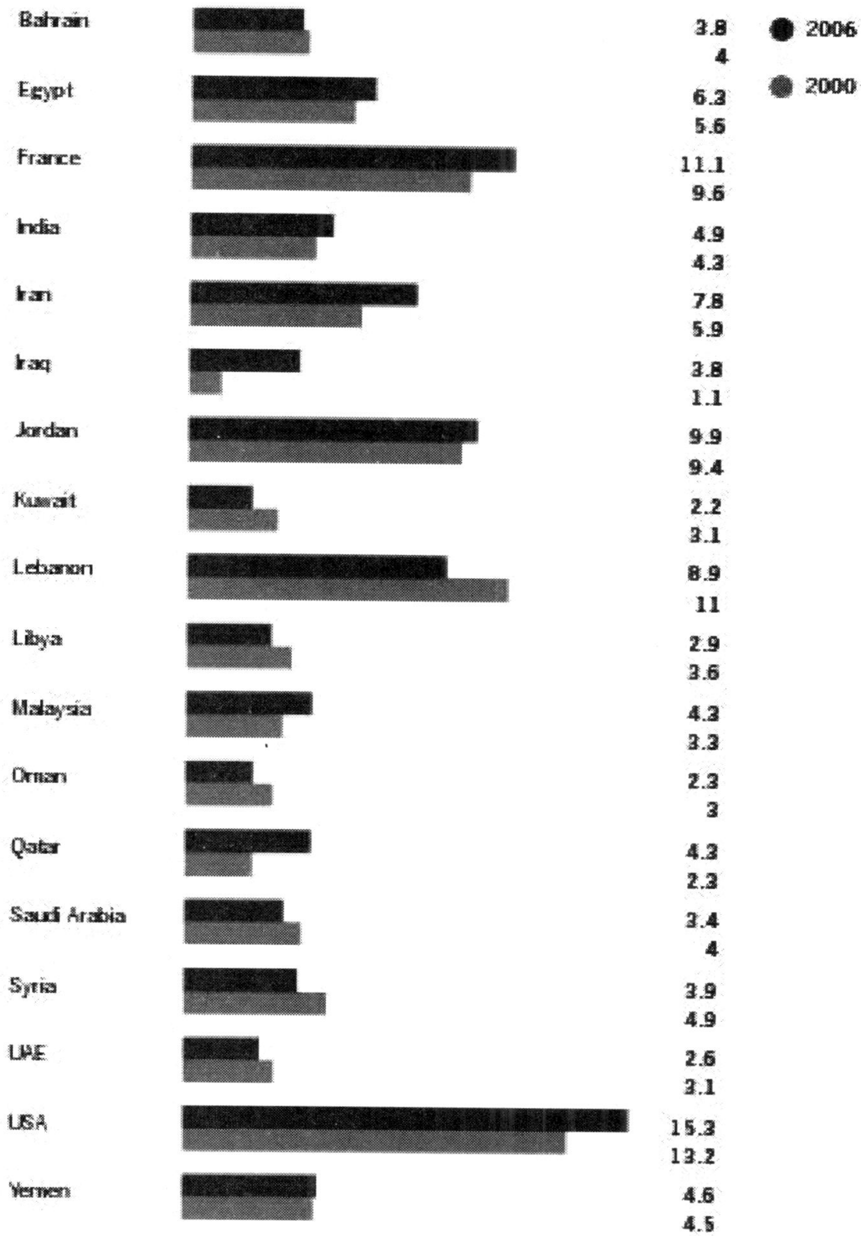

Source: b World Health Organisation (WHO).

Private Prepaid Plans as Percentage of Private Expenditure on Health (%)

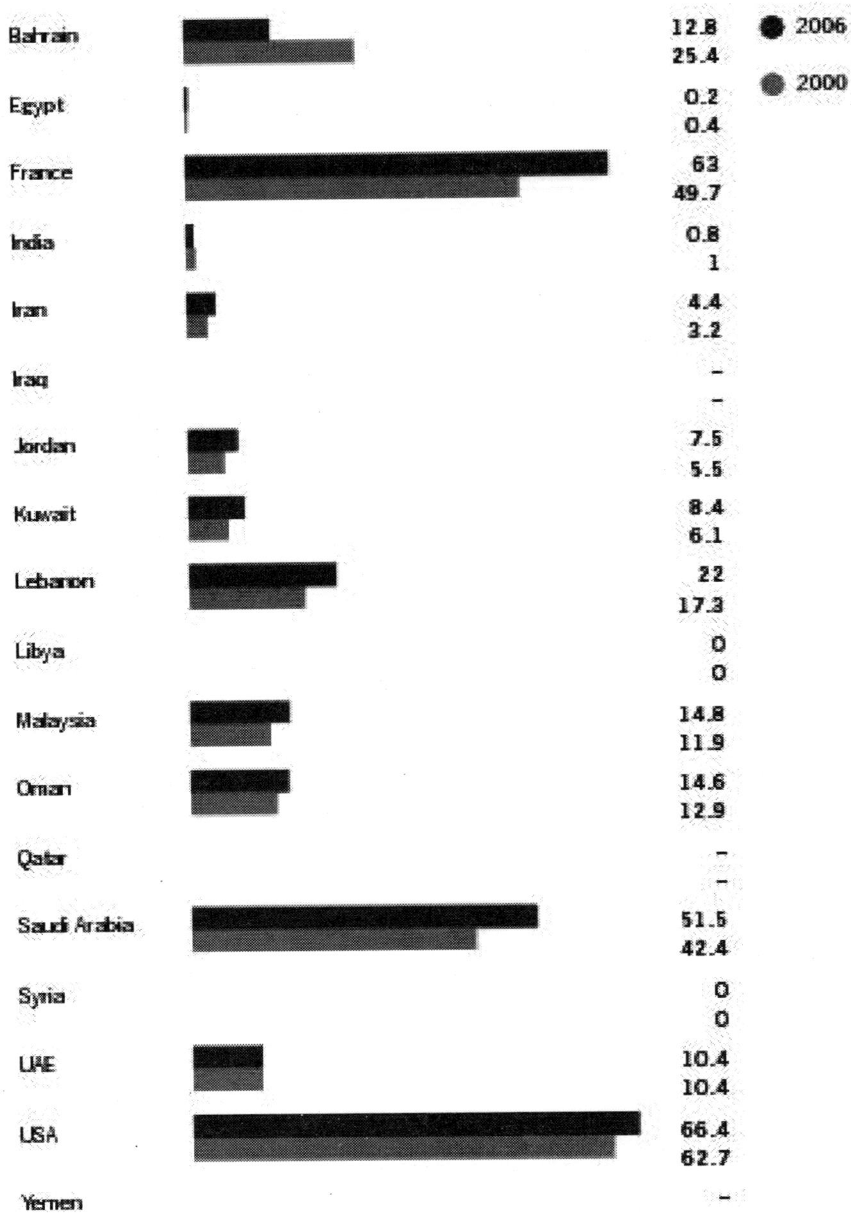

Source: b World Health Organisation (WHO).

The breakdown of facilities is as follows:

(1) Ministry of Health Facilities

These serve the general public and are located in both the large cities and the small towns throughout Saudi Arabia.

(2) Military Hospitals

These serve members of the Saudi Arabia armed forces and members of their families, according to the branch of the military in which the individual serves.

Saudi Arabian National Guard (SANG)

SANG is the branch of the military that is involved with defence against external threats and internal threats. SANG has four hospitals which provide care to the soldiers of the Saudi Arabian National Guard and their dependents:

- King Abdulaziz Medical City, Riyadh (650 beds, formerly the King Fahad National Guard Hospital);
- King Abdulaziz Medical City, Jeddah (350 beds, formerly the King Khalid National Guard Hospital);
- King Abdulaziz Medical City, Dammam (100 beds);
- King Abdulaziz Medical City, Al Ahsa (300 beds); and
- The Saudi Arabian National Guard also operates clinics in Riyadh and Taif.

Saudi Arabian Ministry of Defence and Aviation (MODA)

MODA provides defense against primarily external threats. It includes the Saudi Arabian Army, the Royal Saudi Naval Forces, the Royal Saudi Air Force and Royal Saudi Air Defence. MODA operates nine hospitals which provide care to the soldiers of MODA and their dependents:

- Riyadh Military Hospital Al Kharj, Riyadh (1,000+ beds);
- Prince Sultan Cardiac Centre, Riyadh (150+ beds);
- North West Armed Forces Hospital, Tabuk (350 beds);
- King Fahd Military Medical Complex, Dhahran (316 beds);
- Armed Forces Hospital at King Abdulaziz Airbase, Al Khobar (280 beds);
- King Fahad Armed Forces Hospital, Jeddah (200+ beds);
- King Faisal/King Fahad Hospital, Khamis Mushayt (total 258 beds);
- Al Hada Hospital, Taif (500+ beds);
- Hafr Al-Batin Armed Forces Hospital, Hafr Al-Batin (300 beds); and
- Wadi Al-Dawassir Hospital, Wadi Al-Dawassir (100 beds).

(3) Ministry of the Interior

This serves members the ministry of the interior, including the police and customs collectors.

Security Forces Hospital, Riyadh (500 beds), serves the Ministry of Interior personnel.

(4) Referral Hospitals

Every citizen is eligible to go to the referral hospitals for specialized care. These facilities include:

- King Faisal Specialist Hospital and Research Centre, Riyadh Site (700 beds);
- King Faisal Specialist Hospital and Research Centre, Jeddah Site (250 beds);
- King Khalid Eye Specialist Hospital, Riyadh (360 beds); and
- Sultan Bin Abdulaziz Humanitarian City, Riyadh (300 rehabilitation beds).

(5) Private Facilities

Here are just a few of the private facilities in Saudi Arabia:

- For-Profit: Saudi German Hospital, Jeddah; Dr. Erfan and Bagedo Hospital, Jeddah; Kingdom Hospital, Riyadh;
- Saudi ARAMCO Hospital, Dhahran (480 beds); serves employees of the oil company Saudi ARAMCO, and their family members;
- Social Insurance Hospital, Riyadh (GOSI) (300 beds);
- Royal Commission Hospitals, which serve employees and their family members of the Industrial cities located at: Jubail, on the east coast of Saudi Arabia; Yanbu, on the west coast of Saudi Arabia;
- SAAD Medical Centre, Al Khobar; and
- Soliman Fakeeh Hospital, Jeddah (800 beds, and the largest private hospital in Saudi Arabia; it is contracted to Saudi ARAMCO).

APPENDIX

HOSPITALS IN MIDDLE EAST

Egypt

1. Ain Shams University Hospital, Cairo, Egypt.
2. Al Shorouk Hospital, Mohandeseen, Egypt.
3. Al Moukawileen Al-Arab Hospital, Autostrade, Nasr City, Egypt.
4. Al Nada Hospital, Manial, Egypt.
5. Anglo-American Hospital Zohoreya, Zamalek, Egypt.
6. Anglo American Hospital, Zohoreya, Egypt.
7. As Salam International Hospital, Maadi, Egypt.
8. Arab Contractors Medical Centre, Nasr City, Egypt.
9. Behman Psychiatric Hospital, Helwan, Egypt.
10. Cairo Medical Cente, Heliopolis, Egypt.
11. Cleopatra Hospital, Heliopolis, Cairo, Egypt.
12. El Salam International Hospital, Maadi, Egypt.
13. "French" Kasr El Aini Hospital, Kasr El Aini, Egypt.
14. Giza International Hospital, Pyramids, Egypt.
15. Heliopolis Hospital, Heliopolis, Egypt.
16. Intertility Clinic, Maadi, Egypt.
17. Italian Hospital, Abbassia, Egypt.
18. Kasr El Aini Hospital, Egypt.
19. Magdy Hospital, Dokki, Egypt.
20. Misr International Hospital, Dokki, Egypt.
21. Nile Badrawi Hospital, Maadie, Egypt.
22. Shalaan Surgicentre, Mohandeseen, Egypt.

Jordan

23. Jordan Dental Centre, Al-Asdiqa' Centre, Jordan.
24. Dr. Ali Zayni's Dental Centre, Amman, Jordan.
25. Eye Specialty Hospital, Jordan.
26. Jordan Hospital, Amman, Jordan.
27. Specialty Hospital, Amman, Jordan.

Kuwait

28. Al-Ahmadi Hospital, Al-Ahmadi, Kuwait.
29. Al-Salam Hospital, Al-Dasmah/Ben Aid Al-Qar, Kuwait.
30. Al-Jahra's Hospital, Al Jahra City, Kuwait
31. Ibn Sina Hospital, Shulaibikhat, Kuwait.
32. Al-Nahra'a Hospital, Ministry of Public Health, Jahra'a, Kuwait.
33. University of Kuwait, Safat, Kuwait.

34. Al-Rashed Hospital, Al-Salmiyah, Kuwait.
35. As'ad Al-Hamad Dermatology Centre, Khaldeyah, Kuwait.
36. Kuwait Health Sciences Centre, Kuwait.

Lebanon

37. Dar Al-Ajaza Al-Islamia Hospital, Beirut, Lebanon.
38. Maharishi Health Education Centre, Lebanon.
39. Sahel General Hospital, Beirut, Lebanon.
40. Home Care Lebanon, Badaro, Beirut, Lebanon.
41. Al-Koura Hospital, Al-Koura, Lebanon.
42. American University of Beirut Medical Centre, Beirut, Lebanon.

Palestine

43. Al Ahli Hospital, Hebron, Palestine.
44. Arab CARE HOSPITAL, Jerusalem, Palestine.
45. Harb Heart Centre, Ramallah, Palestine.

Saudi Arabia

46. Abha General Hospital, Abha, Kingdom of Saudi Arabia.
47. Al Hada Hospital, Kingdom of Saudi Arabia.
48. Al Hammadi Hospital, Riyadh, Kingdom of Saudi Arabia.
49. Al-Nour Hospital, Makkah, Kingdom of Saudi Arabia.
50. Asir General Hospital, Abha, Kingdom of Saudi Arabia.
51. Damman Central Hospital, Damman, Kingdom of Saudi Arabia.
52. Dr. Erfan and Bagedo Hospitals, Jeddah, Kingdom of Saudi Arabia.
53. Dr. Soliman Fakeeh Hospital, Jeddah, Saudi Arabia.
54. Dr. Sulaiman Al-Habibi Medical Centre, Riyadh, Kingdom of Saudi Arabia.
55. King Abdulaziz University Hospital, Riyadh, Kingdom of Saudi Arabia.
56. King Fahad Hospital, Riyadh, Kingdom of Saudi Arabia.
57. King Fahad Hospital, Gizan, Kingdom of Saudi Arabia.
58. King Fahad Hospital, Jeddah Kingdom of Saudi Arabia.
59. King Fahad Hospital, Madinah, Kingdom of Saudi Arabia.
60. King Faisal Specialist Hospital and Research Centre, Riyadh, Kingdom of Saudi Arabia.
61. King Khaled Hospital, Haiel, Kingdom of Saudi Arabia.
62. King Fahad National Guard Hospital, Riyadh, Kingdom of Saudi Arabia.
63. Security Forces Hospital, Riyadh, Kingdom of Saudi Arabia.
64. King Khaled Eye Specialist Hospital, Riyadh, Kingdom of Saudi Arabia.

65. King Khaled University Hospital, Riyadh, Kingdom of Saudi Arabia.
66. King Khaled Hospital, Najran, Kingdom of Saudi Arabia.
67. Maternity and Children's Hospital, Damman, Kingdom of Saudi Arabia.
68. Maternity and Children's Hospital, Jeddah, Kingdom of Saudi Arabia.
69. Maternity and Children's Hospital, Madinah, Kingdom of Saudi Arabia.
70. Prince Salman Hospital, Riyadh, Kingdom of Saudi Arabia.
71. Prince Sultan Cardiac Centre, Riyadh, Kingdom of Saudi Arabia.
72. Riyadh Armed Forces Hospital, Riyadh, Kingdom of Saudi Arabia.
73. Sultan Bin Abdulaziz Al-Saud Foundation, Kingdom of Saudi Arabia.
74. Health Ministry for Gulf Cooperation Council, Riyadh.
75. The Saudi Dental Society, Riyadh.
76. King Fahad Medical Hospital, Riyadh.
77. Dr, Aleissa Clinics-Derma, Riyadh.
78. Prince Salman Centre For Disability Research, Riyadh.
79. The Psychiatric Specialized Polyclinic, Riyadh.
80. Al-Salama Hospital, Jeddah.
81. Dr. Erfan and Bagedo General Hospital, Jeddah.
82. Ghassan N. Pharaon, Jeddah.
83. Juffali Help Centre, Jeddah.
84. Al Doha National Dispensary, Dammam.
85. King Abdulaziz University/Scientific Research Council, Jeddah.

Syria

86. New Medical Centre, Damascus, Syria.

Let us look at some of the well known hospitals in the middle east:

King Fahad Specialist Hospital—Dammam

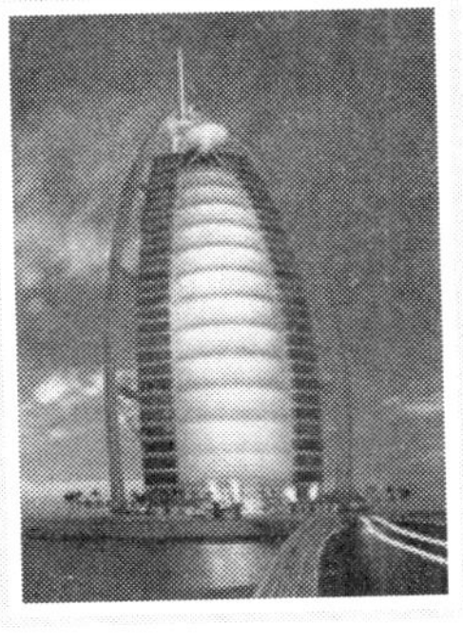

King Fahad Specialist Hospital is located in Dammam, Eastern Provine of Saudi Arabia. It is a tertiary hospital and it is a Ministry of Health Hospital. The capacity of KFSH is 640 beds and it is equipped by the latest technology .

KFSH in Dammam source for its staff from all around the World. All consultant physicians, Senior Nursing staff and Senior Paramedics must be qualified from North America and Western countries.

KFSH in Dammam provide competitive salary and great benefits to its staff. In addition, employees are housed in hospital compound which it is well furnished, has swimming pools, gym, tennis, volleyball, basketball and other entertainment facility.

King Abdulaziz Medical City—Alahsa

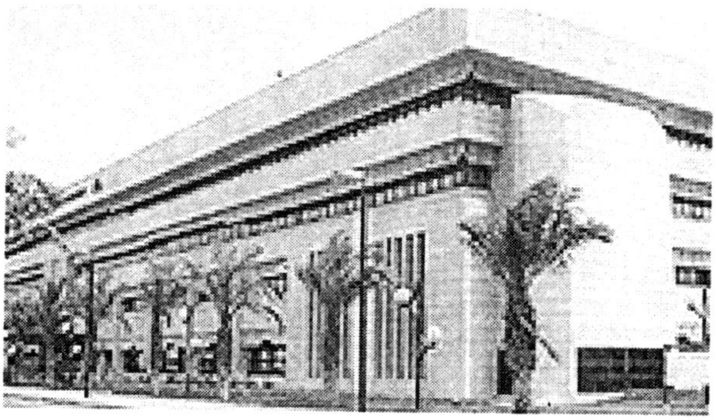

Construction of King Abdulaziz Medical City, Alahsa was completed on June, 2002. It has 300 beds capacity and it provide primary, secondary and tertiary medical services to national Guard personnel and their dependents in the Eastern Province of Saudi Arabia.

King Abdulaziz Medical City—Dammam

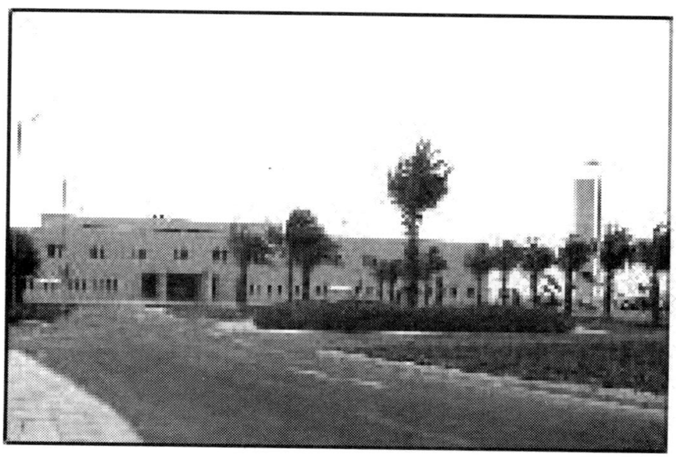

King Abdulaziz Medical City in Dammam construction was completed in June, 2002. The hospital has 100 beds capacity. It is equipped with the latest state of the art medical equipments and recruit its staff from all around the World.

King Abdulaziz Medical City—Jeddah

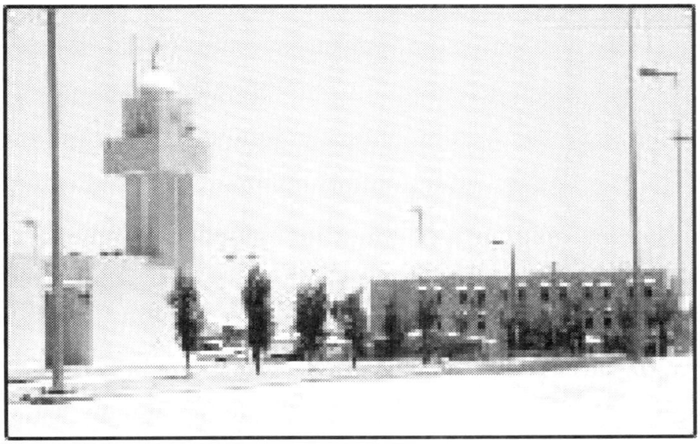

King Khalid National Guard Hospital in Jeddah was founded in July, 1982. In year 2001, King Khalid National Guard Hospital became part of King Abdulaziz Medical Cities. King Abdulaziz Medical City, Jeddah is a tertiary type of hospital and its mission is to provide state of the art medical services to National Guard personnel and their dependents in the Western Region of Saudi Arabia. KAMC in Jeddah has around 350 beds.

King Abdulaziz Medical City—Riyadh

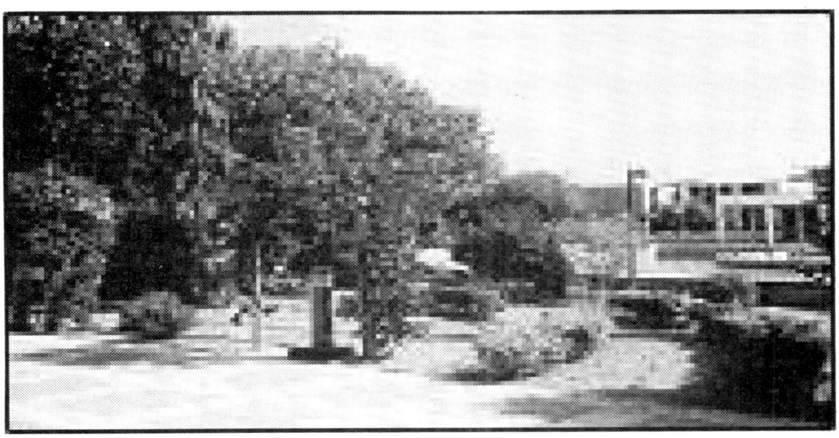

King Fahad National Guard Hospital in Riyadh commenced its operation in May, 1983. In year 2001, King Fahad National Guard Hospital became part of King Abdulaziz Medical Cities. King Abdulaziz Medical City in Riyadh beds capacity is 691. Since many years KAMC in Riyadh recruit its staff from many countries all around the World. Many physicians, nurses and paramedics are recruited from North America, Western Europe, Australia and South Africa. KAMC in Riyadh is a tertiary type hospital and conform to the highest International medical Standard.

Sultan Bin Abdulaziz Humanitarian City

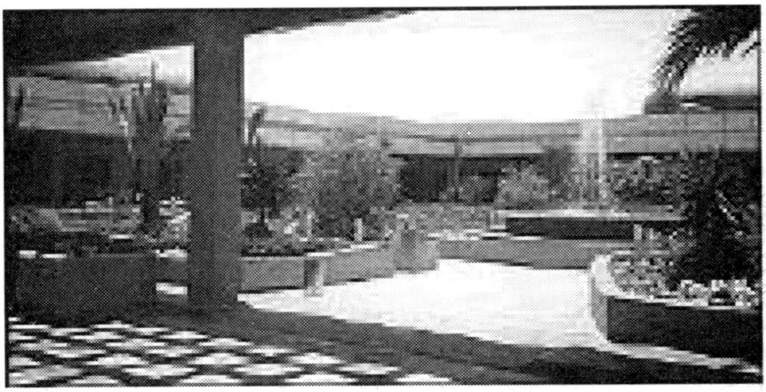

Sultan Bin Abdulaziz Humanitarian City (SBAHC) is a 400 bed rehabilitation hospital which was open on October, 2002, to provide inpatient and outpatient rehabilitation medicine. The city is located north of Riyadh in the Banhan area, Saudi Arabia.

The patients are provided with the highest quality of medical services by well experienced medical staff, nurses, and rehabilitation specialist. SBAHC objective is to be a worldwide centre of excellence in rehabilitation, providing the highest standards of international health care in Kingdom of Saudi Arabia

Zayed Medical Hospital

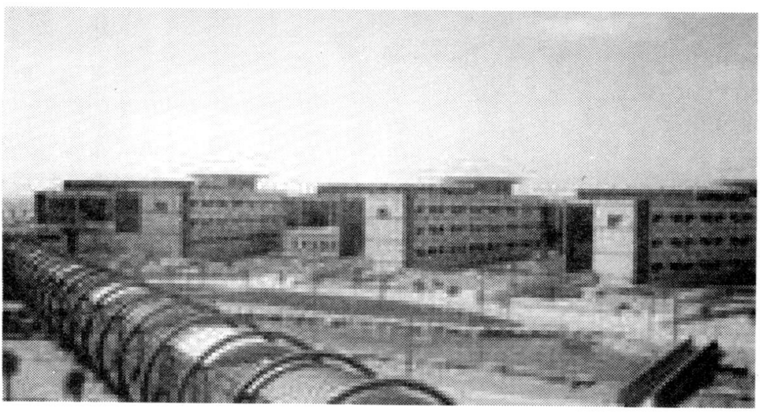

Zayed Military Hospital (ZMH) is located in Abu Dhabi, the capital city of the United Arab Emirates (UAE). ZMH is the only military hospital in the United Arab Emirates. ZMH has 365 beds capacity and provide medical services to more than 100,000 people.

ZMH is a tertiary type hospital and its departments are equipped with the most modern equipment.

Habib Medical Centre, Dubai Health Care Centre is forecasted to be commissioned for operation by the end of year 2006 (HMC at DHCC). HMC at DHCC will be equipped with the state of the art of medical equipments in all departments. Its main goal is to provide excellent medical services to patients and to become a referral centre for the entire Middle East region.

Dr. Sulaiman Habib Medical Centre, Dubai Health Care Centre

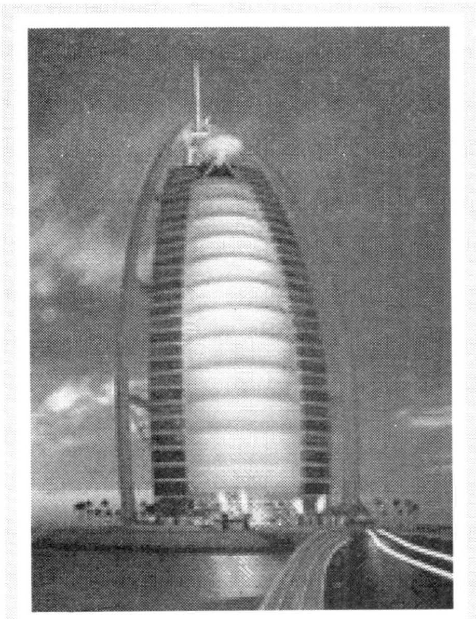

HMC at DHCC will be able to provide treatment for 800 patients per day and will adhere to international standards from initiating the construction of the building to provision of all phases of medical services to patients.

Department of Tourism Dubai City

Saad Specialist Hospital (SSH) was opened in year 2001. SSH main goal is to provide high quality of medical services to the local community. SSH provide modern tertiary medical services mainly to the Eastern Province population and to the Saudi population in general.

SSH is located in Al Khobar in the Eastern Province of Kingdom of Saudi Arabia. It is located within few miles away from Demmam and Dhahran.

SSH was built and constructed according to the highest international standards and it is accredited by Joint Commission International (JCI).

Saad Specialist Hospital consists 600 beds hospital.

King Faisal Specialist Hospital and Research Centre in Jeddah (KFSHRC)

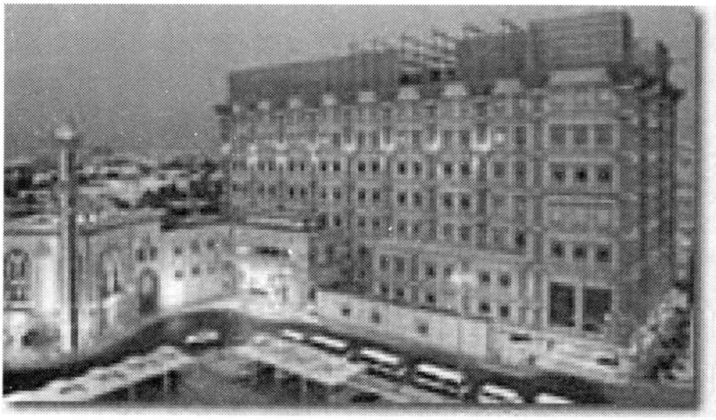

King Faisal Specialist Hospital and Research Centre in Jeddah (KFSHRC), commenced providing medical services to Jeddah city and to the Western Region of KSA in March 2000. It is 200 beds hospital equipped with the most modern medical equipment and medical technology available at present time. KFSHRC recruits many of his medical, nursing and paramedical staff from North America and Western European countries.

The hospital is accredited by Joint Commission International (JCI).

KFSHRC is located on the coastal city of Jeddah on the Red Sea. City of Jeddah is a cosmopolitan city and it is the second largest city in KSA. It has 2 million population. In Jeddah, you will find modern shopping malls, variety international cuisine and many luxurious hotels spread all around the city.

King Fahed Medical City (KFMC)

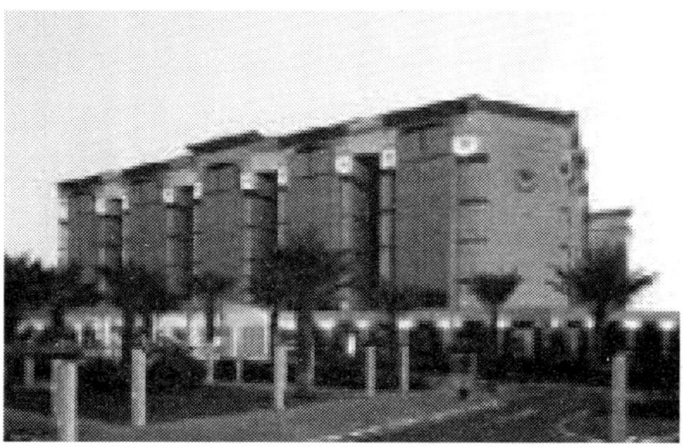

King Fahed Medical City (KFMC) was commissioned for operation in year 2005. KFMC is located in Riyadh, Kingdom of Saudi Arabia. KFMC occupies an area of around 500,000 square meters in the capital of Saudi Arabia.

King Fahed Medical City considered one of the largest health care facility in the region and contain state of the art modern facilities with the following hospitals:

Pediatric Hospital: 246 beds capacity
Maternity Hospital: 236 beds capacity
General Hospital: 460 beds capacity
Rehabilitation Hospital: 150 beds capacity

KFMC has an excellent housing complex with recreation facilities for its employees. International employees are housed in villas, apartments and housing units.

King Fahed Military Medical Complex (KFMMC)

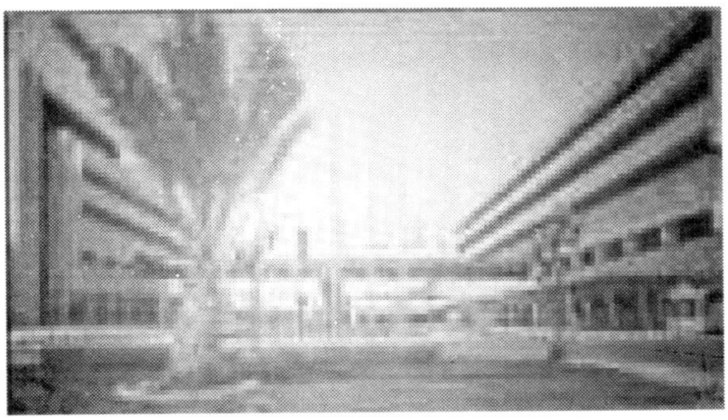

It is a little more than 300 beds, which provide primary, secondary and tertiary medical services. It is located in Dhahran. Its medical equipment contains the latest technology for expatriate staff, it is according to the Western standards and it contains recreational facilities. Furnished housing is provided for all staff.

King Fahed Military Hospital, Jeddah

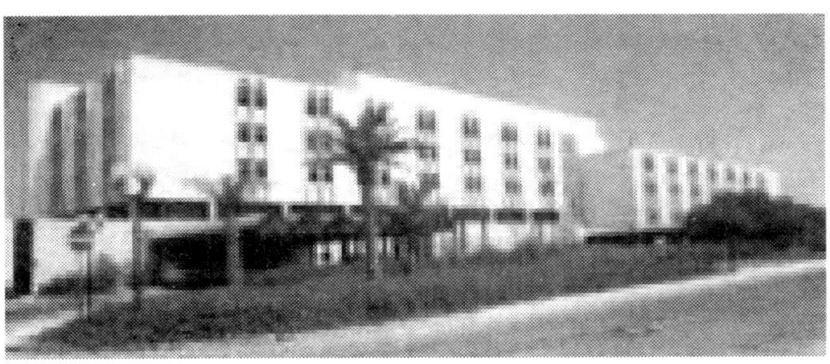

King Fahed Military Hospital in Jeddah is a 250 beds acute care centre providing medical care for Saudi Arabian Military personnel and their dependents. The hospital provides excellent housing facilities for its staff. It is located in Jeddah, a city of 2 million populations.

King Khalid Eye Specialist Hospital, Riyadh

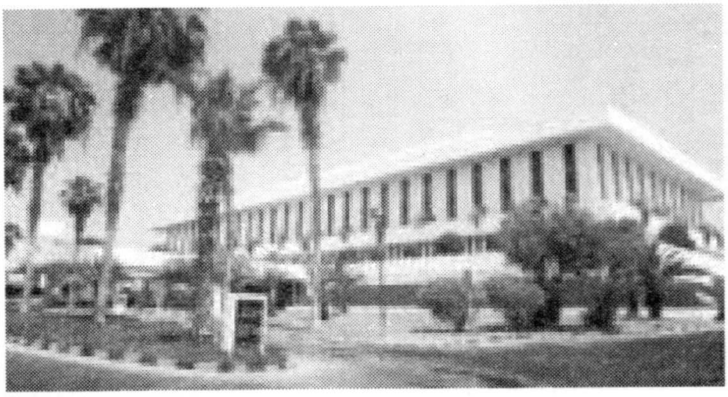

The King Khalid Eye Specialist Hospital (KKHESH) is the largest eye hospital in the Middle East. Among the services offered by the hospital are Cataract Surgery, Corneal Grafting, Optometry, Clinical, Psychophysical and Electro Physical Laboratories, Ultrasonography and Pharmacies.

There are 12 fully equipped operating theaters and 17 bed recovery rooms. The hospital provides excellent furnished housing for its staff. KKESH is located in Riyadh, the Capital of Saudi Arabia.

The Riyadh Armed Forces Hospital (RAFH)

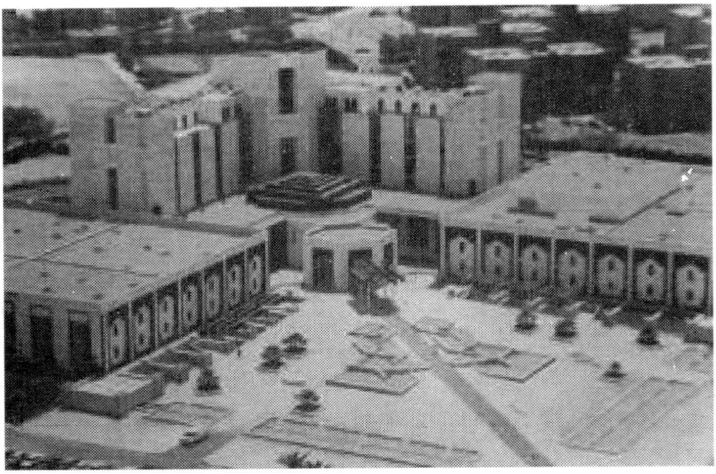

It is located in Riyadh City, which is the capital of Saudi Arabia. The RAFH Hospital is approximately 770 beds. In addition to providing excellent care for patients, RAFH is heavily involved in training and educating Saudi Nationals. Furnished housing is provided for all staff.

Abdul Latif Jameel Rehabilitation Hospital and Specialty Clinics

Abdul Latif Jameel Hospital and rehabilitation and Specialty Clinics is a non-profit hospital which provides excellent medical providing rehabilitation programs, neurological rehabilitation, musculoskeletal rehabilitation, artificial limbs, rheumatic rehabilitation, chronic diseases, sport injuries and various children programs. The Hospital is located in Jeddah a city of 2 million populations. The hospital is a 10 minute drive from the Red Sea and 45 minute drive from Mecca (the Holy city for Muslims).

Armed Forces Hospital at Al-Hada, Saudi Arabia

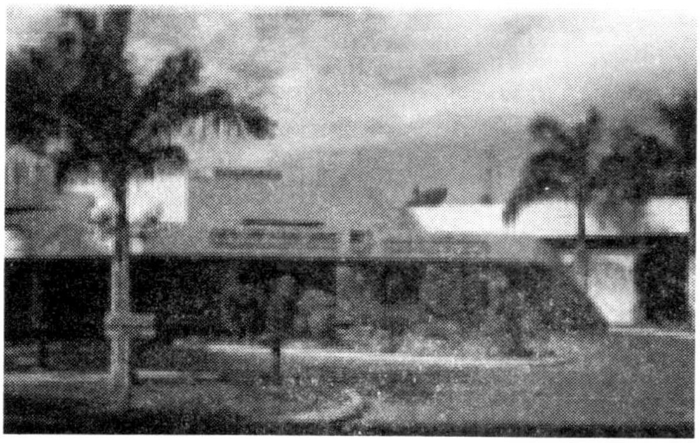

The Armed Forces Hospital at Al-Hada is a 350 bed Hospital. This provides primary, secondary and tertiary medical services to the Saudi Arabian Military, personnel and their dependents. This facility is equipped with the latest technology in Western Countries. Housing for expatriate is located inside the Hospital's complex and it is within walking distance from the Hospital. The Hospital's complex contains excellent recreational facilities for its staff.

The hospitals location is unique, it is a 45 minute drive from Mecca (the Holy city for Muslims), a 15 minute drive from Taif (population 300,000), and 2 hour drive from Jeddah.

The Rehabilitation Centre in Taif, Saudi Arabia

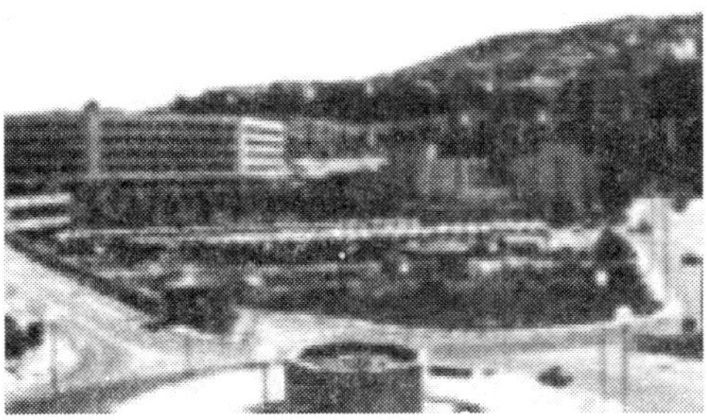

The Rehabilitation Centre in Taif is a 100 bed Hospital facility which provides high quality medical rehabilitation programs to military personnel and their dependents. The Hospital is located in Taif, a 300,000 population.

Prince Sultan Bin Abdulaziz Humanitarian City

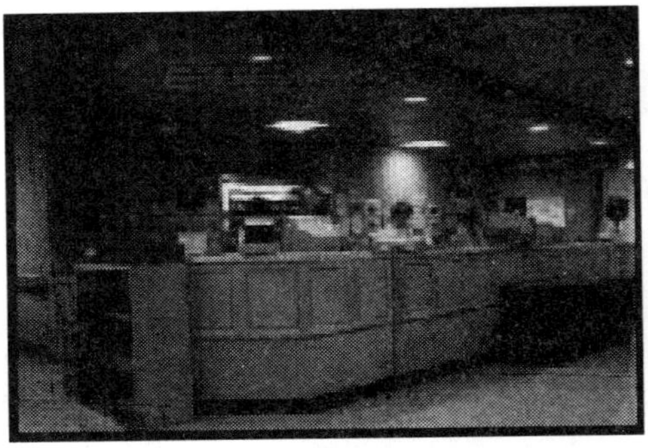

Prince Sultan Bin Abdulaziz Humanitarian City is located in Riyadh, Saudi Arabia. It was opened in year 2002. This facility is specialized in the provision of rehabilitation medicine. It is funded by the Prince Sultan Bin Abdulaziz Foundation.

The city is located around 30 km. north of Riyadh, Saudi Arabia.

Mughrabi Hospital and Medical Clinic Centres in Saudi Arabia and Gulf States.

There are more than 18 hospitals and centres for the diagnosis, treatment and surgeries of the eye diseases.

It has more than 45 years experience and it is considered the pioneer in the provision of medical treatment for patients with eye disease in the Middle East and Africa. Mughrabi Hospital is the first institution to utilize modern technology from western countries.

All medical consultants at Mughrabi hospitals and clinics hold the highest certification and degrees in the world. For instance;

College of Bascom Balmer for Ophthalmology;

Wellmer College for Ophthalmology at John Hopkins University;

Louisiana College.

Al-Mughrabi Hospital and Centres are located in all major cities in Saudi Arabia and Abu Dhabi. In Saudi Arabia Mughrabi Hospitals are located in the following cities:

1. Jeddah
2. Riyadh
3. Mecca
4. Demmam
5. Madinah
6. Taif
7. Khammis-Mushayf

Majority of Mughrabi Hospitals and Centres provides, Ophthalmology Ear, Nose, Throat and dental medical services.

Mughrabi Hospitals and Centres provide the following procedures and services:

1. Glaucoma Unit
2. Cornea, External Eye Disease Unit
3. Vitro, Retina Unit
4. Cataract Unit
5. Retroactive Surgery Unit
6. Pediatric Ophthalmology Unit
7. YAG Laser
8. Argon Laser

International Medical Centre (IMC), Jeddah, Saudi Arabia

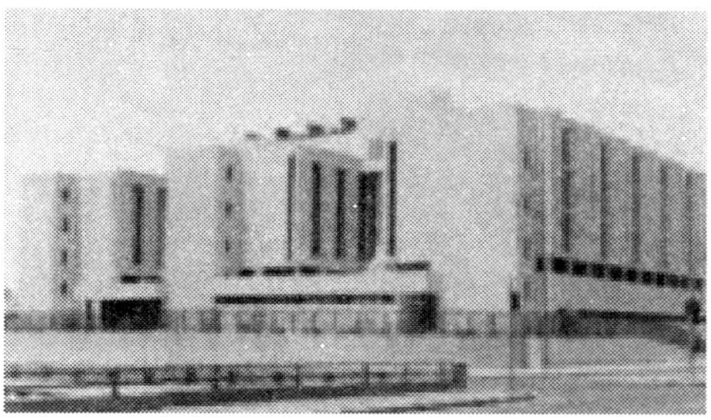

The International Medical Centre (IMC) is a 300 bed private multidisciplinary hospital with several centre of excellence clinics in Jeddah, Saudi Arabia. (KSA) IMC is affiliated with the Cleveland Clinic Foundation in Ohio, USA. It is targeted to open in February, 2005.

IMC will provide an "world class" holistic healing environment through the efficient well designed infrastructure, advanced technology equipment, sourcing and retaining competent physicians/surgeons, nurses, paramedics and support staff from across the globe; and through the continuous support of the management team, and the board of directors.

Key management staff at IMC is Harvard educated/trained and other American educated/trained professionals. IMC will offer competitive salary and benefits package to ensure the employment of highest quality staff. IMC will make a difference in health care paradigm in the Middle East.

Employees and their families will enjoy comfortable living in Jeddah on the Red Sea. Jeddah is a cosmopolitan and the second largest city in KSA known as gateway to holy cities of Makkah/Madinah.

Jeddah has a population of 2 million. In Jeddah you will find modern shopping malls, water sports, golf, equestrian clubs, museums, sea-side resorts, variety of international restaurants, international schools, active professional societies, and many world class 5 star hotels.

Tawam Hospital, Al-Ain, United Arab Emirates

Tawam Hospital is a governmental hospital and it is operated by special budget from The Ministry of Health of UAE. It was commenced for operation in 1979. Tawam hospital has capacity of 477 beds and it is a referral/tertiary type of hospital.providing medical services to to the national population. It is located within 90 minutes drive from Dubai and Abeu-Dhabi cities.

Tawam Hospital is a teaching hospital and affiliated with the medical school of UAE University.

Tawam Hospital is the referral centre for oncology, neurosurgery, and pediatric surgery in UAE.

Tawam Hospital is known for having an excellent reputation in the Middle-East for the provision of high standard of patient services.

The North Western Armed Forces Hospitals Program, Tabuk

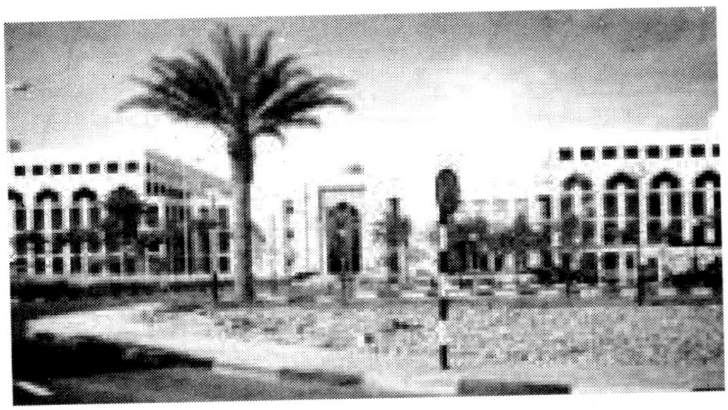

The North Western Armed Forces Hospitals are located in Tabuk city. It is considered as the northern western Saudi Arabia gate to Jordan and other neighbouring countries in the Middle-East. The city is famous with its agricultural production, mainly fruits and vegetables.

Tabuk is located 2200 feet above sea level and has moderate climate in comparison with other Saudi cities climate. It has numerous supermarkets, restaurants and hotels with international standard. Tabuk city has an airport.

The North Western Armed Forces Hospitals:

A — The North Western Armed Forces Hospital has 350 beds capacity. It is considered as tertiary type of hospital and has all major specialties and sub-specialties.

B — King Khalid Armed Forces Hospital:

Its capacity is around 100 beds and provides medical services for pediatric, psychiatric, isolation and outpatient services.

Housing Facility

North Western Armed Forces Hospitals has an excellent housing facility for all categories of staff. The hospital is located within walking distant from housing units. Physicians are provided with villa type housing units.

Recreation Facility

Recreation facility is provided to all employees. This includes swimming pools, games room, weight lifting room, tennis courts, volleyball, basketball, and many more.

APPENDIX

CONCEPT OF DISEASE IN MIDDLE RAST

(a) Disease is considered a mark of imperfection or weakness that reflects on the entire family even to the extent that family members might be unmarriageable. Disabilities and mental disturbance are the most prominent elicitors of 'ayb-oriented behaviour. Arab culture holds an expectation of perfection, particularly physically.

(b) *Perception of mental illness*: Punishment from God for the sins of the individual or his family, touched by jinn (usually perceived as malevolent spirits), or ridden by the devil. Mental illness is shunned. It is not uncommon to see a reluctance to send a disturbed family member to an asylum or for treatment out of desire not to recognize and disclose the problem.

(c) *Non-recognition of chronic disease*: Stigma, 'ayb-oriented. Chronic diseases like cancer, diabetes are considered hereditary and reflect on the whole family. There is also a fear of reducing the marriage-ability of children by disclosure of these kinds of illnesses.

(d) *Belief in unseen forces*: Arabs from the Middle Ages theorized about the germ theory and it is well established within our consciousness. However, there is also an acceptance that unseen forces may cause disease such as jinn, by the evil eye. While jinn are feared as malevolent and capricious spirits that may cause illness and other evil, the evil eye can best be understood in the context of fearing the envy of others which may also be the cause of sickness or even death.

(e) *Deep seated respect for age and expertise*: *Respect increases with age and authority*: Doctors do receive a great respect and trust. Arab patients submit to that authority without questioning. This contributes to the low rate of medical-legal cases among Arabs. Perception that the doctor is incompetent or not trustworthy will not result in an open confrontation/discussion with the doctor, but instead will result in non-compliance with his directions.

(f) *Alternative healing*: A long tradition of treatment exists in the Arab world. The Arabs have a system of healing tradition that is over 3,000 years old, including herbalism and conception of the body as a unified system composed of interacting humors. While the Western approach is to look for the smallest particular cause, the Arab system looked for the imbalance in the body as a whole. Problems like gastrointestinal disorders, fevers, headaches, orthopedic difficulties, and fractures all have a well-established traditional approach for their alleviation. Bonesetters are considered better than orthopedic doctors in the Middle East. Traditional mid-wives are well skilled in the Arab World.

(g) *Concept of time*: In Arab culture, time is not linear and is not constricted in the way that it is in the West. Not tomorrow at 9:30 AM but insha'Allah (God-willing) I'll see you before lunch. Lateness is accepted and anger about it is not understood.

(h) *Arab family structures*: Extended family structure is the most common form for Arab families. There are four types of family organization: nuclear (mother, father and children found in the minority of Arab households), extended (which may also include grandparents, aunts, uncles, and cousins), hammula (3-4 extended families) and qabila (4-5 hammulas).

(i) *Role of the family in decision making*: The consideration of the welfare of the family takes precedence over individual considerations. Indeed, the American focus on individuality is seen as verging on pathological behaviour in the Arab world. Because of the supremacy of the family, decisions are more likely to be made collectively in Arab families. Both the considerations of the family and the individual are carefully weighed. Older males, the patriarchs, of families may be asked to make health decisions for an individual family member. This role of the family complicates informed consent and confidentiality issues.

(j) *Position of men, women, children, elderly in the family*: Men's power and influence is in the external realm, while women control the internal matters of the household. Elderly enjoy final power and respect for consultation and guidance. Children are not participants in family decisions and are expected to be obedient to the family elders.

(k) *Marriage*: Premarital sexual relations are considered shameful, dirty, and sinful. Marriage is a prerequisite for respect and consideration as a mature member of the society.

(l) *Health risk behaviour—smoking, diet, exercise*: Arab culture is supportive of many risk behaviours that are not considered within the context of good health. Smoking is considered both part of manhood and of generosity. Cigarettes are offered like tea and coffee as a matter of hospitality. The Arab diet in the Arab World is considered to be healthy with a tendency toward high fiber, lots of fruit and vegetables, and fresh daily preparation of food. Meat is emphasized as good, but is generally restricted by cost. It is not a part of Arab consciousness to consider diet as a contributor to bad health. Similarly, Arab lifestyle is active due to the nature of life activities (70% rural, family visits, and walking).

Consequently, aerobics and exercise machines are considered foreign and silly. However, after immigrating to the United States, The Arab diet and lifestyle changes. The consumption of meat, snacks, fat, and sweats increases while the amount of exercise declines leading many Arab Americans, especially the elderly, to suffer from obesity, high cholesterol, and other related illnesses (Hassoun 1995).

(m) *Primary health care access in the Middle East and preventive service utilization*: Health services and education are free and accessible in the Arab countries, but quality varies. This is why the rate of medical insurance is very low, since it is not thought of as a requirement for health care. Medical services are generally only sought when the individual is acutely sick. A doctor who does not perform some invasive procedure (injections, clinical tests) or does not prescribe medications is considered incompetent.

(n) *Political and social background—Organizational structures and affiliation*: Arabs in the United States have a variety of national differences compounded with a wide variety of political, social and religious underpinnings.
Also, social stratification exists along class and urban/rural/ refugee camps.

Health Tourism in Israel

Israel is a major medical tourism destination primarily due to its worldwide reputation for high quality health care and world-renowned medical facilities. Complicated treatments and procedures that would be unavailable in other countries are available in Israel at reasonable prices, including orthopedic surgeries, oncology and cancer treatments, fertility and IVF treatments and neurosurgery. Patients from Eastern Europe, the Middle East and Africa are drawn to Israel's quality health care services. Americans (mostly of Jewish ancestry) and Western Europeans come to avail themselves of high quality medical treatment at a very reasonable cost.

Health Care System in Israel

Israel's high standards in health care services, top-of-the-line medical resources, ultra-modern hospitals and health care facilities, and a very high specialist-patient ratio makes the Israeli health care system one of the most advanced and innovative anywhere in the world. Israel's reputation as a health care leader in various fields of medicine is unquestionable.

There are around 70 general hospitals and medical centres in Israel, the majority of which are owned and operated by the government and non-profit organizations.

The Israeli Ministry of Health is responsible for the control and management of health policies in the country, including the standardization and implementation of health regulations among the various hospitals and health centres in the nation.

The Ministry of Health also regulates the qualification and certification of Israel's doctors and other medical professionals, some of whom have developed a reputation that is known throughout the world. Many of Israel's physicians and health practitioners have emigrated from

European and American countries and are well-trained and adept in Western medicine and procedures. Most Israeli medical practitioners put a high emphasis on further education, enabling them to become experts and super-specialists in their chosen medical fields.

Top Hospitals for Medical Tourism in Israel

- *Tel Aviv Assuta Hospital—Tel Aviv*

  This newly constructed privately-owned medical centre was opened to the public in 2009 and is now considered as the most advanced health care facility in the Middle East. Medical tourists can stay in private rooms equipped with cable TV, Wi-Fi internet connections and excellent room and personal assistant services. The medical centre is owned and operated by the Assuta Medical Group, which includes 5 hospitals and 7 other medical centres in the country.

- *Haddasah University Medical Centre—Jerusalem*

  Hadassah Medical is a non-profit organization which operates two hospitals in Jerusalem—Hadassah Ein Kerem Hospital and Hadassah Mount Scopus Hospital, both are advanced tertiary care hospitals who serve thousands of medical tourists annually.

- *Herzliya Medical Centre—Herzliya*

  Established in 1982, the Herzliya Medical Centre is a privately-owned hospital that offers technically advanced medical facilities and services, including complex heart surgeries, neurosurgeries and endoscopic procedures. The medical centre is also the first medical institution in Israel to receive full accreditation and certification from Blue Cross Blue Shield of America for medical tourism treatments, procedures and other services.

- *Tel Aviv Sourasky Medical Centre—Tel Aviv*

  This ISO-certified health facility is the major health care provider in the Tel Aviv area and is ranked as the third largest hospital in the country. Established in 1899, the centre houses a complex of three hospitals, a teaching hospital, a research centre, and a 5-star hotel that caters to international patients and medical travelers.

- *Browse our list of hospitals in Israel*

Common Treatments done by Medical Tourists in Israel

Hospitals and health care facilities in Israel offer top of the line procedures and services for medical travelers, including complicated medical procedures and treatment which include but are not limited to the following:

- Oncology

- Orthopedics
- Cardiology
- Cardiac Surgery
- Neurosurgery
- Neurology
- Ear, Nose and Throat Surgeries
- Endocrinology
- Gastroenterology
- General Surgery
- Pediatrics
- Urology
- Plastic and Aesthetic Surgery
- Ophthalmology
- Vascular Surgery
- Bone Marrow Transplants
- Pulmonology.

Cost of Medical Treatments in Israel

The following are cost comparisons between Medical procedures in Israel and equivalent procedures in the United States and the UK:

	US Hospitals	*Israel*	*Average Savings*
Fertility Treatments			
IVF Treatments	$16,000-$20,000	$5,000-$6,000	68%-70%
Medical Procedures			
Heart Bypass	$120,000-$130,000	$20,000-$35,000	73%-83%
Hip Replacement	$41,000-$43,000	$35,000-$40,000	6%-14%
Bone Marrow Transplant	$240,000-$260,000	$100,000-$120,000	53%-58%
Knee Replacement	$38,000-$40,000	$20,000-$30,000	25%-47%
Eye Surgeries			
Cataract Surgery	$5,000-$6,000	$3,500-$4,000	30%-33%
Plastic Surgery			
Face Lift (Rhytidectomy)	$7,500-$9,500	$6,500-$7,500	13%-21%
Breast Augmentation (Mammoplasty)	$5,000-$8,000	$3,500-$4,000	30%-50%
Complete Liposuction (Lipoplasty)	$4,000-$6,500	$2,000-$3,000	50%-53%
Nose Surgery (Rhinoplasty)	$5,500-$6,500	$4,000-$5,000	23%-27%
Botox (Facial Region)	$500-$1000	$350-$450	30%-55%
General and Cosmetic Dentistry			
Dental Implants	$3,000-$4,000	$1,000-$1,500	62%-67%

	UK Hospitals	*Israel*	*Average Savings*
Medical Procedures			
Bone Marrow Transplant	£140,000-£150,000	£60,000-£70,000	53%-57%
Plastic and Reconstructive Surgery			
Face Lift (Rhytidectomy)	£6,500-£7,500	£4,000-£4,500	38%-40%
Breast Augmentation (Mammoplasty)	£3000-£5000	£2,000-£2,500	33%-50%
Breast Reduction	£3000-£5000	£2,000-£2,500	33%-50%
Botox (Facial Region)	£340-£400	£250-£350	10%-40%
General and Cosmetic Dentistry			
Dental Implants	£1800-£2500	£600-£1000	60%-67%

Malpractice and Liability Laws in Israel

In Israel, a medical practitioner can be charged with malpractice if he or she has acted negligently during the treatment of a patient, or if he intentionally neglected to treat a patient. Several law firms in Israel have placed their focus in this growing field, as malpractice cases are much more complex and would require ample evidence and the backing of professional opinion before any claims compensation are awarded. Patients requiring assistance for malpractice and liability claims in Israel, can seek the services of these professionals and law firms. They have ample experience and technical expertise in this field. Malpractice cases can also include diagnosis failures, misdiagnosis, failure to render the correct treatment, and unreasonable delay before treatment is rendered.

Pros

- Israel hosts some of the most highly qualified and experienced doctors and surgeons in the world.
- The presence and availability of sophisticated medical technology, some of which were developed and perfected in Israel.
- The leading hospitals offer world-class medical facilities and equipment.
- Compared to Western countries such as USA, United Kingdom and Germany, costs of medical treatment in Israel is relatively low.
- English and Russian are widely spoken by medical personnel

Cons

- Prices of medical procedures are high compared to medical tourism destinations such as Asia and South America.

- The ongoing conflict with Palestine and other Arab countries is a cause of concern to tourists coming to Israel.
- Service levels at public hospitals are poor. Private rooms are scarce and the nurse/patient ratio is low compared to other medical tourism destinations in Asia.

Traveling to Israel

There are several major airline carriers traveling to Israel directly from all major cities in Europe and America. Most Arab countries do not have a direct flight to Israel, but can be reached through Amman, Jordan.

Average Estimated Travel Time in Hours

From/To	*Israel*
Moscow	4
St. Petersburg	5
Bulgaria (Sofia)	2
Romania (Bucharest)	3
Cyprus (Nicosia)	1
Greece (Athens)	2
Jordan	1
UAE (Dubai)	3
Georgia (Tbilisi)	2
Ukraine (Kiev)	3
New York	12
Los Angeles	16
London	5

Entry and Exit Requirements to Israel

Israel has made arrangements and agreements with 65 countries whereby citizens from these countries will no longer require a visa to enter Israel. The only requirement is a valid passport. Here is a list of these countries.

Most African, Asian and Arab countries need to apply for a Visa through the Israeli embassy in their country.

Statistics of Medical Tourism in Israel

Thousands of medical travelers have visited Israel in the last few years to avail themselves of the sophisticated health care and medical procedures that this country has to offer. In 2006, approximately 15,000 foreign nationals entered the country specifically for various medical treatments. Approximately 50% of these visitors were medical tourists from Russia and Eastern Europe.

Most of these patients came for medical procedures that were not available or were very expensive in their home countries, including heart surgeries, oncology and cancer treatments, bone marrow transplants and fertility treatments—Israel records the highest number of procedures performed compared to anywhere else in the world. 65% of medical visitors coming to Israel have undergone various medical treatments whilst the other 35% availed themselves of cosmetic and aesthetic surgeries and treatments.

2

Health Tourism in Middle East: Understanding Ethos of the Locals

Unequal economy, unequal care, unequal health spending and unequal health care services bring nothing but unequal challenges for each country. On the whole, people are healthier, wealthier and live longer today than 30 years ago. There have been significant improvements in access to water, sanitation, communicable diseases and antenatal care. There have never been more resources available for health than now. However, there are other trends that must not be ignored. First, the substantial progress in health over recent decades has been deeply unequal, with convergence towards improved health in a large part of the world, but at the same time, a considerable number of countries are increasingly lagging behind or losing ground, as reported by the World Health Organization.

The health care system worldwide is observing significant issues arising from a shift in diseases, an increase of non-communicable and chronic disorders, Baby Boomers and an aging population, a fragmented health care system, commercialization of health care and increases in the cost of care while countries are facing a shrinking health care budget. Moreover, there is very little anticipation and slow response by authorities to tackle such challenges. Many government bodies are engaged in the management of diseases, and are not at all close to the prevention programs, which presents a major problem. The growing reality is that many individuals present with complex symptoms and multiple illnesses, which challenges service delivery to develop more integrated and comprehensive case management.

As per the World Health Organizations recent report, there are five common shortcomings of health care delivery worldwide.

Inverse Care

People with the most means—whose needs for health care are often less—consume the most care, whereas those with the least means and greatest health problems consume the least. For instance, 5% of the US Population spent almost half of the health care spending. Public spending on health services most often benefits the rich more than the poor in high- and low-income countries alike.

Impoverishing Care

Wherever people lack social protection and payment for care is largely out-of-pocket at the point of service and they can be confronted with catastrophic expenses. Over 100 million people annually fall into poverty because they have to pay for health care that they cannot really afford in the first place.

Fragmented and Fragmenting Care

Changing the perspective on access to one framed in terms of ensuring comprehensive, effective and efficient health care highlights the problems associated with the fragmentation of care delivery. The excessive specialization of health care providers and the narrow focus of many disease control programs discourage a holistic approach for the individuals and the families they deal with and do not appreciate the need for continuity in care. Health services for poor and marginalized groups are often highly fragmented and severely under-resourced while development aid often adds to the fragmentation.

Unsafe Care

Poor system design that is unable to ensure safety and hygiene standards leads to high rates of hospital-acquired infections, along with medication errors and other avoidable adverse effects that are an underestimated cause of death and illness.

Misdirected Care

Resource allocation clusters around curative services at great cost, neglecting the potential of primary prevention and health promotion to prevent up to 70% of the disease burden. At the same time, the health sector lacks the expertise to mitigate the adverse effects on health from other sectors and make the most of what these other sectors can contribute to health.

Global Health care Structure

Let's have a look on health care challenges in each country:

Health care in US

Although nearly two trillion USD a year is spent on medical care, many people are receiving more care than they need, many are receiving less than they need and many are receiving the wrong kind of care.

The United States spends the most money on medical care of all advanced industrialized countries, but it performs more poorly than most on many measures of health care quality. The US scores 33% worse than the best country on mortality from conditions amenable to health care, that is, deaths that could have been prevented with timely and effective care.

Health care in UK

Government takes the burden of providing Health care Services through the world's biggest health care workforce—NHS. Only 10% of the population has private insurance coverage. Lack of personalized services, funding shortage and staff severity are key challenges which leads to high waiting times for treatment.

Health care in Canada

Canada's health care system is funded by both the federal government, and by the provincial and territorial governments. Patient waiting times, overall health care funding, shortages in personnel and improvement of medical technology are key areas which need improvement in the country's health care system. Some argue that Canada's health system should include home and long-term care. There is also criticism about the difference in health care coverage in difference provinces.

Health care in Japan

Japan has a system of universal health coverage, although individuals may receive coverage relatively differently. It can be divided into two broad categories: National Health Insurance and Employees' Health Insurance. Membership in either program is compulsory. There is also a national health program for people over 70, which is funded by contributions from the two main plans. The Japanese social system as a whole is expected to struggle in the future, as its population of young working citizens will increasingly be outnumbered by elderly retirees. Preventive measure to control common health issues are under criticism. In Japan, hospital stays are two to three times longer than in the West. Access to health care system is also a concern in Japan.

Health care in South Africa

South Africa's health system consists of a large public sector and a smaller but fast-growing private sector. Although the state contributes about 40% of all expenditures on health, the public health sector is under pressure to deliver services to about 80% of the population. The standard of health care delivered varies from province to province. With less resources and more poor people, cash-strapped provinces like the Eastern Cape face greater health challenges than wealthier provinces like Gauteng and the Western Cape. Government has controlled Malaria and other regional diseases, but controlling and managing AIDS is still a big challenge for the South African health care system.

Health care in Germany

Most Germans receive health care coverage through the public health insurance plans, which are funded from contributions of employers and employees. Currently, the rate is 15% of the net income which is compulsory deducted to the insurance system. Though quality and variety of health care services in Germany is one of the best in the world, the German health care system suffers from a lack of competition, insufficient or inappropriate care, shrinking revenue and an aging population.

Health care in France

WHO ranked France number one for Health care services, but high health care funding is a serious concern for the country. Concern is constantly rising about keeping health care expenditure under control by taking several measurements to control cost of insurance and fixing treatment costs.

Health care in Gulf Countries

Health care in GCC (UAE, Oman, Saudi Arabia, Bahrain, Qatar and Kuwait) has a higher demand than supply. Economic growth coupled with population growth is far higher than health care infrastructure growth. Currently GCC spent almost $12 billion USD on health care which will increase to $60 billion USD in just the next few years.

Health care conditions are getting worse as many health care diseases are increasing above 200%. Chronic and affluent disorders, along with genetic disorders are key challenges for the Arab world. Though GCC governments have initiated huge health care investments, lack of resources leads to lack of operational outcomes which cause several GCC nationals to opt for health care services abroad. Lack of health care trust within national the health care system presents a unique challenge in this part of the world.

Health care Globally

The global health care struggle for affordability, accessibility, availability and quality of care is apparent. Fragmented health care systems, commercialization of health care, unequal economies, health care resource shortages, aging populations, chronic health disorders and a lack of prevention programs are key factors behind struggling global health care challenges.

What's Future of Global Health care Crises?

There is no upfront blueprint solution for global health care crises. Certainly, primary health care with a focus on prevention programs can bring relief, but health care challenges are beyond reform or available solutions. Every country presents unique challenges which require unique solutions and no global reform would work to cure health care blues. Though collective experience with globally shared learning and understanding could be utilized more productively, and it would certainly bring better results, health care systems would still continue to struggle for many more years to come. Needless to say, prevention should be the prime focus of any health care system or reform.

Health care industry in the developing nations has been experiencing brain drain since the 70's. Health care professionals, especially doctors and nurses, from countries like India, Philippines, Thailand, and China etc migrate to countries like the US and the UK in search of better pay packages, better working environment and better lifestyles. This usually happens when the native country is unable to provide competitive remunerations. Brain drain creates a shortage of health care professionals and may increase the number gap between the patients and the health care professionals. As a result, the native countries do not have enough doctors and nurses to provide health care to the local people of their country. In the Philippines, for every two doctors who graduate from a medical school, three leave for foreign shores, resulting in a net loss of one doctor every year. To counteract it, the Government has started promoting medical tourism. In the past few years, the brain drain in Malaysia has intensified, with a dire shortage of specialists in public hospitals. The country has about 20 percent of the doctors working abroad as nurses.

Industry experts feel that medical tourism may eventually be able to mitigate the phenomenon of brain drain with foreign patients travelling back to their native countries. These health care facilities catering to foreign patients have world class facilities and provide the highest standards of care. Treating a foreign patient is more profitable than treating a domestic patient. Since revenue from the foreign patients are more, the health care agencies are able to provide better salaries and attractive packages, better than those facilities that cater to the domestic population. As more and more people from the developed countries start coming to the developing nations for medical care, the health care professionals may be attracted back to the native countries, thus reversing the brain drain. Many governments are working towards promoting medical tourism in their country to reverse the brain drain.

Medical tourism may claim to reverse external brain drain but may replace it with internal brain drain with health care professionals moving from the public sectors to the corporate ones. Those health care facilities that cater to the medical tourists not only provide world class facilities to the patients, but also a better working environment to the health care professionals. Health care professionals earn much more in these hospitals when compared to the Government-run hospitals. As a result, more and more health care professionals choose to work in corporate establishments rather than in public hospitals. This internal brain drain may leave the public hospitals with less doctors and nurses than what are required for a hospital to function. For example, Thailand experienced the replacement of external brain drain with internal brain drain in 2007 due to the higher pays provided at Bumrungrad. This brain drain was one of the reasons for the Bangkok government being unable to provide one doctor per 1,800 citizens for public health. In India, 59 per cent of India's practitioners are located in cities, and especially metropolitan ones. Medical tourism may intensify this gap with more health professionals attracted to large urban centres, and within them, to large corporate-run specialty institutions.

A research done by the World Bank showed that many countries are hit by internal brain drain, and the impact is more in countries who already have a shortage of nurses and doctors. However, the research also suggests that countries with higher numbers of health care professionals may not be hit hard due to the surplus of resources. Internal brain drain in these countries could be alleviated by reforms in medical education policies.

Medical tourism may be an answer to the brain drain in many developing countries and the governments should take leverage of their potential as medical tourism destinations to bring their trained professionals back into the country. Government policies should be modified to make the maximum use of medical tourism to attract medical tourists and facilitate easy access to medical care for foreigners. This modification needed includes not only the health care industry, but is equally needed for the tourism policies regarding providing medical visas. Profitable associations need to be made between the health care and tourism industry to promote medical tourism and provide a memorable experience to the medical tourist. However, considering the risk of internal brain drain, appropriate policies should also be formed to take maximum advantage of medical tourism without getting the adverse effects of it. Medical education policies should be reviewed in order to ascertain uniformity in the distribution of health care professionals and services.

The health care system abroad, more so in developed countries, is tagged with flaws. Medical tourism promoting countries are encashing these flaws by swaying the foreign patients, showcasing quality health care services at affordable cost.

The industry is growing rapidly because health care crises of the developed world become factors of the growth of the industry. When questions of the health care cost, lack of availability and need of arise, medical tourism answers immediately by providing affordable, accessible and available care. (See Appendix attached to this chapter 'Health Tourism in Middle East').

Blues

Medical tourism could serve as an interim solution until health care crises stabilized in the developed world, but this is only possible if medical tourism should not fall under the crises itself. I am afraid that the growth of medical tourism business is gradually sprouting to elicit contention. The major issues that bring in this second wave in the industry include education regarding the industry, awareness and availability of authentic information, legalization of the system, quality/transparency in operations, ethical aspects, need of a two-way street health system, need for good networking/communication, and the need for one world—one organization—one team.

What is the Perception of Medical Tourism?

The concept of this 'Generation Next Health Holidays' are still undercover among few people, which demands creating awareness about the medical care available abroad. Few are clouded with the misconception that it is a mere tourism or trip. Surgeons and Insurance companies alike hate the word "Tourism" in "Medical Tourism". They take it as a casual industry focused on tourism.

They must be made aware that in Medical Tourism the treatment remains the core focus with tourism as a complimentary. 'Information overload' created by innumerable quack blogs, websites and new so called "news" sites are responsible for the unreliable, unauthentic and fraudulent online information. Medical tourism is poorly portrayed due to the word of mouth by ignorant spreading of only the cons, while carefully masking the pros to suit their own business interests. This can be overcome by keeping the potential health care seekers informed about the official and responsible associations dedicated for Medical Tourism related affairs. Making the medical tourism market accessible to travel agents and health tourism websites exclusively recognized by governmental organizations can majorly resolve this issue with high revenue generation. Thus, misrepresentation of this industry can be dragged out for lack of depicting its clear picture.

Medical tourism facilitators must be educated about Globalization of Health care, regional health care crises and development, evaluation and monitoring of Medical Tourism Related Solutions. They must also be educated and trained about the regional, cultural and language differences, and health care ethics. This will enable them to recognize the cultural sensitivity for attracting patients especially from countries like Middle East.

Inside the Package—Quality and Transparency

Standardization and transparency in medical outcomes and quality care is a must in health care globalization. Safety and quality are of primary concern for potential patients considering medical services abroad. Every medical tourism destination claims to offer high quality service. However, the transparency in many aspects remains a query. In the developed countries health and medical regulatory laws ensure quality. There is little way of knowing an overseas facility or physician has the same quality. Internet claims certainly are highly dubious. Current health care accreditation programs might assure quality health care services but there is no one health care accreditation program dedicated specifically for international patient safety.

Critical issues like pre-operative check up and lack of post-operative follow-up care may involve unexpected complications or side-effects. There is an additional risk is of long flight journeys after the surgery which might lead to thrombosis or embolism. In such cases, the original doctor will be unavailable for rectifying the problem and in turn falls over the shoulders of the health care system within their home country. Understanding of post-operative care in medical tourism is still a challenge. The increasing demand for health care services from foreigners is being captured by corporate hospitals to increase their profits with a hike in prices. Besides, there exists a wide difference in this pricing between the hospitals in few countries. Health care services for foreigners might seem cheaper, but not necessarily for the locals. Excess glamorization of health care with the hospitals offering five star ambience and services is becoming more and more out of reach to sustain the "value for money". Serious concern is that the excessive and unjustified importance is given more for packaging than services in medical tourism promotion.

Unethical advertisements are flaunting on the web. Marketing traps could harm the entire industry if not addressed immediately. There lies a need of ethical marketing practice within international and national boundary. Therefore, the health and medical regulatory laws in medical tourism countries need to be transparent with standards of proper certification or accreditation of Medical Tourism providers and facilitators. They should adhere to standard guidelines to provide the best value and quality practice. The pricing issue can be handled with the concept of 'price banding' to provide consistent prices for different therapies and surgeries, which must be legalized by the government, along with accreditation. Additionally, hospitals can get certified on limiting high charges to foreigners as part of a dual pricing-system while offering lower prices to domestic patients.

Advertising health tourism must be done in a more professional way by the doctors visiting foreign countries, tourist companies, foreign travel agents, and international websites of government tourism. These strategies can minimize the issues of transparency and create a positive picture about the quality standards in the minds of foreign visitors.

Out of the Boundary Challenges—Out of the Box Solutions

Delivery of health care services for international patients comes with lots of cultural, ethical and legal challenges and complexity. There is no set service definition or scope of work for such segment. For instance, an international patients' service desk with a comprehensive patient feedback system and proactive follow-up might help in gaining confidence of patients but many hospitals do not provide proper interpreter services, there is not much thoughtfulness about professional health care interpreters. Having non-health care interpreters' agents certainly increase the chances of miscommunication. So far regulating and accreditation bodies have thought only about patient safety programs through developing quality health care services but out of the box solutions require for international patient considering ethical, legal and cultural challenges.

An Eye on Malpractice—Need for Legalization

Medical tourism is viewed as a solution by various medical associations and government authorities but itself is a reason for arising issues due to lack of formal legalization in the industry. Unlike local patients, foreign patients are left with hardly any access to local courts or medical boards in case of any violations due to poor malpractice laws. This is a challenge for both the industry and corporate health care service providers. Hence, it needs an acceptable legal approval officially from the respective authorities—Government, Insurance companies and corporate buyers.

There should be constant support and compensation for health care seekers travelling abroad from developed countries like UK and the US in case of any medical malpractice. Patient health care financing can be a step ahead offering for under developed countries. Patients must not be allowed to travel abroad unless health care services are unavailable, inaccessible, or unaffordable within their health care system. This can broadly change the industry scenario in terms of abating these legal issues.

Contention of 'Medical Apartheid'

Medical Tourism government authorities in many countries are trying to capture the profit by giving high end priority to the foreign patients neglecting the domestic patients. It is widening the gap and decreasing equity in offering health care for local patients, bringing in the two-tiered system of the 'have' and 'have-nots'. Balancing this local demand *vs.* global demand is of prime concern and it still remains a challenge to maintain quality on both sides. Health care must be affordable, accessible and available in home country and the priority is to be given for the residents.

Reinforcing Synergy

Finding a platform for bi-lateral communication within the health authorities, B2B opportunities between the medical tourism providers and insurance companies, and the two sectors—health care and tourism is challenging. There are many B2B providers, health authorities and insurance companies, but there is a need of more business to consumer relations communication, B2C events and interaction and platform for non-commercial networking. Many Medical Tourism events are appearing on calendars, but not many are focused on industry related issues and challenges. Medical tourism is in quest of a platform from which regular connections could be established to educate the consumer. Mutual marketing tactics between the health tourism industry and the foreign Insurance companies is another area to tackle. Marketing the medical tourism concept to the developed countries by state intervention is challenging, as it requires international tie-ups with Health Authorities and Insurance providers.

Coordination between Coordinators

The need of the hour is coordination between medical tourism stakeholders with intense knowledge exchange program between medical tourism promoting countries, medical tourism related association, regulating or accrediting bodies and global health care associations. Synergetic efforts would protect the interest of the medical tourism industry, in the view of ultimate objective of delivering quality health care services to patients.

Sole Entity for Sole Authority—One World, One organization, One team

Most of the issues arise in executing the health tourism activities is due to the different regulations, different standards and different laws existing to govern this industry. There is a need for one sole authority/ organization to set direction, objectives, mission and role. This helps in regulating and managing medical tourism effectively with active participation of Health care Leaders, Insurance Providers, and Corporate Buyers. Hence, one world—one organization—one team will strengthen the destination to set-up uniform standards and legalization of health care.

Medical tourism is definitely on the way to 'The Edge' in terms of growth but not without controversies. To set back its related issues and avoid hindrance in its burgeoning pace, every medical tourism destination must identify, analyze and implement the mitigating strategies for touching that niche in the industry. For this, the basic key note remains- "A complete quality concierge service is all it takes to make them smile and bow". Let us work together for one world—one organization—one team.

- Almost 70% of Americans search for medical information online.
- Over 113 million Americans search for health information online.
- Most Americans now gather information online through search engines such as Google, Yahoo and Bing.
- Keeps business flowing by advertising online in the Health Tourism Magazine.
- Advertise to your target audience and get more "bang" for your buck, because of the reduced costs of advertising online.
- Reach thousands of potential clients, employees, industry participants and other important publics.
- Generate inquiries and sales leads from health care professionals, buyers and sellers.
- Increase your "Brand Name" reputation throughout the country in Health Tourism Magazine.
- Educate the world on your organization, what you provide, and why it is unique.
- Use the Health Tourism Magazine to communicate the vision of positively improving the health and wellness of people today.

The demand for health tourism is growing in the Gulf. Why?

There are several factors contributing to the growth of medical travel from the Gulf Co-operation Council countries to other destinations. The GCC is witnessing a rapid population growth rate combined with an aging population and an acute shortage of qualified medical staff and bed capacity. A report from consultancy McKinsey, published last summer, estimates that over the next 20 years treatment demand in the region will rise by 240 per cent. In particular, cardiovascular disease will experience a steep increase (419 per cent), as will diabetes-related ailments (323 per cent). The medical establishments in the Gulf are not equipped to handle these numbers. So there is a real need for the governments to send their nationals to be treated abroad. People also choose to travel abroad for medical treatment, even if local expertise is available, to avoid waiting lists or because of lower costs.

Is the Middle East considered a key market for hospitals trying to attract foreign patients?

Yes. The Middle East is one of the few areas in the world where the government pays to send its nationals to be treated abroad.

What do you estimate the value of the health tourism business from the GCC to be?

It is very hard to estimate what the overall size of the industry is in the region. There are unconfirmed reports that the industry in the Gulf was worth about $10 billion in 2008. Overall, the amount of money at stake in the global medical tourism market is huge. McKinsey estimates that the industry was worth $60 billion in 2006 and that it will reach $100 billion by 2012.

Which countries or regions tend to attract the most patients from the Middle East?

According to McKinsey, 58 per cent of GCC patients go to North America for treatment, 32 per cent go to Asia, eight per cent go to Europe and the remaining two per cent go to other countries in the Middle East.

What sort of medical treatment or surgery is most in demand?

The main categories of treatment in demand right now are cardiovascular, diabetes, sense organ diseases and cancer treatment. Of course, these figures are easier to track than elective and non-essential surgeries that are basically done by and paid for by individuals, because it is usually the government or the insurance companies that pay for them. Elective surgery procedures, where a person would elect to visit another country and combine their vacation with a surgical procedure, are usually of a cosmetic nature.

A number of health tourism projects are planned for the Gulf, for example, Bahrain's Dilmunia Health Island. What are their prospects?

Each project will have to be studied on a case-by-case scenario, but what we can say for sure is that it takes a lot of work to convince potential patients to come to the Gulf region for treatment. We have seen some initiatives launched in the last five years, notably in Dubai's Health Care City, Bahrain's Dilmunia and some other projects in Saudi Arabia. I would like to see these projects succeed, but I think we still have a long way to go.

Can the Gulf become a medical tourism destination in its own right?

In the long-term, yes. There are some centres of medical excellence in the region and we can build on that to attract international patients. The region is already a popular tourist hub for Europeans, Arabs, Asians and North Americans and we can build on this brand recognition. However, I have to stress that this is a long-term project and it needs the partnership of the public and private sectors.

Can the Gulf compete with cheaper health tourism destinations, for example India or Thailand?

Yes we can. You cannot have a medical tourism positioning strategy based on being the cheapest. Singapore for example is much more expensive than India. However, they do not position their medical tourism offer as the cheapest, but as one of the best in the world. South Korea, a recent entrant into the health tourism segment, has been very successful in attracting patients from the GCC recently and they are far more expensive than Thailand and India. I don't think that the Gulf would want to position itself as a cheap medical tourism destination, but rather create a niche market within the health tourism segment.

You're organizing the World Health Tourism Congress in Durban next year. How many participants from this region are you expecting?

We anticipate more than 700 delegates to attend and about 20 per cent of those will be from the Arab region. Now in its fifth year, the World Health Tourism Congress has established itself as the biggest annual global event for medical tourism in the world. We focus on bringing together the destinations that tend to be "exporters" of medical tourism—sending patients to other countries for treatment—with the "importers" of medical patients in a business-to-business format. We invite all decision-makers from the GCC health ministries so they can meet with hospitals and clinics from all over the world. It makes their job of searching for the best hospitals and best treatments in the world much easier.

At this time there are more people living on this small planet than have ever lived before—all with a need for proper health care, sanitation, food, and a decent quality of life. The rationing of health care and the numbers of patients per day has placed great pressures on physicians and health care providers. While people have started going to Dubai and other centres for treatment from outside world, traditionally Arabs have been visiting several destinations in the world, including India, in search of good medical treatment. "Medical tourism", people visiting the gulf only for medical care, is a new phenomenon. Thus, it is imperative for the physicians who treat the Arabs in their host countries or go as expats in Gulf countries to man their medical cities, to be acquainted with their cultural practices. Understanding the Middle Eastern health environment, the cultural perceptions of health and illness, and the social factors that interplay in the patient's personal decisions are essential for the betterment of health service provision to this population.

Who is an Arab?

The term Arab is associated with a particular region of the world. Almost all of the people in the region extending from the Atlantic coast of Northern Africa to the Arabian Gulf call themselves Arabs. The classification is based largely on common language and a shared sense of geographic, historical, and cultural identity. The total population of the Arab world is approximately 230 million in 22 nations. there are 10 Arab countries in Africa (Morocco, Mauritania, Algeria, Tunisia, Libya, Sudan, Somalia, Eritrea, Djibouti and Egypt) and 12 countries in Asia (Iraq, Jordan, Lebanon, Syria, Kuwait, Bahrain, Qatar, Oman, United Arab Emirates, Saudi Arabia, Yemen, and the people of Palestine). Despite the national boundaries, the Arabs view themselves as a unified entity. Arabs are not homogeneous with respect to religious belief, but include Christians, Jews, and Muslims. The large majority of Arabs are Muslim (92%), however, in total the Arabs comprise only about 17% of the Islamic population worldwide (with other substantial populations in Indonesia, Malaysia, South Asia, Iran, Central Asia, Turkey, and Sub-Saharan Africa). The religion of Islam is closely associated with Arab identity because of the origin of Islam in the Arabian Peninsula and the fact that the language of Arabic is the sacred language of the Holy Qur'an. Since, fertility is high in the Arab world while so are many negative health indicators such as IMR (infant mortality rate), but no statistic is consistent throughout the Arab world.

Understanding Islamic Socio-Religious Behaviour

A Muslim is literally "one who submits to the will of God". The system of Islam was established in the 7th century A.D. The Prophet Muhammad, who lived in the 7th century AD, is considered the final prophet and the messenger of the final universal law for all humanity in all subsequent times. The sacred scripture, the Qur'an, is considered by Muslims as pure Divine revelation and as such is the ultimate source for the judgment of human behaviour. Islam is a complete way of life—a social, economic, spiritual and political system and it is outlined in array of practices of daily life. These practices range from spiritual actions like prayer and meditation, to washing, eating, dress, economic activity, rules for war and peace, relationships and roles in society, family interactions, marriage, birth, and death.

The Islamic norm for politeness includes not making definite assertions about the future e.g. this disease is curable—the Muslim will invariably add In-sha Allah—God-willing. Muslim tends to perceive bold assertions about the future as arrogant disrespect for God's will. Many doctors perceive the Muslims as fatalistic in their acceptance of bad health outcomes. Muslims may sometimes be resistant to the idea that their disease is the product of a carcinogen or risk behaviour rather than the result of Alah's Will.

Dietary Restrictions

Consumption of pork is entirely forbidden by Islam. This has presented ethical issues in modern times, as some medical products are produced through pigs and other animals. For example, genetic research has developed the ability to produce medically usable forms of insulin in pigs. Lard, gelatin, and some forms of non-soy lecithin, are pork products that are generally widespread in processed foods. Because of the prominence of these products in prepared foods, the Arab Muslim patient is often wary of hospital meals. Most Muslims consume meat that is specially slaughtered viz. halal meat. For Muslims, alcohol may not be consumed in any form—as beverage, in cooking, or in non-emergency medication. Consumption of alcohol among Muslims is considered shameful.

Modesty and Gender Separation

Generally male/female interaction in Islamic societies is limited to the family unit and is explicitly defined by Islamic law. Gender separation is generally observed in public interactions, including separation within adolescent and adult hospital wards. It is generally inappropriate for non-family members of the opposite sex to approach for conversation. Handshakes between non-related men and women are considered improper. Eye contact is frequently avoided. The male doctor may not have eye contact with female patient. The female patient might not look directly at the male practitioner when speaking or the male patient might not look directly at the female practitioner when speaking. In general, same-sex providers should be made available if possible and examinations in front of other individuals should be avoided. Strong modesty norms make issues that are related to reproductive health embarrassing.

Arab society has developed a philosophy of life that includes traditional values:

(1) A feeling of dependency on God.
(2) The fear of God's punishment on earth as well as in the hereafter.
(3) A deep-seated-respect for tradition and for the past.
(4) Politeness to all and generosity if something is lost or goes wrong, for example, death, etc., the Arab would not stop to examine the causes for the loss, but will merely sigh philosophically, 'this is the will of God'.

Similarly, they believe that all children are born simply because God willed it. No child is born without his 'ruzq' (wish) being sent down from heaven with him. Indeed, to practice birth control is to oppose the will of God.God is interested In his everyday behaviour, he will be punished for his 'bad acts', and rewarded for his 'good'. Consequently, if he commits a sin or undertakes a move which might be construed as sinful, he will expect punishment e.g. a traditional Arab may report that two days after he had committed adultery, one of his sons drowned.

Arab family system and Health Care

Four types of family units are found in the Middle East. The first and most simple structure is the nuclear unit, which consists of the father, mother, and offspring. The second familial unit is the 'aila (the extended family) or the joint family. It consists of father, mother, unwed children, as well as wedded sons and their wives and children, unwed paternal aunts, and, sometimes, unwed paternal uncles. In short, this unit is composed of blood relatives plus women who were brought into the kinship through marriage. The third type of blood kinship unit is the hammula, or clan. It consists of all individuals who claim descent from the same paternal ancestor. The social, psychological, and economic security of the individual stems from membership in the extended family and this membership is the primary motivating factor for the decision-making of the individual. Women do not add their husband's name to their own after marriage. All members of a hammula identify and relate themselves to one another in a very systematic way. For example, a young man refers to every one of his fellow young men of the hammula as ibn 'anim, or "paternal first cousin". The same for every one of the young women referring to each other as bint 'amm, or "paternal female cousin".

The feeling of kinship is so strong that the easiest way to insult an Arab is to curse one of his relatives. This norm has a great deal of bearing of health behaviour.

Caution for health professionals

It is important for a health professional not to rush his or her contact with the client. One should be careful on how to express admiration for any female member of the family. An appropriate comment would be, "what a nice child" or "you have a nice wife" with regards to a spouse, which would be taken in a positive manner by the individual. A health professional should seek to establish a relationship of trust with the entire family, not just the patient. For Arab patients, it should be understood that the family's presence is highly emotionally important. Once this trust is developed, the family can play an important supportive role in health therapy and place much weight on the physician's opinion.

Many Arabs live on a diet that is largely seasonal in the Middle East. They consume a high fiber intake of fruit and vegetables locally grown in the summer and dried beans and pulses in the winter. Meat is considered a luxury and is consumed infrequently, except the rich. They also encounter foods that are more often processed and high in fat. This is predictive of rising rates of diabetes, cardiovascular diseases, and certain cancers that did not previously affect these individuals.

Respect is conferred on the individual by having a large number of successful children. For the women, the first birth is viewed as an important initiation into womanhood. The position of mother holds a great amount of respect among the Arabs. The typical supporting participant for the woman in delivery is the mother, sister, sister-in-law, or mother-in-law. Families might request the hospital to provide a female ob/gyn to supervise the delivery; this implies that those families do not wish to have any male staff in the birth room. Breastfeeding is traditionally encouraged within Arab societies. Islam exhorts women to breast feed her child for two years. The same is the advice from international health agencies.

Bury the dead quickly and with utmost respect and dignity

For Muslims, prolonging a person's life in this world with no possibility of further action is seen as futile and an interference with the person's passing to Allah. Arabs view the dead as having returned to God. The tradition exhorts Muslims to bury the dead quickly and with utmost respect and dignity At death, the body is cleaned and perfumed by the family and wrapped in a simple white garb. Muslims believe that at birth and death, every human is equal. Autopsies are often refused and Arabs consider them disrespectful to the dead. Death is an occurrence that is viewed as a community obligation in which all community members must participate. Wailing and gasping is a common reaction in grieving. If the patient who dies is young, the grieving process requires more time and significance. The death of young parents who leave small children behind is particularly traumatic with the loss of the children's primary support system. Similarly, the death of a child is a tremendous loss that is surrounded by extensive grieving.

Sources

Abraham, S.Y. and N. Abraham, 1981. The Arab World and Arab Americans: Understanding a Neglected Minority. Detroit: Wayne State University Centre for Urban Studies

Abraham, S.Y. and N. Abraham, 1983. Arabs in the New World: Studies on Arab-American Communities. Detroit: Wayne State University Centre for Urban Studies

ACCESS Cultural Museum. 2651 Saulino CT., Dearborn, Michigan. Open for viewing during most regular business hours.

Al-Qudsi, S. "The Health Sector of a High Fertility Region: The Arab World", in Teebi, A.S., Farag, T.I., eds. Genetic Disorders Among Arab Populations., 1997. New York: Oxford University Press.

Deeb, M.E. and Sayegh, L.G. "Population Dimensions in the Arab World", in Teebi, A.S., Farag, T.I., eds. Genetic Disorders Among Arab Populations., 1997. New York: Oxford University Press.

Good, B. and M. Del Vecchio Good, 1982. "Patient requests in primary care clinics", In N.J. Chrisman and T.W. Maretzki eds. Clinically Applied Anthropology., Boston: D. Reidel.

Helman, A.G., 1997. Culture, Health, and Illness. Third Edition. Boston: Butterwoth Heinemann.

Hahn, R.A., 1995. Sickness and Healing: An Anthropological Perspective. New Haven and London: Yale University Press.

Hamarneh, S.K., 1983. "The Life Sciences" In The Genius of Arab Civilization: Source of the Renaissance. Second Edition. J.R. Hayes. Editor. Cambridge: The MIT Press pp. 173-200.

Hammad, A., 1989. Effectiveness and Efficiency in the Management of Palestinian Health Services. Ph.D. Thesis. University of Manchester. Jan. 1989.

Hassoun, R.J., 1995. A Bioanthropological Perspective of Hypertension in Arab-Americans in the Metropolitan Detroit Area. Dissertation. University of Florida, Gainesville. UMI Microfiche.

Ingstad, B. and S.R. Whyte, 1995. Disability and Culture. Berkeley: University of California Press.

Johnson, in Michigan Department of Public Health, 1995. Minority Health in Michigan. Lansing: Michigan.

Kleinman, A., 1981. Patients and Healers in the Context of Culture. Berkeley: University of California Press.

Kulwicki, A., 1990. Cardiovascular and Diabetes Survey.

Michigan Department of Public Health, 1988. Minority Health in Michigan: Closing the Gap. Lansing: Michigan.

Naff, A. Becoming American: The Early Arab Immigrant Experience, 1985. Carbondale and Edwardsville: Southern Illinois University Press.

Savoie, C., 1995. Environmental Health Director of ACCESS.

Teebi, A.S., 1997. "Introduction", in Teebi, A.S., Farag, T.I., eds. Genetic Disorders Among Arab Populations., 1997. New York: Oxford University Press.

United Nations Development Program (UNDP) 1993: Human Development Report. Investing in Health. Oxford University Press, New York.

APPENDIX

HEALTH TOURISM IN MIDDLE EAST

The Middle East has unique dual position in the Medical Tourism Industry. On one hand, the region's well-developed hospitals are preparing to capture the international market for elective procedures while on the other, international health care organizations are tapping into GCC's affluent society in search of highly sophisticated and advanced health care services unavailable within the GCC. The Middle East is a region that spans southwestern Asia and northern Africa. It has no clear boundaries, sometimes it is also referred as Middle-Eastern. Arabian Peninsula or Gulf Corporate Council is most affluent area in Middle East. GCC countries include Saudi Arabia, Qatar, Kuwait, Oman, Bahrain and UAE.

The rise of medical tourism provides an opportunity for the Middle East, which so far has made few inroads in the sector. From many years, a top priority for medical providers around the world have attracted medical tourists from the Middle East, now the trend is gradually reversing as the Middle East is seeking to attract medical tourists where the cost of health care and delays in getting treatment have risen sharply.

Health care Demand

Health care demand in the Arab world is under significant pressure as GCC spent just 2-3% of GDP on health care. The health care demand in GCC is growing rapidly. McKinsey estimated that GCC health care spending would increase five fold in next year from currently $12 billion to $60 billion. This demand will continue growing until new strategies on the part of government and private health care players come into play.

Although GCC health care systems are far better than they were 20 years ago, many residents remain unsatisfied with the availability and quality of care at government-run hospitals and clinics. Government agencies mostly lack the managerial skills needed to run health care facilities, and cash incentives alone have not been enough to attract specialists to treat the rising numbers of people with ailments such as heart disease and cancer, stated in report by McKinsey.

Key drivers for the growth in health care demand are population growth, limited investment and increase in affluent health disorders. A recent report suggested that Arabians suffer from more than 900 chronic health disorders. In United Arab Emirates, diabetes prevalence rate is above 20 percent, which means one out of five is diabetic.

Today GCC population is 35 million. By 2015, the size of the population will increase at a compound annual growth rate (CAGR) of around 3.0 percent, one of the highest in the world. As a result, total GCC population in 2025 will be almost twice the size it is today.

In 2008, a report done by ExHealth revealed above 50% people in UAE are overweight mainly because of sedentary lifestyle. Health care disorders will increase by 20% in next few years because of poor preventative measures and lack of understanding.

There is lack of super specialty services in GCC especially above tertiary level care. Emergency health care services are still challenge for GCC as not many private hospitals are prepared to handle cases.

Middle Eastern Patients

If the current trends continue and if GCC countries do not take immediate measure, patients from GCC will continue traveling for medical services, providing opportunity to medical tourism stakeholder of west and Asia.

Arabs from GCC spend billions of dollars on health care outsourcing. Saudi Arab alone sent more than 200,000 patients in 2008 abroad for medical treatment. UAE spent over billion dollars on health care outsourcing. Together, all Arab patients from Arabian Peninsula have willingness to travel outside of UAE.

A recent survey done by the national newspaper reveal that 70% UAE population would prefer to travel outside if they get serious illness. The GCC market is willing to travel. In fact, they travel abroad just for common health checkups. The market has affordability, and most importantly, the government sponsors the medical cost in most of the cases.

Considering all evaluations, it is believed that GCC is within undersupply today; tomorrow they may have enough supply, but still affordability will be a big question because of inflation and several other factors. There is great need of coordinated efforts from government and private sector to reverse the trend till then international health care providers can land a hand to provide health care services to struggling GCC Health care.

At a recent roundtable held at the World Medical Tourism and Global Health care Congress in Los Angeles, health leaders from the UAE noted that inbound health care is a large an opportunity in the Middle East as outbound. Undersecretary of Health He Nasser Khalifa Al-Budoor of the United Arab Emirates stated, "A very important topic under scrutiny was the economic and qualitative benefits of medical tourism to a country's population and the positive impact medical tourism exerts on health care quality within a specific country and region".

"We are looking at a lot of collaboration. Our recent health reform was intended to strengthen the health systems in Dubai which will assist us going forward. We are here to strengthen medical tourism," added Laila Al Jassmin, CEO of the Clinical Support Services Sector for Dubai Health Authority.

Understanding the Outbound Target Market

When health care providers intend to serve GCC market, their prime target could be Arab patients. Providers can build a successful brand if they just provide personalized care to Islamic Patients. Many health care providers consider Arab patients demanding, but my last ten years of experience in Middle East helped me to realize that if we understand Islamic patient requirement, we can make Arab patients happy very easily.

Regrettably, companies spend most of their money on advertisements and promotion; they do not spend on cultural consultancy services. Understanding culture is one of the key component in serving medical tourism industry.

If a health care provider would like to extend personalized service to a Muslim or Islamic patient, the below suggestions could be very helpful. Implementation of below guidelines would make the stay of a Muslim patient in hospital more acceptable and contented. It would also make sure that the care being provided was of the highest quality possible for Muslim patients. The recommendations cover aspects of clinical care, food services, religious observance and visiting arrangements amongst others.

Food Services

All catering staff should be aware that only halal meat (i.e. meat slaughtered according to religious requirements) must be given to Muslim patients. They should also be made aware that Muslims do not eat pork or any other pig meat and its products e.g. Hand washing before and after meals is particularly important to Muslims. Bathroom facilities are readily available to ambulant patients, however washing facilities should be made available to bedridden patients at meal times.

Clinical or Nursing Care

It is preferable for a female Muslim to be cared for by females and a male Muslim by males. This is most important during confinement when strict privacy is very essential. Only female health workers should be present. Exposure should be kept to a minimum. The position of delivery should be discussed and the woman given the choice.

Present medical examination techniques should be modified where possible so that as little of the patient is exposed as possible, whilst not inhibiting the medical procedures. Facilities should be provided for male circumcision if required.

Alcohol

Alcohol and any other intoxicating substance are prohibited in Islam. Where a choice exists, medicines containing alcohol should not be used. In emergencies, this rule does not apply if an alternate drug is not available, but this should be explained to the patient. If the medication is necessary, then Islam permits its use.

Forms

In most circumstances informed consent must not be only in English. It must be verbal as well as written in their own language so that the issue is fully understood. In circumstances where the patient has difficulty communicating in English, a professional interpreter should be arranged.

Maternity Services after delivery

The placenta (which is part of the baby) should be offered to the parents for disposal by burial in accordance with Islamic tradition.

After Death

The face and indeed the whole body of the deceased must be covered by a sheet. The body must be handled as little as possible. Muslims believe that the body 'feels' pressure and pain numerous times more than that applied. Muslims also believe that the soul remains close to the body until burial. The body must be handled with utmost respect only by a person of the same sex. Relatives may wish to pray close to the body or in a room close by. Islam prohibits post-mortems. However, the statutory laws of the country must be followed with respect to post-mortems.

Fasting in the month of Ramadan

Fasting is compulsory for all healthy, adult Muslims on reaching puberty. Every individual is responsible for his or her own fast. Fasting begins an hour before sunrise and ends at sunset. It is a total fast with abstinence from any food or drink. Smoking is not allowed. Gargling is acceptable as long as no fluid goes down the throat. Besides fasting in Ramadan, some Muslims also keep optional fasts. Fasting is a purification inwardly and outwardly. Exempted from fasting are pregnant, lactating or menstruating women, the ill and travelers.

Visiting the Sick

Strong emphasis is placed on the virtues of visiting the sick. The sick Muslim is usually happy to receive many visitors. It is a requirement of the family members of the sick Muslim to notify as many people as possible of the illness. This is usually done by the close relatives.

Above are just few basic tips provided by authorities, as this helps in understanding Islamic patient needs.

Marketing

As marketing guru Kotler writes, "What should our aim be with customers? First, follow the Golden Rule of Marketing: Market to your customers as you would want them to market to you. Second, recognize that your success depends on your ability to make your customers successful. Aim to make your customers better off. Know their needs and exceed their expectations. Organizations must view the customer as a financial asset that needs to be managed and maximized like any other asset. Tom Peters sees customers as an "appreciating asset." They are the company's most important asset, and yet their value is not even found in the organization's books.

Turkey has seen a boom in the number of hospitals accredited by the US-based Joint Commission International (JCI). "With 33 JCI-accredited hospitals, 12 percent of all JCI-accredited hospitals are located in Turkey—

which is more than anywhere else in the world," he noted. Along with this, he noted an increase in the availability of hospital and procedural information in English, such as on hospital Web sites. "What we can now see in Turkey is a robust health care infrastructure, including domestic accreditation procedures," he said.

Turkey's medical tourism potential strong

Woodman notes a recent change in the demographics of medical tourism, saying that while in the past it was the rich who traveled abroad to save on procedures like nose jobs and tummy tucks, today's health tourist is of another variety. "You now see members of the middle and upper working class traveling abroad for medical procedures—because they've realized that you don't have to drift into financial ruin for an operation. Not everybody can afford $45,000 to $60,000 for a new hip or knee, or a quadruple bypass operation—but they can probably scrape together $15,000," he said.

But with an issue such as health, it boils down to more than cost, Woodman noted, explaining Turkey's strong points in terms of quality and service provided. "Turkey's superior health care infrastructure and relatively short flying times are attracting an increasing number of European, North American and Middle Eastern patients. Well-known for its rich heritage, breathtaking beauty and Mediterranean flair, it is easy to see why an estimated 200,000 medical tourists each year are choosing to have their procedures in Turkey," Woodman said, noting Turkey's proximity to many patients when compared to places like Thailand and Malaysia. "In Turkey, patients can receive American-style care at JCI-accredited hospitals for prices ranging from 30-80 percent less than out-of-pocket expenses they'd have to pay in the US."

In addition, the factors that draw traditional tourists to the country—the history, sights and tourist stops—are also important to medical tourism. More and more facilities are looking into the connection between wellness and post-operative care, Woodman noted. "Turkey has a lot going for it both on the clinical/procedural side and in terms of health care maintenance," he said, noting the trend toward focus on medically supervised spas and recovery centres.

A final important quality that Turkey can boast in terms of medical tourism, Woodman says, is simple: experience. "Two millennia ago, wealthy Greeks were traveling here for baths and spas," he said, noting also, viewed from one perspective, medical tourism is at the end of the day still a form of tourism. Turkey has experience in tourism and in making tourists feel welcome and that their trip was worthwhile, providing high-level service, he notes. "Medical tourism is the same thing, essentially—making patients leave this place feeling that they've had a good time and come away with a bargain."

"Turkey has a good shot at positioning itself in the medical tourism world—it is in a central location, not to mention the sheer number of JCI hospitals there, a history of tourism, the service provided, and references," Woodman said.

Facts on medical tourism in Turkey

Medical tourists traveling to Turkey come from Europe and the Middle East in addition to Russia and countries in the former Soviet bloc for a variety of reasons, including both cost and the quality of care in their home countries. The hot spots for medical tourism in Turkey are the urban centres of Istanbul, Azmir and Ankara, in addition to alternative medical and spa centres scattered throughout Anatolia. The main specialties in Turkey drawing medical tourists are bone marrow transplantation, cardiology and cardiovascular surgery, dentistry, genetics, neurosurgery, obstetrics/gynecology and assisted reproduction, oncology, ophthalmology, orthopedics, plastic surgery and transplantation. Medical tourism in Turkey grew by 40 percent between 2007 and 2008 and according to Woodman, projections estimate that private and public Turkish medical establishments will make around $8 billion in 2015 by serving 1 million foreign patients.

High cost of health care in North America and Europe

With rising health care costs and hospital waiting times in North America and Europe, the global medical tourism sector has been booming in recent years, especially in Asia, where countries such as India, Thailand and Singapore can offer medical care for a fraction of the price that it would cost in the US. Until recently the Middle East has been a major consumer, rather than a provider, of health care services in this context. Now governments in the region, particularly in the UAE and other GCC countries, are hoping to reverse this trend, by building health care facilities that will attract patients from elsewhere. The leading global health care accreditation and certification organization, Joint Commission International (JCI), whose accreditation has become the international gold standard for the quality and safety of health facilities, has now accredited a total of 16 hospitals in the UAE, all of them (with the exception of the American Hospital, Dubai, which was accredited in 2000) in the three years since May 2006. Saudi Arabia now has 20 JCI-accredited institutions, while Jordan and Qatar each have five. These numbers compare very favourably with leading medical tourism destinations such as Singapore, which has 14 JCI-accredited hospitals, and Thailand, which has four. But it is telling that so many UAE nationals still travel abroad for medical procedures rather than have them at home, spending some US $2 billion annually in the process.

UAE has a huge disadvantage in terms of the cost of medical care. For example, the average cost of heart by-pass surgery in the UAE is US $44,000, compared to US $18,500 in Singapore, US $11,000 in Thailand, US $10,000 in India and US $9,000 in Malaysia. Nevertheless, the UAE price tag still compares very favourably with the US $130,000 cost of doing the same procedure in the US, indicating the huge potential that still remains in the medical tourism market.

The UAE has the opportunity and the means to become an important medical tourism destination. India is of course better placed and already has advanced facilities to keep its position as market leader. But the increasingly low confidence of developed countries, namely, the USA and UK, in their country's health care system, is an opportunity for the Emirates. Improving facilities and regulation could attract many medical tourists. Instead, Middle Eastern governments are encouraging public-private partnership (PPP) model, under which a government project is funded and operated through a partnership between the government and one or more private sector companies. The latter raise the finance for the capital investment, in return for which they receive a contract or lease to design and build the facilities and operate services. Government contributions to PPP may also include the transfer of existing assets such as hospitals to a private operator.

All providers will have to work out how to cope with the chronic shortage of qualified medical staff in the region. The payer system must also provide coverage to all citizens. Notably, in Saudi Arabia, Abu Dhabi and Dubai, health insurance is a must for expatriate workers. Bahrain is also introducing the same health insurance requirements for expatriates. A decision must be made on whether the vulnerable will or will not be exempted from financial contributions, or if a minimum universal package should be developed for all. However, it can be achieved throughout the region, given the political will, and with the promise that access to health care services will not be restricted. These assurances can be reinforced by increasing government investment in providing better basic health care services, focusing on public health policy, disease prevention and expanding primary care coverage, while gradually carrying out insurance coverage for specialist secondary and tertiary care.

Some Countries offer a basic package that covers the main health problems and offer it at a low cost or for free for the less well off. Meanwhile, extra packages including more services and benefits are available at a premium for those who can afford it. Health care systems can only work in an environment policed by credible, independent and efficient institutions which provide transparent rules and foster competition. This illustrates the need for a robust regulatory system, whose main objective should be the protection of patients. To achieve this, governments should implement and enforce improved standards for all aspects of health care, ranging from structural requirements for facilities to standards of care and staff qualifications, and perhaps even to limits on the fees that can be charged for certain procedures. The system must also have a mechanism for monitoring provider performance and allow the discontinuation of the services of the non-performers. Transparently and effectively enforcing standards and dealing firmly with low-quality providers, as Dubai did with its cosmetic surgery clinics in 2008, will build confidence among patients.

Success may require the creation of a public insurance system in parallel with the private one, to cover the higher-risk and lower income sections of the population that might otherwise be unable to get cover in a completely free-market system with only private insurers.

Medical city model is catching the fancy of Arabs

Numerous countries are taking the opportunity to enhance their marketing programs, working as a team by setting up health care clusters and medical cities. What's this we hear about lower patient inquiries and cut backs in marketing spending? Have we no faith in the balance of economics? What happens when employees lose jobs? The first problematic expense for a laidoff employee is health care. In many countries where many employees enjoyed employer paid health care programs, now one is faced with paying the actual cost of the program their employer provided them with. This can range from $100 to $1000 per month. How many unemployed workers can foot a bill this high? Likely not many and, accordingly, the number of uninsured and underinsured persons go up.

What about the credit crunch? Employers typically use credit each month to support their overhead costs, paying cash only for those types of expenses requiring cash payment, such as health care premiums. With credit companies and banks reducing their extension of credit lines, employers have to spend cash for previously credited items on their balance sheets. Now employers cut back on or eliminate their health care plans altogether. The number of uninsured and underinsured persons goes up.

What does this mean for medical tourism? More and more patients will be looking for alternative means for their more essential elective procedures such as orthopedics, bariatrics and cardiac care. If there was ever a time to spend your marketing dollars wisely, the time is now.

Many countries have taken this opportunity to expand their marketing programs, seizing the recession as a chance to work together and to get the biggest bang for their buck through setting up health care clusters and medical cities. Why not look to your government for financial assistance to promote your country and increase tourism revenues?

The Medical Tourism Association recently completed a Middle Eastern Tour to Israel, Jordon and Dubai. MTA announced the opening of its Tel Aviv Office to a group of 70 health care providers and government representatives at a conference sponsored by Israel Scientific Instruments, its partner in the region. ISI organized the free MTA conference as an educational seminar about market opportunities in the US, health care cluster development, and strategic market development in furtherance of the MTA's primary educational directive.

The opening of the Tel Aviv Office is designed to facilitate the development of medical tourism to the region though member management and to address the considerations of the region unique to that part of the world.

Following the event, the MTA delegation moved on to Arab Health in Dubai where it exhibited at the event which hosted thousands of exhibitors from all over the world representing the best of international health care.

The 2009 MTA initiatives were developed through its Dubai Office which is located in Dubai Health Care City. Dr, Prem Jagyasi will be spearheading the MTA Certification Program with the top quality health care facilities in Dubai for certification of facilitators and international patient departments. The Dubai office is responsible for coordinating all MTA member programs amongst the regional offices throughout the Middle East and the Gulf Coast Countries.

Jordon Hospital, under the patronage of His Excellency the Prime Minister Engineer Nader Al Dahabi held the first MTA and Jordon International Medical Tourism Congress of over 150 health care providers and government officials January 30 to February 2, 2009. Amongst the topics held were: The Business Case for Medical Tourism, What Works and What Does Not, Branding, Marketing and the Role of Medical Tourism Facilitators. The conference was well received with a very positive conclusion of the high potential for Jordon in the medical tourism industry.

In this issue, we are taking a look at some of these marketing opportunities, starting with our feature on the Ethnic Employee. Evaluating the most costeffective platform must begin with an understanding of your largest market segment. We take a look at the Future of Medical Tourism and the rise of Medical Tourism in Europe with a special piece on HCA International Hospitals in the UK, dispelling some of the myth about UK health care.The launching of the Medical Tourism Magazine website has been a great success. The goal of the online version of Medical Tourism Magazine is to obtain readership from hundreds of thousands to eventually millions. info@medicaltourismmag.com

History of health care development and Islamic medicine

One of its most famous scholars was Hunayn ibn Ishaq, who eventually translated the entire canon of Greek medical works into Arabic, including the Hippocratic oath. Later a director of the House of Wisdom, Hunayn also wrote at least twenty-nine original treatises of his own on medical topics, and a collection of ten essays on ophthalmology which covered, in systematic fashion, the anatomy and physiology of the eye and the treatment of various diseases which afflict vision. The first known medical work to include anatomical drawings, the book was translated into Latin and for centuries was the authoritative treatment of the subject in both Western and Eastern universities. Others prominent in Islamic medicine were Yuhanna ibn Masawayh, a specialist in gynecology and the famous Abu Bakr Muhammad ibn Zakariya al-Razi—known to the West as Rhazes. According to a bibliography of his writings al-Razi wrote 184 works, including a huge compendium of his experiments, observations, and diagnoses with the title al-Hawi, "The All-Encompassing."

A fountainhead of medical wisdom during the Islamic era, al-Razi, according to one contemporary account, was also a fine teacher and a compassionate physician, who brought rations to the poor and provided nursing for them. He was also a man devoted to common sense, as the titles of two of his works suggest. The Reason Why Some Persons and the Common People Leave a Physician Even If He Is Clever, and A Clever Physician Does Not Have the Power to Heal All Diseases, for That is Not within the Realm of Possibility.

The scholars at the House of Wisdom, unlike their modern counterparts, did not "specialize." Al-Razi, for example, was a philosopher and a mathematician as well as a physician and al-Kindi, the first Muslim philosopher to use Aristotelian logic to support Islamic dogma, also wrote on logic, philosophy, geometry, calculation, arithmetic, music, and astronomy. Among his works were such titles as An Introduction to the Art of Music, The Reason Why Rain Rarely Falls in Certain Places, The Cause of Vertigo, and Crossbreeding the Dove. Another major figure in the Islamic Golden Age was al-Farabi, who wrestled with many of the same philosophical problems as al-Kindi and wrote The Perfect City, which illustrates to what degree Islam had assimilated Greek ideas and then impressed them with its own indelible stamp. This work proposed that the ideal city be founded on moral and religious principles from which would flow the physical infrastructure. The Muslim legacy included advances in technology too. Ibn al-Haytham, for example, wrote The Book of Optics, in which he gives a detailed treatment of the anatomy of the eye, correctly deducing that the eye receives light from the object perceived and laying the foundation for modern photography. In the tenth century he proposed a plan to dam the Nile. It was by no means theoretical speculation; many of the dams, reservoirs, and aqueducts constructed at this time throughout the Islamic world still survive.

Muslim engineers also perfected the waterwheel and constructed elaborate underground water channels called qanats. Requiring a high degree of engineering skill, qanats were built some fifty feet underground with a very slight inclination over long distances to tap underground water and were provided with manholes so that they could be cleaned and repaired.

Agricultural advances are also part of the Muslim legacy. Important books were written on soil analysis, water, and what kinds of crops were suited to what soil. Because there was considerable interest in new varieties —for nutritive and medicinal purposes—many new plants were introduced: sorghum, for example, which had recently been discovered in Africa.

The introduction of numerous varieties of fruits and vegetables and other plants to the West via the Islamic empire was, however, largely the result of the vast expansion of trade during the Golden Age. This trade was vital; in the central lands of the 'Abbasid empire natural resources such as metals and wood were scarce, and increases in urban populations had outstripped the capacity of the agricultural system to support them. The 'Abbasids, therefore, were forced to develop extensive and complicated patterns of trade. To obtain food, for example, Baghdad had to import wheat from Syria and Egypt, rice from the Fayyum in Egypt, southern Morocco, and Spain, and olive oil from Tunisia. Called "a forest of olive trees," Tunisia exported so much olive oil that its port of Sfax was called "the port of oil."

To obtain scarce metals the 'Abbasids had to turn elsewhere. They imported the technologically advanced "ondanique" steel from India, for example, and then processed it at such famous centres of weapons manufacture as Damascus and Toledo, both of which cities won fame for their blades. The 'Abbasids also imported iron from Europe, tin from the British Isles and Malaya, and silver from northern Iran, Afghanistan, and the Caucuses. For gold, once the vast quantities in the treasuries of the conquered countries were exhausted, they turned to several sources. One was the gold mines of the Hijaz which were reopened around 750, reworked for about four hundred years, and then, in 1931, explored again by Karl Twitchell, who was searching for minerals in that area on behalf of King 'Abd al-'Aziz of Saudi Arabia.

For these necessities the 'Abbasid traders exchanged a wide variety of products: pearls, livestock, paper, sugar, and (a specialty of the Islamic world) luxurious cloth. The traditional cloths were wool and linen—the latter an Egyptian specialty since ancient times—but cotton, which was introduced into upper Iraq about the time of the Prophet, later spread with Islam around the Mediterranean, to Syria, North Africa, Spain, Sicily, Cyprus, and Crete.

The cloth trade produced a number of auxiliary exports: gold and silver thread for embroidery, gum from the Sudan for glazing, and needles, looms, and dyestuffs. Closely connected with the trade in dyestuffs was the trade in medicines, an offshoot of 'Abbasid advances in medicine and the spread of hospitals in all major Islamic cities. As scientific research and translation of medical texts from India and possibly even China expanded the earlier pharmacopoeia, ingredients for medicines were brought from all over the known world and also re-exported.

Because the religious, political, and military achievements of the Islamic period loom so large in the history of the world, the extraordinary cultural, scientific, technological, and commercial achievements are frequently obscured or overlooked. Yet these advances were, in fact, of enduring significance to mankind as a whole. The destruction by the Mongols of many of these achievements and of much of what the Muslims had accomplished by the end of the Golden Age was a tragic loss for the world as a whole.

Dr, Ashraf Kamel has not felt the economic crisis as most entrepreneurs have in Dubai. Since the Egyptian-born urologist set-up the German Medical Centre in Dubai Health Care City (DHCC) free zone in May 2005, Dr, Kamel and his team have treated almost 12,000 patients, with the team growing from an initial half a dozen doctors to 20 professionals. "We are attracting patients from Egypt to Afghanistan", the Managing Director of the German Medical Centre told AMEInfo.com.

The $1.8 bn-valued DHCC is the world's first health care free zone, allowing owners of hospitals, medical schools or recreational centres to own up to 100% of the entity. These entities can also hire staff regardless of their nationality and keep 100% of the generated profits.

The DHCC has grown each year, receiving over 200,000 patients up to last year, with global brands such as Harvard Medical School, Boston University, Mayo Clinic, Moorfields Eye Hospital, AstraZeneca, Johnson and Johnson and Novartis based there. DHCC is home to 5,000 health care professionals, 90 out-patient clinics, two hospitals and over 100 commercial and retail services. The Medical Community, occupying an area of 4.1 million square feet, focuses on clinical services for disease treatment and prevention, while the Wellness Community occupies 19 million square feet.

Travelling for treatment

However, not every clinic in Dubai has been as successful as the German Medical Centre. In fact, the entire health care sector in the GCC is still in its infancy. According to Kathe Mullally, Director Licensing at DHCC, over two thirds of UAE residents prefer to get treatment abroad.

While Westerners tend to visit doctors back in their home countries, locals are opting for operations anywhere—as long as they are convinced of the quality. Preferred destinations for Emiratis and Arab expats are clinics in India, Thailand, Germany, the UK and North America. Hospitals in Bangkok even hire Arabic-speaking nurses and service staff, in order to attract GCC nationals. The global medical tourism industry is estimated at $60bn annually.

Ironically, the Gulf countries are not lacking in health care staff. The GCC and the UAE in particular benefited from a mass exodus of Iraqi doctors who left their country during the UN embargo in the 1990s and in the wake of the US-led 2003 invasion. Excellently equipped and well-financed, the sector simply lacks know-how and customer-oriented service. "A state-of-the-art operation room does neither mean high standards nor does it automatically lead to the required know-how", says Dr, Gerald Zimmermann, an orthopedic specialist and visiting doctor at the German Medical Centre.

Increase in obesity

Typical health problems in the GCC are diseases associated with 'wealthy' societies such as obesity, cardiac attacks and diabetes. Kuwait's Body-Mass-Index, the world-wide accepted indication for obesity is as high as in the USA and in West-Samoa. This is the result of one of the highest living standards in the world and because of neglecting sports and cardio-vascular activity and overindulging in fast food.

According to Abu Dhabi Ministry of Health, diabetes mellitus accounts for 75% of deaths among UAE nationals and 31% among non-nationals. One in four UAE residents is diabetic. Osteoporosis is another severe problem among the elderly. "Because men and women likewise protect their skin against the strong sunshine in this part of the world throughout their entire lives, their bodies often cannot produce enough

Vitamin D, which is an essential ingredient for stable bone development", explains Dr, Zimmermann.

Moreover, there are fields where the GCC is lagging behind industrial states. "This region lacks specialism in neurosurgery and neurology", Dr. Kamel says. In other segments, there is an excess supply. Driving down Jumeirah road, one has the impression that there are more beauty surgeries based in Dubai than dentists.

Expansion of medical facilities

The good news is that new medical centres are mushrooming in the region, leading to competition and hopefully better services. "We are currently examining opportunities outside the UAE and we would be ready to expand", says Dr, Kamel. Qatar is currently finalizing Hamad Medical City (HMC) in Doha. This complex would be made up of three hospitals with a total bed capacity of 1,100, to be executed over phases at a total cost of QR 3.2 bn.

The Saudi German Hospital Group, owned by Saudi tycoon Al-Bartajee is setting up a new hospital in Dubai, comprising 300 beds. Saudi German Hospitals Group is considered the largest private Health care company in the Mena region. It plans to open at least five hospitals per year in the region during the next five years, creating 50,000 jobs in the sector.

Spill-over effects will be felt in the form of higher spending in the establishment of research and development, internationally compatible medical curriculaes and the exchange of know-how. Dubai has already established another free zone, the Dubai Biotechnology and Research Park (DuBiotech), for research, development and the production of pharmaceuticals. DuBiotech has attracted 48 business partners (as yet), among them leading brand names such as Amgen, Merck-Serono and Pfizer.

A cure is good, but prevention is better. Awareness programmes to teach young people about breast cancer or Aids, topics which have been taboos for quite a while in the Middle East, are also steps into the right direction.

Working in the Middle East

HCL International launched our Middle East business in early 2007 and since then have won contracts with major Public Health Authority Boards and Private clients throughout the region. With a particular focus on contracts in the UAE; HCL International staff are either based in the region or have travelled extensively ensuring a sound knowledge base of the region and the opportunities currently on offer. With a dedicated team managing the entire recruitment and relocation process, you can be assured your journey to the Middle East will be as smooth as possible.

Benefits of working in the Middle East:

Aside from living in one of the most prosperous regions in the world, health care professionals will benefit from working with state of the art equipment and with some of the best specialists across the globe.

You will enjoy a tax free salary, with salaries starting from AED5025 per month. Hospitals also offer some fantastic benefits, differing slightly between each Middle East location and depending on your profession. These include:

- 30-42 calendar days annual leave, plus approximately 14 days public holidays,
- Free accommodation (villa) or an apartment allowance,
- Annual furniture allowance or one off furniture allowance,
- Monthly water and electricity allowance,
- Monthly transportation allowance,
- Educational allowance for your children,
- Medical Insurance (yourself, spouse, up to 3 children under 18 years),
- End of Service: One months salary for each year worked,
- Free Flight home once a year, and
- Hospitals offer excellent courses and development for doctors as they are supported by major universities such as Harvard, etc

LIVING AND WORKING IN THE MIDDLE EAST

The United Arab Emirates (UAE) is situated in the Middle East. Because of its physical location, the United Arab Emirates has become economically prosperous and politically successful. It is now perceived very positively around the world as a forward-thinking, advanced nation, offering its habitants a refreshing and cosmopolitan lifestyle. Not only does the region offer varying landscapes—from built up cities, to barren deserts with 700 km of coastline, the Middle East benefits from hot summer months (April to September) with temperatures ranging from 50 Degrees Celsius and warm sunny days with average temperatures of 26 Degrees Celsius throughout November and March. It is no surprise it is fast becoming a popular destination for travellers and holiday makers.

Huge investment has recently been given to further development within both Dubai and Abu Dhabi. Spectacular, uniquely designed leisure/shopping Centres and accommodation are all part of this commercial growth. In addition to Dubai's development is 'Dubai Health Care City' which will benefit from 1000 clinics, treating the region to a wide host of medical facilities. This highlights the Middle East's focus on providing some of the best health care offered in the world.

Further highlights:

- Health care provision in the UAE is of a very high standard.
- Health care organizations benefit from state of the art equipment

- Some of the worlds leading specialists are brought into the UAE to share their knowledge and expertise.
- There is a low crime rate even within the major cities of the UAE.
- Airports are highly accessible with good international connections to Europe, America, Australasia and the Far East.
- All hospitals provide a free bus and taxi service from your compound to your work site to cover all of your shifts.
- Free accommodation is normally provided close to the hospitals however each hospital is slightly different.
- The population in 2006 was 1.3 million with anticipated growth to 2.6 million by 2010.
- 75% of the UAE workforce comes from countries outside the UAE.
- The official language of the UAE is Arabic. The other main languages spoken are English and Hindi. Within the Hospitals, the main language spoken is English.
- Habitants benefit from a tax free lifestyle.

HCL International's main clients are based in Dubai and Abu Dhabi. This is in direct response to our candidates' requests for where they would most like to relocate. These two major cities are only 150 km apart and are perhaps the most liberal of the Emirates; with expats living a fantastic lifestyle and benefiting from a truly cosmopolitan way of life. In Dubai, it is estimated that only 8% of the population are locals. If you want to work with health care professionals from all over the globe, have access to the very best equipment and standards of care and enjoy a tax free sunshine filled lifestyle, let HCL International take you to the Middle East

Greater need to promote medical tourism in KSA

In spite of a rapidly developing health care sector, which includes world-class medical centres and some of the most modern and state-of-the-art facilities in the world, the Kingdom has yet to make its mark in the booming medical tourism industry. A greater paradox lies in the fact that the nation's own citizens often look outwards when it comes to medical help for some specific problems. However, according to Dr. Sami Badawood, Director for Jeddah Health Affairs, the number of such people are less than they used to be, and more people, particularly from Gulf countries, are coming to the Kingdom to receive medical care.

Speaking exclusively to Saudi Gazette, Dr. Badawood talked about the government's initiatives to boost medical tourism, which includes five-year plans to develop medical cities in Jeddah and related workshops that are in progress.

"The number of people going abroad for medical treatment has decreased by around 20 to 30 percent over the last three years. This is because of two reasons. One, the global economic downturn, and two, the fact that better medical services are now available in the Kingdom itself," he said.

Admitting that there has not been enough marketing for the Kingdom's heath sector as the government "pays more attention to services to nationals," Dr. Badawood said there are strategic plans afoot and that special attention is being given to build a brand for medical tourism in Jeddah, the country's commercial hub and gateway to the Two Holy Mosques.

"The strategic five-year plans seek to develop medical cities in Jeddah that will have concentrated medical services, similar to those in other countries, and this will attract people," he said, stressing that more private sector investment and cooperation with specialized companies is required.

Jeddah's summer festivals also attract tourists from different regions, and medical tourism is at a peak time at this time of the year with a dramatic increase in the number of patients seeking appointments.

Jeddah's medical tourism, if promoted alongside tourism in Jeddah, which has 40 hospitals and a whole array of mushrooming private clinics, can reap the benefits from its association with the tourism industry.

"A workshop between the Ministry of Health and the Jeddah Governorate is scheduled to boost medical tourism in Jeddah. Formal conclusions from this gathering will be forwarded to the SCTA (Saudi Commission for Tourism and Antiquities)," said Dr. Badawood.

Medical tourism, in view of the huge economic potential that it offers, is reportedly the fastest growing outbound tourism sector in the Middle East.

Recent research conducted by author Josef Woodman suggests that the Middle East, Saudi Arabia in particular, is one of the fastest growing markets for an industry that already attracts over three million tourists a year. And it's no surprise that Saudi Arabia, like other Middle Eastern countries, such as, Jordan and the UAE, is gearing up to meet this growing demand by launching initiatives to establish itself as a top-notch cost-effective destination for the medical tourism market.

Korea, Malaysia, Thailand, India and the Philippines are attractive places for patients from the Middle East to visit as medical tourists. According to Dr. Badawood, there is no need to travel abroad for medical treatment for common problems. Those who seek treatment overseas may need transplants as "donors are not easily available here," or may be taking advantage of the availability of "natural resources in some East European and South Asian countries."

"Some countries have a reputation for certain treatments, such as rehabilitation, sports surgery, etc. Some patients also travel to seek second opinions," he added.

It can be assumed that the health industry, like most other industries, sees an increase in business during the Haj and the Umrah season, and this could well be one way to market the country's medical tourism. However, "We do not utilize the Haj and Umrah for promoting medical tourism. There is no connection between the two areas," said Dr. Badawood.

He said the most popular medical services for which people come to the Kingdom include: pediatric and obesity treatments and eye surgery.

Dr. Srinivas Rao, a Jeddah-based plastic surgeon, said that around 100-150 international patients annually seek treatment at his clinic, and that the most sought after cosmetic surgeries are nose reshaping and tummy tucks. Nowadays, he said, local doctors attempt to convince patients to undergo treatment in the Kingdom. "Although cosmetic treatment in the Kingdom is relatively expensive, if an individual travels abroad for treatment it may cost him more as the overall expenditure of travel, hotel, food, etc., outweighs the costs that he would incur for the same treatment in Saudi Arabia," he explained.

"There is a general feeling that doctors here are not competent enough. In every country, about 10 to 20 percent of doctors may not be good, but this cannot be generalized," said Dr. Rao. "Expat doctors are not allowed in government hospitals unless there is an emergency. Expat patients are not seen in government institutes and most of them postpone their treatment, surgeries, etc., till they visit their home countries," Dr. Rao said.

He said that there are appointment problems, and that one can have to wait for six months to see a doctor. "The other reason why individuals travel abroad is social stigma. Patients fear that their relatives who live here will learn that they have undergone cosmetic treatment," he added. He said that if the treatment takes place outside the country, one cannot contact the doctor often as the physical distance between the doctor and the patient poses a communications problem.

Diagnosis and overall care

Zahid Eskander, a Saudi national and father of a 12-year-old girl who has juvenile rheumatism, took his daughter to the southern Indian state of Kerala for alternative treatment (massages, herbs). He says that it took six months for doctors here to even diagnose the disease.

"Doctors here were unable to diagnose her condition. They even scared us by saying that our daughter had a very dangerous brain disease, while some others claimed she suffered from myopathy (a muscular disease). And during the six months that we had to go around to different doctors, her joints suffered permanent damage and now her leg is 80 percent damaged," said Eskander.

He said after researching about Kerala on the Internet, he found that the place has "good resources, and is inexpensive when compared to the cost of the same treatment in Dubai and Bahrain."

Eskander's daughter is undergoing medical treatment in Jeddah, but her parents decided on alternative treatment as "it has no side effects, and there is no harm in trying it till she turns 16 as doctors say they can operate on her only then".

"In Kerala," he said, the whole system is very organized, the hospital has a computer room, library, and the patients are taken out for tours and made very comfortable."

This overall patient care is perhaps what the medical sector here lacks.

"Given the option, most would choose to go abroad for treatment rather than stay here. While it is true that Saudi Arabia does have some great medical facilities and doctors, it lacks overall patient care. There is more to treating a disease or ailment than facilities, doctors and medicine. What seems to be missing is that a patient should be treated with proper follow-up care, educational materials, group support, and other patient treatments that are available in other parts of the world," said Ann Tamimi, (Nzingha), an American Muslim married to a Saudi and a mother of a child with Down Syndrome. She said she is unable to find proper facilities for physical therapy, occupational therapy and speech therapy, and that there is a complete lack of understanding when it comes to home care with pediatric patients, including the elderly. "I take my son to a very good physical therapist. However, it is such a sterile environment that my child dreads going every week. Broken cheap toys, dull colours, and equipment that looks like it was designed to cage an animal rather than to treat a child," said Nzingha, adding that it is difficult to find educational facilities with trained staff for children with disabilities.

She said that medical care should be an individual choice, which would include Saudi women, "who usually can't determine what medical care they will receive (male guardians do)". "If a person feels more comfortable being treated in another country then that should be considered, as the overall health is needed in order to fight disease or deal with disabilities. For example, it is better for a person's health to have a positive attitude in which he feels secure and has faith in his doctor than to be negative in outlook or unsure of his doctor's abilities, which is an aspect of care that I believe the Kingdom is not taking into account," Nzingha said.

Cost comparison

Nzingha said that cost-wise, Saudi Arabia is much cheaper for quality treatment. "For example, my father's many medications cost him over $3,000. However, the same medications in Saudi Arabia cost us only $800. A recent hospital stay for my father who had an accident cost us about $3,000 for a week's stay at Saad Hospital. The same would have run anywhere from three to four times more in the US," she said.

According to Dr. Rao, cosmetic treatment (average cost—SR20,000 to SR40,000) is expensive in the Kingdom as compared to other countries, such as India (approximately SR8,000), and Egypt and Lebanon, "where it is half the cost of what it is in the Kingdom".

A humanitarian cause

The National Guard Health Affairs (NGHA) in Riyadh is known worldwide for its efforts of separating conjoined twins. Majority of these separations have been performed by Dr. Abdullah Al-Rabeah, Minister of Health, who is an orthopedic surgeon. The complex surgeries on twins who come from all over the world are performed as humanitarian acts with no costs to the families.

To date, 23 sets of conjoined twins have been successfully separated in the Kingdom under the sponsorship of King Abdullah, Custodian of the Two Holy Mosques.

Last month, a multidisciplinary team headed by Dr. Al-Rabeah performed a lengthy surgery on a set of Moroccan twins who shared a liver and pancreas, and the upper part of their intestines. The separation was carried out in seven phases.

The twins were brought from Morocco on the instructions of King Abdullah, who is personally involved in supporting conjoined twin operations. Other sets of twins who have been operated on in the Kingdom have come from countries, such as, Egypt, Poland, Philippines, Malaysia, Sudan, Yemen, Morocco and Iraq.

Scope for improvement

On ways to boost medical tourism in the Kingdom, Dr. Rao remarked that it "depends on the participation of the private sector and the reputation of the institution and individual doctors, both of which are built up over the years. Moreover, advertising by the authorities plays an important role".

Recently, the Ministry of Health announced the creation of a new Clinical Revision department to improve medical performance and reduce medical errors, as part of an overhaul of the ministry ordered by Dr. Al-Rabeah.

Dr, Iqbal Musani, consultant pathologist and director Al-Jedani Group of Hospitals, said: "There is no doubt that the Kingdom's health sector is fast developing and this is particularly in specialized fields, such as, stem cell research and infertility treatment, where a lot of work is in the offing".

"Development in the health sector is very fast, but there is always room for improvement," said Dr. Badawood. But as Dr. Musani puts it: "It's something like this: Home food is more hygienic and tastier than restaurant food, but still people, out of the habit of wanting to try something new, tend to eat out."—SG

3

Health Care and Health Cities in Qatar and other Gulf Cooperation Council (GCC) Countries

Health tourism has been an increasing problem for too long, from the Middle East with many people opting to go abroad for medical care, even for superficial procedures such as cosmetic or dental surgery. When it comes to more complex issues, the GCC countries have to send people abroad and this can cost millions. If a citizen needs bypass surgery, the government would have to spend money to not only send the patient abroad, but also their family and this means massive expenditure and as a result, a lot of money leaving the country. In its quest on a complete makeover of the fundamental health care system, the Gulf Cooperation Council countries comprising Bahrain, Kuwait, Oman, Qatar, Saudi Arabia and the United Arab Emirates are undergoing an unprecedented change in its Health care systems to provide state-of-art medical services at an affordable, easy to access manner. The World Bank estimates the total health care spending in GCC countries will reach US $60 billion in 2025 from its modest spending of US $12 billion currently. GCC has in recent years achieved overall life expectancies, reducing infant mortality rates, overall death rates and other important health indicators. However, despite its tenacious measures the service is still in need of significant overhaul to cater to the demands of the ever escalating GCC population along with increasing standards of living. The objective of these countries in improving health care standards is to promote health tourism from other countries to GCC countries, as well.

(See Appendix I, attached at the end of the book on page 254 for comparison of middle east medical cities with south-east Asian medical cities that have excelled in the field of health tourism from far and near.)

Lifestyle ailments on the rise in GCC; Alpen bank, Dubai

The GCC population, currently at about 38 million, is growing at one of the fastest rates in the world. Qatar, Bahrain, and the UAE have been most proactive in this regard, by providing concrete incentives to attract private investment, including commitments to reimburse a minimum number of patient visits to such hospitals, even if the number of patients is less," said the report.

High prevalence of diabetes, obesity cardiovascular diseases, and cancer diseases has been found in this region. 'These ailments along with a high prevalence of smoking coupled with changes in health insurance regulations have led to an increase in the demand for health services in the region.' Thus, Health care demand and spending are on the rise in the GCC Countries. 'No other global region faces such rapid growth in demand with the simultaneous need to realign its health care systems to be able to treat the disorders of affluence'. 'In the GCC, estimates from various sources indicate around 75 to 132 hospitals are planned for construction with a total bed capacity of around 20,000 to 25,000 beds. As per a high-level analysis done by experts, there is a bed requirement of around 400,000 to 450,000 beds in the MENA (Middle East and North Africa) Region by the year 2018.' However, acute shortage of skilled manpower and dearth of private investments are the key obstacles in the GCC health care system.

"The GCC health care industry is poised for unparalleled and consistent growth accompanied by a fundamental shift in the industry structure, infrastructure quality, payer model and funding options," said Tommy Trask, Executive Director and Head of Equity Research at Alpen. The GCC health care industry is expected to grow threefold to $47 billion to $55 bn in the next 10 years, Alpen said, but asserted that this growth will not be possible until the governments clear some roadblocks. Low private sector participation, sub-optimal health infrastructure availability and acute shortage of human resource for all medical services are major obstacles for growth in the industry. "GCC needs to develop a strong professional health care workforce. unless the governments take strong initiatives to overcome the undersupply of health care professionals, the reform efforts will be rendered ineffective. Medical education and training of a paramedical workforce present a major opportunity for private players to establish a footprint in the region," report said. Moreover, treatment of lifestyle ailments calls for establishment of super specialty hospitals with state-of-the-art facilities, further necessitating higher private sector participation," it added. The bank estimated the size of the GCC health care services sector at about 46 million treatments in 2008. It emphasized on the need for an independent regulatory body to oversee the sector. Currently, the ministry of health is both regulator and major provider of health care services. More international investments—both direct and institutional will be available once sound and independent regulatory bodies are established." The investment bank, however, expressed satisfaction over the pace of construction of new hospitals. "Per capita health care spending in the GCC was $631 in 2006, below the global average of $716. The US and the UK registered per capita health care spending of $6,719 and $3,332 respectively in the same period," it said.

Indian connection; Aster is a brand name to reckon with

DM Health care, a US $300 million group and one of the largest health care service providers in the region, introduced their new corporate brand identity "ASTER" today. Aster will be integrating the hospitals, clinics, diagnostic centres, and pharmacies of the Group, spread over 90 locations in 5 countries. Commenting on the occasion, Dr. Azad Moopen, Chairman, D.M. Health care, said, "We dedicate ourselves to achieving excellence in health care, with a conviction that a society is as healthy as its people and its achievements as high as its aspirations. Mr.Ameer Ahmad, Director, Oman Operations said in a short span of 10 months 21,000 patients have been treated at the Al Raffa hospital, Muscat (now Aster Hospital) and the group aims to replicate the success with the introduction of 'ASTER'. Health care is now considered a sunshine sector, which has proved to be recession proof in turbulent times. The GCC and Indian health care markets together are projected to grow to a whopping US $150 Billion by 2020 from the present US $45 billion. 'Aster' is the Greek word for star, and is a popular flower associated with vibrancy, colour, popularity and abundance. The new identity embodies these attributes and the Group's promise to enrich life with love and care. Aster will bring alive the expertise, the value, the technology and best medical practices and emerge as a premier health care provider in the Middle East and India.

Dr. Azad Moopen also announced a sizeable investment in a unique CRM initiative—for its existing and growing customer's. It will seamlessly offer comprehensive health care through all ASTER verticals. Benefits will include accessibility and convenience under one window-medical history, priority appointments and reminders, online chat with our consultants and online purchase of medicines. This initiative is in keeping with the DM health care philosophy of bringing 'Health care for all' closer to our customers. It will also offer special privileges for patients needing tertiary care intervention in our high end hospitals in GCC and our associate hospitals in India.

DM Health care has emerged as a gateway to good health with its various CSR initiatives like health camps, Breast cancer awareness campaigns, etc. In partnership with the MIMS Charitable Trust, DM Health care has created the 'Save the Little Hearts' foundation, aimed at providing free surgical treatment for underprivileged children with congenital heart diseases in UAE and Kerala, India. Diabetes prevention and management will be another focused initiative by the Group across GCC countries. Aster vertical will continue to foster these initiatives and support philanthropic ventures.

Health care market in MENA region expanding

The health care market in the Middle East and North Africa (MENA) region presents a complex, diverse and rapidly changing picture, rich in opportunities for foreign companies and institutions. The region has built some of the world's most advanced medical facilities. At the same time, there is a need for improved primary health care services, and some countries such as Yemen and Sudan are still struggling to bring down infant and maternal mortality rates.

Improvements in health indicators are altering population structures and disease patterns. There have been huge drops in infant mortality rates, and life expectancy has risen. According to the 2009 Arab Human Development Report issued by the United Nations Development Programme, life expectancy across the Arab world averages nearly 68 years, up from 52 in 1970-75. But there are major variations: the UAE enjoys the highest figure, of 78 years, while in Yemen and Sudan life expectancy is only 61.5 and 57 years respectively, and Iraq 58—the same as in 1970-75. The overall population growth rate in the Arab world has fallen from 2.6 per cent in 1970-75 to 1.9 per cent in 2005-15. But this is still one of the highest growth rates for any region, increasing the pressure on health services.

The proportion of the population over the age of 65 is rising. An Economic and Social Commission for West Asia report on aging in Arab countries notes that the number of people in the Arab world aged over 65 doubled from 5.7 million in 1980, to 10.4 million in 2000, and is expected to hit 14 million in 2010 and 21.3 million by 2020. There are increases in the incidence of age-related diseases such as heart disease, cancer and dementia. Lifestyles featuring fast-food diets, a lack of exercise, and a high incidence of smoking are also changing disease patterns. Obesity is rocketing, helping push up rates of Type 2 diabetes; in the UAE, an alarming 20 per cent of the population is diabetic.

The cultural connection in health

Persistently high rates of marriage between first cousins and other close relatives maintain the incidence of genetic diseases, such as the potentially fatal blood disorders thalassaemia, sickle cell disease and hemophilia, and a variety of other physical and mental abnormalities. It is estimated that one-in-12 of the population of the UAE is a thalassaemia carrier. Survival rates for those afflicted by congenital disease are increasing, thanks to improved medical care, placing an additional burden on health budgets. Due to religious and social pressures against abortion—even if antenatal testing finds fetal abnormalities—the preferred approach to reducing incidents of disease is through genetic screening. Mandatory pre-marital genetic testing of couples has been introduced in a number of countries. In December 2009, Qatar became the final Gulf Cooperation Council (GCC) state to make such tests compulsory for all national and expatriate couples planning to marry in the country.

A report by management consultants McKinsey predicts that total GCC health care spending will increase fivefold, from $12 billion in 2007 to more than $60 billion by 2025. By then, the demand for hospital beds will have soared to 162,000, up from 114,450 beds in 2015 and 68,000 in 2006. Over the next two decades the population of the GCC is expected to double and the number of people aged 65 and over to rise sevenfold. The report warns that government-run hospitals and clinics are "ill prepared for a rapidly growing and aging population, as well as for the rise in chronic diseases such as diabetes" and advocates changes in government policies and regulations to encourage private health care.

GCC countries look at Britain and beyond

Some of the best-known names in the UK health field have set-up GCC operations. One magnet for such institutions is the Dubai Health Care City (DHCC), the world's first health care free-zone, in which Dubai's strategic collaborator is Partners Harvard Medical International. Moorfields Eye Hospital NHS Foundation Trust founded a branch in DHCC in 2007, and Imperial College of London has established a diabetes centre in Abu Dhabi, wholly owned by the Abu Dhabi government's Mubadala Development Company. The centre collaborates with MEHD on the treatment of patients with diabetes-related eye complications. Great Ormond Street Hospital for Children has had an office in DHCC for the past three years to complement and support its treatment services in London. Kuwait is looking to Britain for help in expanding and developing its health care system. During an October 2009 visit to London, Kuwaiti Health Minister Dr, Hilal al-Sayer signed a memorandum of understanding (MoU) with Guy's and St. Thomas's NHS Foundation Trust. Syria's Ministry of Health reached an MoU with Britain's Department of Health in 2008. Syria is in the throes of fundamental health care reform and plans a number of health care cities and other centres of excellence. It is also redesigning the public health system to accommodate imbalances, such as only a fifth of the rural population having ready access to public health services. Several UK universities and institutions have negotiated training and supply contracts with Syrian partners. Lebanon's $600 million pharmaceutical and health care market—the largest in the Arab Levant and expanding at 6 to 7 per cent a year—is a magnet for UK exporters who have about 5 per cent of the market share. Iraq is a difficult, but potentially rewarding, market as it tries to restore its health system. The Cornish health consultancy M.J. Medical was appointed in mid-2009 as lead design consultant on a $400 million project to build three 400-bed teaching hospitals in Baghdad, Diyala and Diwaniya. Libya is also trying to make up for lost time. The Libyan British Business Council was scheduled in February 2010 to take its first-ever delegation of UK health care business leaders to Tripoli to explore trade and investment openings.

By the time it is completed in 2012, the multi-billion-dollar HMC Hospital facility at the Medical City will be the finest centre of medical excellence in the Gulf region, the developers said at the MEED conference. The state-of-the-art project, being managed and supervised by US-based Hill International, is expected to become the leading hospital in the Arabian Gulf and beyond for the treatment of children, women and long-term care as well as rehabilitation. Hill International strategic development senior vice-president, Tim Judge, gave a brief update on the project at the MEED Qatar conference. According to Judge, the hospital project site spanning 44 hectares comprises four different hospitals—Children's hospital, Women's hospital, the Physical medicine and rehabilitation hospital and Skilled Nursing facility. The Children's hospital, having a total built-up area of 75,250 square metres, is a 13-storey structure with a tower block of seven floors each comprising 17 private patient room units. In each unit, there are 12 private rooms, two VIP patients rooms, two isolation rooms and one VIP isolation room.

The hospital will accommodate approximately 250 beds together with an emergency department, radiology, out-patients clinics, in-patient surgical suite and pediatric cardiac catheterization unit. It will also have a surgical intensive care unit, burn, dialysis, cardiac and hydro-therapy units as well as family centre, general medical support and other supporting facilities such as pharmacies, kitchen, laundry and sundry.

The new 10-storey Women's hospital will have a built-up area of approximately 52,000 sqm. It will be a tower block of six patient floors of 3,130 sqm each. The hospital will have a 200-bed capacity with 96 postpartum beds, 68 antenatal beds, 34 gynecology and four ICU beds. A typical 16-bed unit will have 13 private rooms, two VIP patient rooms, one isolation room as well as a head nurse and all in-patients and staff facilities. It will have 16 labour delivery rooms and three cesarean section operating rooms, neonatal intensive care unit, in-patient surgical suite and out-patients surgery and assisted contraception, family medicine unit and pre-admission testing unit. It will also have an emergency department, observation suites, and radiology and out-patient clinic.

The Physical medicine and rehabilitation hospital will have five floors each with two 20-patient room units. Each unit will consist of six private rooms, two isolation rooms, and six semi-private rooms. There will also be an adult hydro-therapy unit consisting of one large pool area, two pool rooms, tub treatment areas, two massage rooms and three in-patient waiting bays. Other sections in the hospital include an out-patient occupational therapy, prosthesis unit, physical therapy and main laboratory.

The skilled nursing facility is a four-storey structure with a total area of 28,000 sqm. The 270-beds facility has three patient floors each with two 44-patient room units split into smaller units. Each unit consists of six private rooms, two isolation rooms and six semi-private rooms. Apart from its main clinic, it also has a multi-functional therapy sections comprising a main gymnasium, activity room, two work areas, speech room, training room, technical area, kitchen and lounge areas. All the four hospitals will share a two-level oval car park accommodating over 1,100 cars. Apart from the completed and fully occupied Supreme Council of Health building, the site will also have other ancillary buildings such as a 80 megawatt central energy plant and staff car park for some 630 vehicles, nurses club, staff club, two mosques and an education centre. There will also be housing units for nurses and married staff. Construction work on the nurses club, education centre and Friday mosque started on January 24, 2010, and the medical city in Bahrain is expected to be complete by 2012.

Health tourism is also on the cards

Medical 'tourism' is a rapidly growing industry and several MENA countries offer cosmetic surgery, elective surgery, infertility treatment and dentistry, their own poor health care standards notwithstanding. Lebanon is a well-established centre, but is facing competition from Morocco, Egypt and Tunisia. Turkey draws an estimated 200,000 medical tourists annually, while Jordan accommodates more than 250,000 patients. The Medical Tourism Association expects medical tourism to earn Jordan $650 million in 2009 and $1 billion in 2012. Dubai's DHCC hopes to win some of the $2 billion tourists from the Gulf are estimated to spend abroad each year, but faces stiff competition on price from Middle Eastern rivals as well as India, Singapore and Thailand.

Hospital Projects in the GCC

Bahrain

King Hamad General Hospital
Al Areen Medical Complex and Serviced Apartments
Organ Transplant Centre

Kuwait

Jaber Ahmed Al-Jaber Al-Sabah Hospital
Sabah Medical Area in Shuwaikh
Health Centre at Bayan Palace

Oman

Psychiatric Hospital at Al Amerat
Cardiac Centre at Sultan Qaboos Hospital
Hospital in South Salalah
Jalan Bani Bu Hassan Hospital

Qatar

Sidra Medical and Research Centre
4 Hospitals at Hamad Medical City—Fit-out Package
Al-Wakra Hospital

Saudi Arabia

Ajyad General Hospital Development in Makkah
440 Clinics in Different Areas of Saudi Arabia
227 Clinics in Different Areas of Saudi Arabia

UAE

Cleveland Clinic in Abu Dhabi
Health Care City on Shams Abu Dhabi
Mafraq Hospital in Abu Dhabi
Medical Tourism in the GCC

Qatar

Bahrain
Kuwait
Oman

Qatar Health care

Qatar is planning to spend about $100 billion (Dh367 billion) on investment and infrastructure projects over the next seven years. The government has revised its current allocations for investment and infrastructure projects, said Shaikh Mohammad Bin Ahmad Bin Jassem Al Thani, Minister of Economy and Commerce. The minister spoke during a seminar on investment opportunities in Qatar recently held in Spain. Hamad medical city is one of these projects.

"Health care is the primary concern for our society in Qatar", he said. It is available in all forms, preventive and curative, to a diverse population without any discrimination. The Ministry of Public Health and Hamad Medical Corporation work in smooth coordination to deliver the maximum benefits in the field of medical care.

Cornell Medical College

Now in its sixth year of operation, Weill Cornell Medical College in Qatar (WCMC-Q) offers young people an unprecedented opportunity to access a world-class medical education in the Gulf region. Cornell is the first American university ever to offer its M.D. degree outside the United States. In the context of Qatar, WCMC-Q is leading the way as the country's first medical school and co-educational higher learning institution. The establishment of the Medical College followed the signing, on January 25, 2001, of an Agreement between Cornell University and Qatar Foundation for Education, Science and Community Development, a private, not-for-profit organization set-up in 1995 by His Highness Sheikh Hamad Bin Khalifa Al-Thani, Emir of the State of Qatar. Teaching started in the two-year Pre-medical Program in fall 2002. The Medical Program opened two years later; the Inaugural Class graduated in 2008. WCMC-Q shares the triple mission of Weill Cornell Medical College in New York City, of which it is a branch: a commitment to excellence in education, patient care and research.

Medical Education

WCMC-Q's unique, integrated, six-year program of pre-medical and medical studies leads to the M.D. degree of Cornell University. With teaching by Cornell and Weill Cornell faculty, academic standards are consistent with those of the University and its Medical College in the U.S. The Pre-medical Program consists of courses in the sciences basic to medicine; humanities, in the form of writing seminars and an introduction to medical ethics; and social science, with students following, via e-Learning technology, the Psychology 101 course taught at the Ithaca campus.

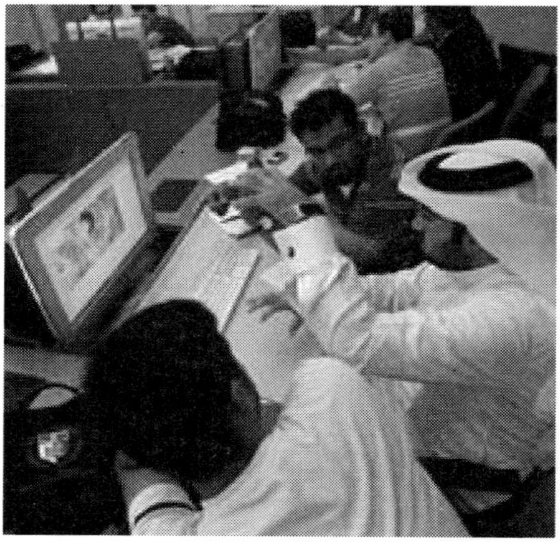

The Medical Program replicates the curriculum taught at Weill Cornell Medical College. This highly motivational program features a variety of learning experiences, including problem-based learning in small groups, seminars, lab work and lectures. It is an important principle of the Program that medical students begin to develop an understanding of the doctor-patient relationship from the first year. Following the signing of an Affiliation Agreement with Hamad Medical Corporation (HMC), a significant part of the introductory clinical courses (Medicine, Patients and Society I and II) occurs in primary health care centres and clinics of HMC. The clinical clerkships in the third year, and electives in the fourth year, will take place in HMC hospitals; there are five such hospitals in the capital city, Doha, with major facilities now under construction in the new Hamad Medical City.

Hamad Medical Corporation (HMC)

The Medical College continues to work closely with HMC, building on the Affiliation Agreement signed in 2004, to educate the physicians of tomorrow in Qatar and the wider region. Established in 1979, HMC is the state health care provider in Qatar. The Corporation manages a network of hospitals and is now undertaking a major expansion, with construction of Hamad Medical City in Doha and additional hospitals elsewhere in the country.

HMC physicians holding Weill Cornell appointments teach medical students during the Medicine, Patients and Society I and II courses, and play key roles in the Clinical Clerkships. A number of fourth year electives are offered in the Corporation's facilities. Collaboration among clinical faculty at Weill Cornell and HMC is increasing. Experts from the Medical College in New York City present Grand Rounds and give lectures at HMC during their visits to Qatar. Set to open in 2011, this state-of-the-art, all-digital facility of approximately 380 beds will be constructed in Education City. Together, the Medical College and Hospital will form an American-style academic medical centre, with clinical programs focusing on women's and children's health, residency training for the graduates of WCMC-Q and biomedical research programs that focus on diseases of concern in the region.

Senior Weill Cornell faculty and staff will collaborate with colleagues in Qatar's National Health Authority (NHA), HMC, Qatar Foundation and Sidra Medical and Research Centre in building biomedical research capacity. This will be carried out at WCMC-Q and HMC, and once the Medical and Research Centre opens in 2011, it too will become a site for clinical and translational research.

Preventive Health Dept. includes Health Education, Communicable disease control and Prevention, Non Communicable disease Control, Environmental health, Occupational Health, Port and Food Surveillance, Central Laboratory and Vital statistics. The aim of this department is "Prevention is better then cure" and it strives hard to deliver this message to the public through its activities.

The three hospitals of HMC

Located in the heart of Doha, the capital city of Qatar, HMC consists of three hospitals: Hamad General Hospital was commissioned in 1982 and since has gained an International reputation as a teaching and referral centre. It is certified by the American Hospital Association and provides medical and surgical sub-specialties to a population of more than 600,000 people. The facility has a capacity of approximately 660 beds and utilizes the most state of the art medical and surgical equipment to keep current with the rapid new development in medicine. The Medical Department provides a wide range of services in: Cardiology, Endocrinology, Nephrology, Gastroenterology, Hematology/Oncology, Neurology, Chest and Pulmonary Disease, Infectious Diseases and Rheumatology, Medical ICU and a Renal Dialysis Unit. On the other hand the Surgery Department has eight operating theatres, a recovery room and the Surgical Intensive Care Unit (SICU). Surgical specialties include General Surgery, Plastic Surgery, Neurosurgery, Orthopedics, Urology, Pediatric Surgery, Ophthalmology and ENT. The Outpatient Department consists of 52 specialty clinics and 15 sub-clinical services. Patients have to get a referral from the Primary Health Centres or an accredited private physician before they can get an appointment at the OPD.

Women's Hospital

It was commissioned in 1988; it provides medical and surgical care to the female population. Its bed capacity is about 330 beds. It boasts a high rate in specialized In-Vitro Fertilization and Neo-Natal care. The number of deliveries is about 10,000 per annum and prenatal mortality rate of about 12.8 per 1000 births. Women's Hospital. Provides a wide range of Obstetrics and Gynaecology services, infertility treatments. This facility also provides services for newborns at a state of the art NICU at three levels: Intermediate, intensive and isolation.

Rumailah Hospital

It was commissioned in 1956 and renovated in 1997; it houses more than 300 beds for Geriatrics and Physical Rehabilitation Medicine patients. The grounds of the Hospital compound also house the Burn and Plastic Unit, Dental Clinic, Special Education School for the handicapped and developmentally disabled, TB Unit, Dermatology and Venereology Clinic. Currently it is a Rehabilitation Centre for physically and mentally challenged adult and pediatric patients. But, this facility also offers a wide range of services as: Ophthalmology, ENT, Dermatology, Dental Services, Geriatrics, TB Treatment Unit, Physical Medicine and Rehabilitation including: Prosthetics/Orthotics, Speech Therapy, Occupational Therapy, Physiotherapy, Special Education, etc. The facility also offers services at Burns Unit, Plastic Surgery, Pharmacy, Outpatients Department, Social Services, etc.

HMC offers many outstanding and attractive staff privileges such as:

- New health care program
- Transportation allowance
- Interest free car/furniture loans
- 30/40 days annual or bi-annual paid leave
- 10% shift allowance
- Educational assistance
- End of Service Benefit
- Air Tickets, All overseas senior staff recruits and their families (up to 3 children under 18 years of age) are entitled to an annual free air passage to their home country. Junior staff recruits are offered free air passage once every 2 years.

Doha hosted the 15th Asian Games. Following completion of the Games, the site was transformed into Hamad Medical City, which incorporates several new health care facilities (totally 1,000 beds), staff housing, and staff recreation.

Hamad Medical City Qatar

Hamad Medical City (HMC), is the second biggest health care development in the Middle East. This $1 billion health care project named after the current ruler of Qatar, Hamad Al-Thani, will include state of the art hospitals, therapeutic facilities, and medical staff residential buildings. It will also include the National Health Authority's offices and a tunnel road access to the complex.

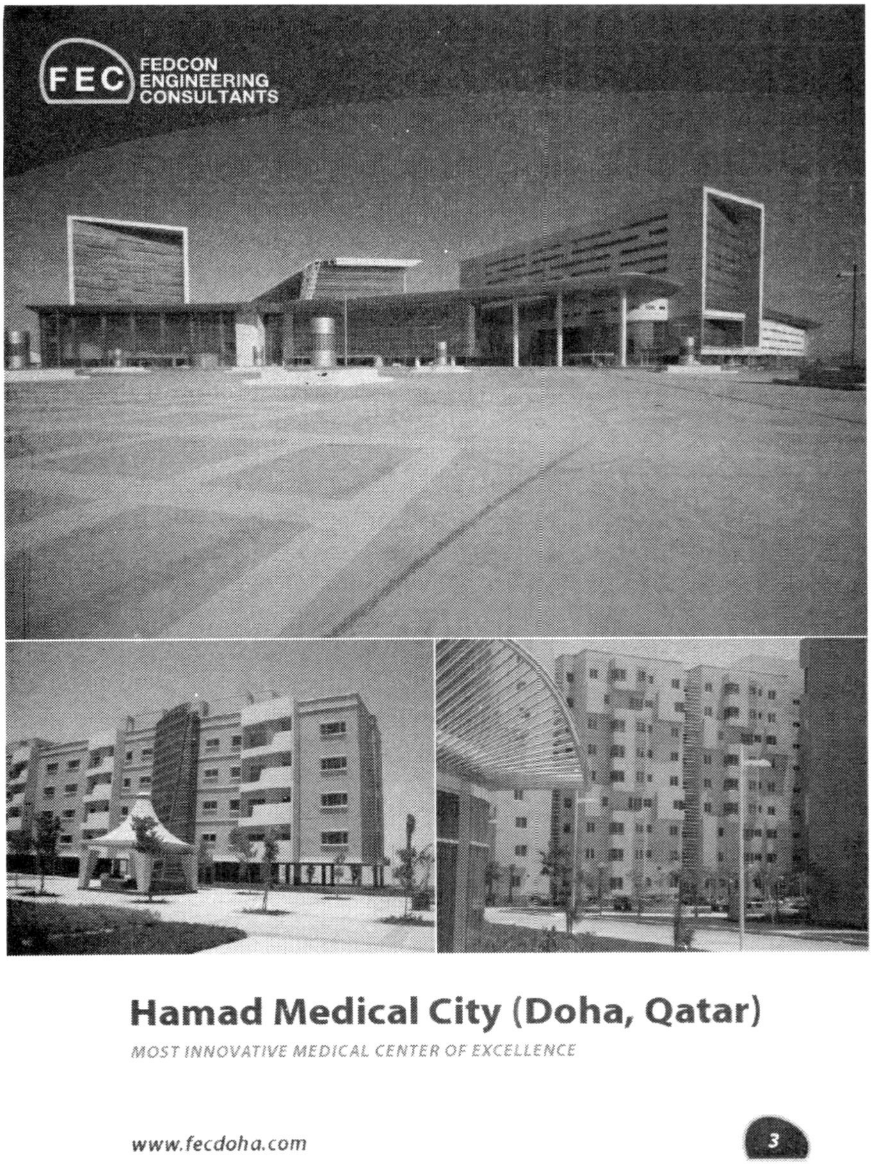

44 hectares comprises four different hospitals

The hospital project site spanning 44 hectares comprises four different hospitals—Children's hospital, Women's hospital, the Physical medicine and rehabilitation hospital and Skilled Nursing facility. The Children's hospital, having a total built-up area of 75,250 square metres, is a 13-storey structure with a tower block of seven floors each comprising 17 private patient room units.In each unit, there are 12 private rooms, two VIP patients' rooms, two isolation rooms and one VIP isolation room. The hospital will accommodate approximately 250 beds together with an emergency department, radiology, out-patients clinics, in-patient surgical suite and pediatric, cardiac catheterization unit. It will also have a surgical intensive care unit, burn, dialysis, cardiac and hydro-therapy units as well as family centre, general medical support and other supporting facilities such as pharmacies, kitchen, laundry and sundry.

The first four levels of each hospital building would be designated for outpatient clinics, operation theaters, pharmacies, support services, management offices, a cafeteria and a mosque. The upper floors would be designated for inpatients. HMC was determined to have the complex built in accordance with the internationally approved American standards. Support services such as storage, laundry and food catering facilities would be situated in the underground levels of the complex buildings. The complex would be provided with 650-car parking lots. Work is being executed round the clock by 7000 construction workers supervised by 126 engineers and architects. By the time it is completed in 2012, the multi-billion-dollar Medical City will be the finest centre of medical excellence in the Gulf region. The state-of-the-art project, being managed and supervised by US-based Hill International, is expected to become the leading hospital in the Arabian Gulf and beyond for the treatment of children, women and long-term care as well as rehabilitation.

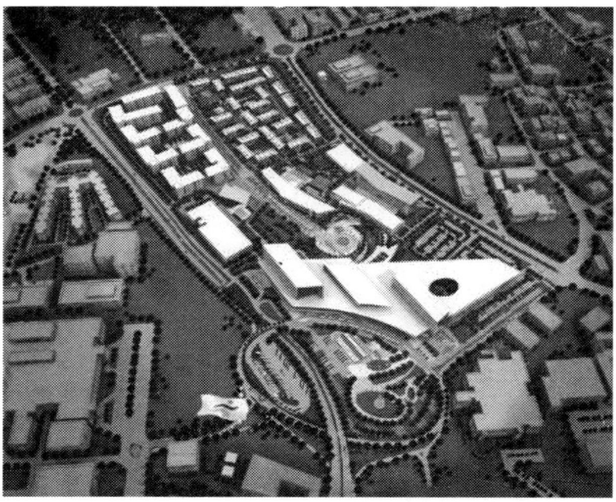

The new 10-storey Women's hospital will have a built-up area of approximately 52,000sqm. It will be a tower block of six patient floors of 3,130sqm each. The hospital will have a 200-bed capacity with 96 postpartum beds, 68 antenatal beds, 34 gynecology and four ICU beds. A typical 16-bed unit will have 13 private rooms, two VIP patient rooms, one isolation room as well as a head nurse and all in-patients and staff facilities. It will have 16 labour delivery rooms and three cesarean section operating rooms, neonatal intensive care unit, in-patient surgical suite and out-patients surgery and assisted contraception, family medicine unit and pre-admission testing unit. It will also have an emergency department, observation suites, and radiology and out-patient clinic.

The Physical medicine and rehabilitation hospital will have five floors each with two 20-patient room units. Each unit will consist of six private rooms, two isolation rooms, and six semi-private rooms. There will also be an adult hydro-therapy unit consisting of one large pool area, two pool rooms, tub treatment areas, two massage rooms and three in-patient waiting bays. Other sections in the hospital include an out-patient occupational therapy, prosthesis unit, physical therapy and main laboratory.

The skilled nursing facility is a four-storey structure with a total area of 28,000 sqm. The 270-beds facility has three patient floors each with two 44-patient room units split into smaller units. Each unit consists of six private rooms, two isolation rooms and six semi-private rooms. Apart from its main clinic, it also has a multi-functional therapy sections comprising a main gymnasium, activity room, two work areas, speech room, training room, technical area, kitchen and lounge areas.

Other hospitals in Qatar

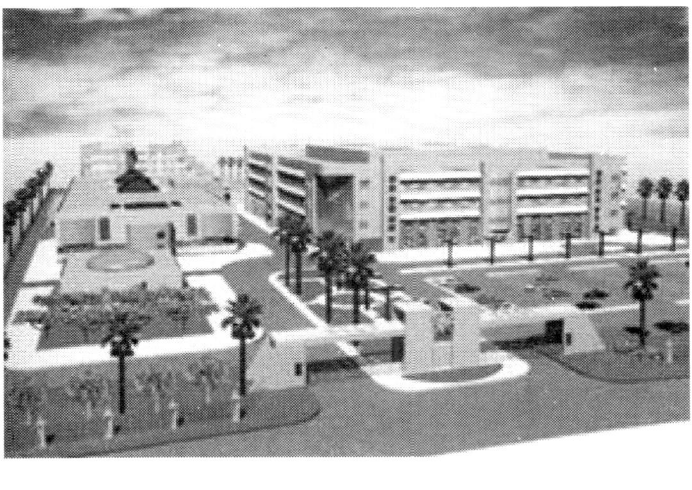

Al-Ahli Private Hospital

The Al-Ahli Hospital is Qatar's first major private hospital and on completion will be one of the biggest private hospitals in the Gulf. A $60 million financing package for the project was arranged in 1999 with QNB being the Lead Arranger. The 250 bed hospital will also have an accommodation block for staff, and is scheduled to open in the second half of 2004.

Two other new hospital projects are also in the design phase; the estimated QR 220 million Southern Area Hospital at Wakrah, with a 200-bed facility, and the estimated QR 100 million Cardiology Hospital at Rumailah, with a 110-bed facility.

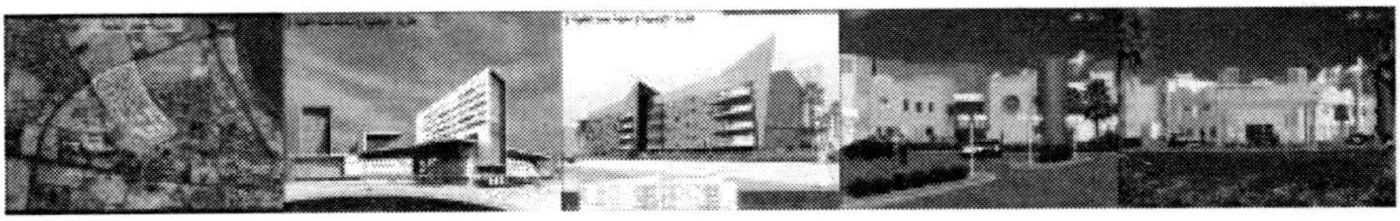

Currently, residents have to pay for public health care, but it is heavily subsidized. Qatar is planning to move towards a system of health insurance, although no plans have yet been announced. In the meantime, to reduce the strain on its health service, Qatar is encouraging the development of the private health sector. People who choose the private sector or purchase private health insurance generally do so for speed and convenience (and to avoid the dreaded bureaucracy!)

For non-emergency treatment your first visit should be to a clinic. A single visit to the clinic costs QR 30/$8. Alternatively, buy a health card for QR100/$25, which covers you for a year.

Sick-Kids Canada signs partnership to develop children's hospital in Qatar

Leaders from Sick-Kids marked the official announcement of the five-year partnership. Sick-Kids has been enlisted to provide advisory services for the development and operation of the new 217-bed, 45,000 square foot children's hospital located in Hamad Medical City, a large, not-for-profit health care complex in the heart of Doha, Qatar's capital city. While in Doha, Sick-Kids staff will provide expert counsel in such areas as pediatric medicine, surgical services, inter-professional practice and education, family-centreed care and research. The partnership will also see staff from HMC travel to Toronto to take advantage of fellowship and learning opportunities at Sick-Kids. As of result of its world-class reputation for excellence in pediatric medicine, Sick-Kids won the contract to partner with HMC over other leading health care organizations in the United States, Europe and Australia.

New Children's Hospital will open in 2012 in Hamad Medical City and is designed according to international best practice standards in pediatric care. Sick-Kids has also partnered with Bloorview Kids Rehab who will share their expertise in rehabilitation and complex continuing care. As Canada's largest pediatric rehabilitation hospital, Bloorview's involvement in the project will be focused on developing services for children who are chronically ventilated and to build rehab capacity as an important element of the continuum of care for children with congenital or acquired disability.

Founded in 1875 and affiliated with the University of Toronto, Sick-Kids is one of Canada's most research-intensive hospitals and has generated discoveries that have helped children globally. Its mission is to provide the best in complex and specialized family-centreed care; pioneer scientific and clinical advancements; share expertise; foster an academic environment that nurtures health care professionals; and champion an accessible, comprehensive and sustainable child health system. HMC prides itself in providing quality and cost efficient health care for all patients regardless of nationality, in line with the State of Qatar's pledge of "Health for All".

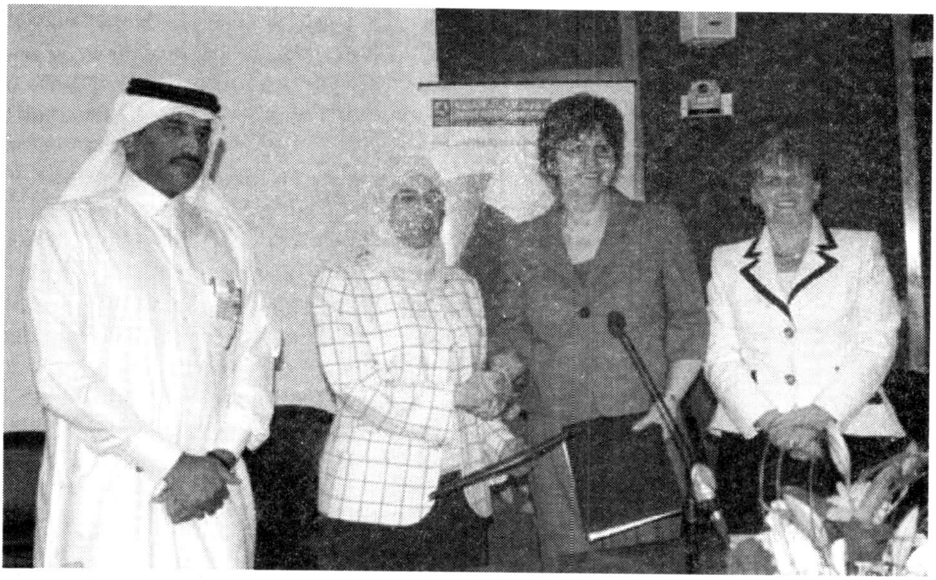

Dr. Abdulla Al Kaabi, Project Director, HMC, Dr. Hanan Al Kuwari, Managing Director, HMC, Mary Jo Haddad, President and CEO, Sick Kids, and Cathy Seguin, Vice-President, International Affairs, Sick-Kids

Kuwait Health care System

The health care system and health conditions have improved dramatically in the years after oil revenues brought wealth to the country. Kuwait's first attempts to introduce a modern health care system date back to the first years of the twentieth century when the ruler, Shaykh Mubarak Al Sabah the Great, invited doctors from the Arabian Mission of the Dutch Reformed Church in the United States to establish a clinic. By 1911 the group had organized a hospital for men and in 1919 a small hospital for women. After the government began receiving oil revenues, it expanded the health care system, beginning with the opening of the Amiri Hospital in 1949. The Kuwait Oil Company (KOC) also opened some small health facilities. In the 1950s, the government introduced a comprehensive health care system offering free services to the entire population. Most of the physicians were foreigners, particularly Egyptians. Nonetheless, improvements in available health care and in public health were dramatic. The number of doctors grew from 362 in 1962 to 2,641 in 1988. The doctor-to-patient ratio improved from one to 1,200 to one to 600. Infant and child mortality rates dropped dramatically; in 1990 the infant mortality rate was fifteen per 1,000 live births. Life expectancy increased ten years in the post-independence years, putting Kuwait at a level comparable to most industrialized countries. In 1990 life expectancy for males was seventy-two years and for females seventy-six years.

By 1990 Kuwait had an extensive welfare program, exceeded perhaps by no other country. Citizens receive free medical services from highly trained practitioners in modern facilities; free education through the university level; subsidized food, housing, utilities, and transportation; and various other benefits. For all this, they pay no taxes: the system is supported by oil revenues from outside the country. The benefits of the welfare system, however, are unevenly distributed among the population.

Owing to Kuwait's small population and the numerous medical facilities in the private and public sectors, long waiting lists are almost unheard of. For specialized treatment, however, it's sometimes necessary to seek medical assistance outside Kuwait, and locals who can afford it often do so. Members of the ruling families and wealthy Arabs invariably have all major operations outside their own territory, particularly in London and American cities. American Mission Hospitals, which used to operate on a part-private (for those who could afford treatment), part-free (for those who couldn't) basis, played an important part in the development of medical services and can still be found today, although they no longer offer free treatment.

Among expatriates, common health problems include alcoholism (particularly among bachelors, owing to loneliness and depression) and respiratory problems caused by sand and dust in the air—a situation exacerbated by continuous building work in most states. Hard work and long hours in often extreme heat can also affect the immune system and compromise the body's ability to counter illness. Expatriates—particularly manual workers—can suffer sunstroke and sunburn. You should be excused work outdoors if the temperature reaches 50°C (122°F), which isn't uncommon at the height of summer, although it's unusual for work to be stopped under these conditions. In the summer, humidity causes added discomfort, with eye infections common. Dehydration is also a threat and is a potentially fatal condition that shouldn't be underestimated—not only by those working outdoors but also by anyone playing outdoor sports, including 'leisurely' pursuits such as golf.

The 'winter' months of October to March, however, bring some of the best weather anywhere in the world, with continuous warm sunshine generating a feeling of well-being and providing the opportunity for a wholesome, outdoor lifestyle. Good weather is also beneficial to mental health, and people in Kuwait tend to be happier and livelier than those who have to cope with cold, wet, depressing climates.

The Kuwaiti Ministry of Health plans to build three integrated medical cities in strategic locations that they cover the whole country and ease the pressure on existing hospitals. The ministry is still studying the proposal and the project is aimed at offering medical services to citizens and residents all over the country. these medical cities would be fully managed by foreign staff, who will be brought in from famous international hospitals, and will help end the trend of sending patients abroad for treatment. Meanwhile, a delegation from the American Cleveland Clinic made a visit to Ahmadi hospital. The delegation toured the hospital to evaluate the level of the medical services and the management status. Khalid Al-Khamees said, "this visit is part of our effort to lift our hospital health care standards and make sure it is managed efficiently according to highest international standards." Evaluation will encompass doctors' performance, staff competency, service level and other activities. Practical solutions will be set-up to expand the hospital, advance the medical services and reduce treatments outside Kuwait.

Kuwait Health Care is comparable to British Health Care?

The systems of health care provision in Kuwait and Britain possess similar properties and characteristics. Both systems of the two countries have a fair distribution of health care facilities in different regions of the country. The health care system of Kuwait ensures the provision of ambulance whenever a patient needs it, just as the health care system of Britain does. In addition, the health care system of Kuwait obtains new tools and devices and uses modern technology in diagnosis and medical treatment. Similarly, the health care of Britain possesses similar tools and devices and, in some cases, manufactures them.

A difference between the systems of health care provision in Kuwait and Britain is the organization of medical departments for particular health problems. In Kuwait, the health care system provides specialized hospitals for most health problems and emergencies, such as rheumatic, gynecology and obstetrics, orthopedics, ophthalmology, dermatology, and burns hospitals. (Al-Sadani, 1998) On the other hand, due to the large area Britain holds, the system of health care provision followed another technique, in which it distributed most of the specialized departments throughout numerous health centres in different regions of the country.

The final and most significant difference between the systems of health care provision in Kuwait and Britain is the source of income that helps provide such services for the citizens. In order to be registered with the National Health Service, there are certain rules and regulations to be followed by the citizens in Britain. Most of these rules and regulations are based on financial support from the citizens to the National Health Service. The majority of funding generates from general taxation, which makes up 82% of the total income. Every citizen is required to pay taxes to back up the health care provision. The NHS national insurance contributions is a second major source of income that adds up to 12% of the total income. The remainder, which sums up to 6%, comes from patients charges for dental treatments and prescriptions. (Ham, 1999) Unlike Britain, Kuwait has an entirely different system in obtaining such income for health care provision.

Accreditation helped Kuwait

Accreditation Canada International helps the national accreditation program for the Kuwait Ministry of Health. The Ministry intends to implement an accreditation program for health care quality and to ensure national standards developed specifically for Kuwait are followed. Earlier this year, three hospitals began piloting the accreditation programme, process and standards. They are two acute care hospitals and one specialist orthopedic clinic. The pilot hospitals established self-assessment teams and are completing the assessment against the relevant standards for their programme area. They need to show that they comply with five patient safety standards.

January 2010 will see Accreditation Canada provide on-site training to 40 surveyors. The surveyors will be selected by the Ministry of Health according to a surveyor system appropriate to the Kuwait accreditation programme structure and the Kuwait context. Accreditation Canada surveyors will mentor the Kuwaiti surveyors and support them in conducting their pilot surveys in February 2010. From March to June 2010, Accreditation Canada will work with the MOH to complete the survey reports for the three pilot surveys, evaluate them, adjust the standards and accreditation process if required, and finalize the programme and process.

There are already two local hospitals with international accreditation from Accreditation Canada; Dar Al Shifa Hospital in Safat and New Mowasat Hospital in Salmiya. The New Mowasat Hospital has launched its first Certified Professional in Health Care Quality (CPHQ) review and study program. According to Dr, Ghada Welwel, a certified professional in health care quality, the program is part of the hospital's objective to enhance the performance of its staff from the executive level to the bottom. She said New Mowasat Hospital is the first hospital in Kuwait to adopt the service quality standards applied by the Canadian board, "Through New Mowasat, the private and public hospitals in Kuwait are working hard to adopt these international standards. In a hospital setting, quality takes on a variety of meanings. It encompasses technical excellence. It is also about patient-centreed approach to care delivered by the dedicated professionals in the hospital. In addition to having the technical and clinical expertise to provide safe and high quality care, it is also critical that the hospital focuses on other factors in a patient's hospital experience. For us to develop high quality services we have to educate the staff on how to provide health care quality."

Dr. Welwel plans to hold an international conference in February 2010 on the quality of patient care and the legal responsibility concerning the health and safety of patients, "Professionals from Europe and the United States are expected to attend this conference. It will be the first of its kind in the Middle East and hopefully it will take place in collaboration with New Mowasat."

Kuwait's health ministry deputy, Dr, Ibraheem Al-Abdulhadi has announced the cabinet's approval for setting up a new 300-bed hospital for alternative medicine and rehabilitation at a total cost of KD 30 m, *Kuwait Times* has reported. The new hospital will include a rehabilitation centre for the disabled, senior citizens' care centres and will be connected to one of the most advanced international centres in the field of alternative medicine. The new hospital will be ready within five years, he said.

Private Health care

No matter what country you decide to relocate to, getting private health care is always a safe option. The quality of national health care fluctuates from country to country. The price of the most fundamental care is often very high and this is supposing you find a suitable hospital or doctor to begin with. Private health care, on the other hand, often adheres to a standardization of service. Consequently, as an expat, it is probably wise to invest in private health care at least until you are completely familiar with the national health system. Getting medical treatment for you and your family without comprehensive health insurance could prove arduous, and no-one wants the hassle of bureaucracy in an emergency. You may even find that the country you are emigrating to has no national health service.

The benefits of private health care include:

- Peace of mind
- Better efficiency and quality of service
- Could save large sums money (possibly thousands of pounds) in the case of an emergency
- A vaster choice of services and practitioners
- No waiting lists or bureaucracy
- Ensures you do not have to settle for local, possibly inadequate or unhygienic, services
- Request an English-speaking doctor/nurse

Will the insurer cover:

- Maternity?
- A chronic illness/condition?
- A country at war?

You will have to weigh-up the costs of such services as private doctors, outpatient medicine, and dental cover. But that's not all. You may also have to decide where you'd like to receive treatment in the case of a serious health problem or injury. Does your adopted nation meet requirements, or would you prefer to return to the UK for treatment?

The United Medical Services group has announced the launch of one of its hospitals here. After years of continuous hard work, the first phase of Al-Seef Hospital which overlooks the tranquil Arabian Gulf was opened. It will offer the latest and most sophisticated in medical technology to citizens as well as residents. The first phase's opening was inaugurated by Sheikh Ahmad Al-Fahad Al-Sabah, Minister for Housing and Economic Development. "Al-Seef Hospital will provide health care by combining modernity and quality. Apart from being a well-designed hospital, it is complete in itself that combines complex health services. We hope that this hospital will provide additional health services that cater to the public," he noted.

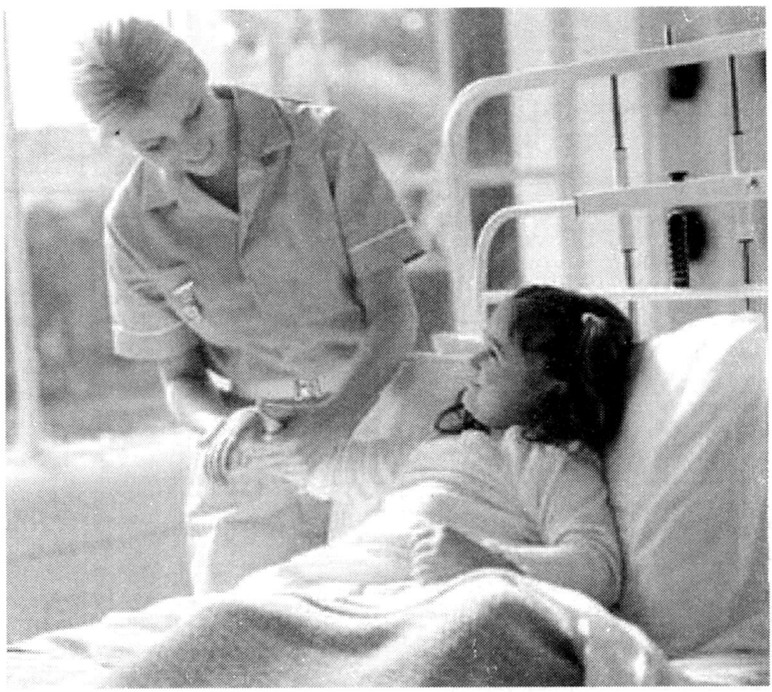

Sheikh Ahmad said that the hospital's management faces a shortage in financial resources. "Although the economic situation isn't at its best, the board of directors and the shareholders of Al- Seef Hospital are keen to execute this project. This reflects their interest in the country's public welfare," he added.

The largest private and most technologically advanced hospital in the Middle East will offer services to the whole family including services in pediatric, obstetrics and gynecology, dental, dermatology, venerology, physiotherapy and nutrition services to name some. In addition, Al-Seef Hospital also has specialized health care units for children and women like the Neonatal Intensive Care Unit (NICU), the Special Care Baby Unit (SCBU) and the plastic surgery unit.

Public health care is liberally provided

The hospitals and other health care institutions in Kuwait never disappoint the patients with its efficient services and treatment procedures. Public health care is provided through a number of clinics and hospitals. The clinics are located throughout Kuwait and can usually be found next to the local supermarket or co-operative. Clinics offer preliminary examinations and routine check-ups and services, and will refer a patient to a specialist where necessary. All public facilities are open to expatriate residents. There are currently five major (general) government hospitals throughout the country, all of which provide an outpatients service. These hospitals are recommended for emergency treatment although not all facilities have obvious emergency entrances. It is advisable to pass by when you are in the area to establish exactly where the entrance is. It will make life a lot less stressful if you ever need to find it in a hurry. Your Civil ID card will need to be produced when visiting the government hospitals for treatment.

Private health care is of a high standard, although it does come at a price. There is an ever-increasing number of private hospitals and clinics in Kuwait, all of which require a patient to register prior to treatment. Your

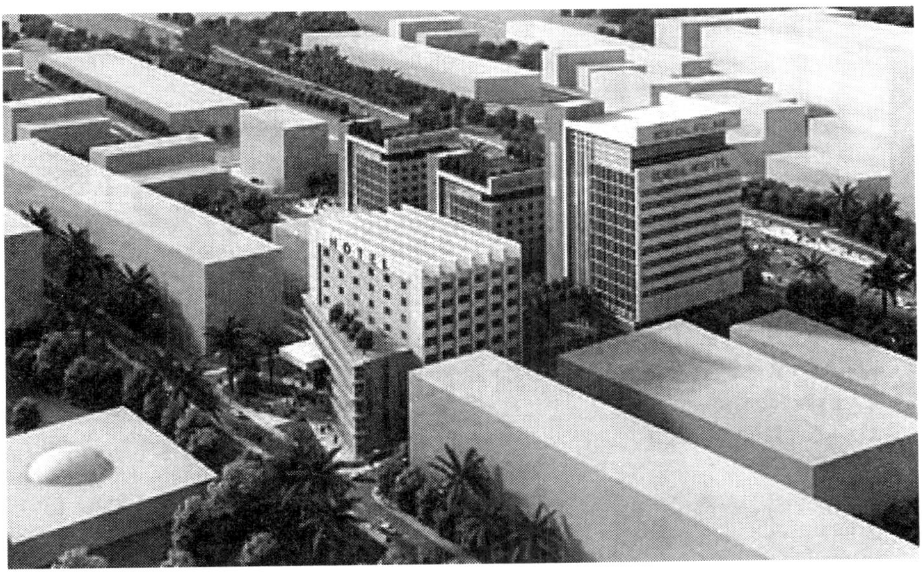

Civil ID card is required (passports are accepted for visitors to Kuwait and new residents yet to receive their Civil ID card). Private medical insurance is not absolutely necessary in Kuwait. However, expatriates generally prefer to be covered by private insurance allowing for the use of private hospitals and clinics where there are more comfortable facilities and shorter waiting periods. English is spoken at both government and private hospitals. Pharmacies are located next to hospitals and clinics and at most co-operatives. A number of night pharmacies are listed in the newspaper on a daily basis. Some government hospitals: Mubarak Al-Kabir hospital in Jabriya, Sabah hospital, Al-Adan hospital, Amiri hospital, Farwaniya hospital.

By order of the Commercial Real Estate Company (CRC), the University Medical Centre Hamburg-Eppendorf (UKE) prepared a feasibility study for a high-capacity hospital in Kuwait. Initially this led to the foundation of a prevention centre: Similar to the Medical Prevention Centre Hamburg, in which the UKE has a share, the hospital will offer a comprehensive four-hour medical examination—including a full-body magnetic resonance imaging scan—in a luxurious hotel environment. A five-year management contract was signed.

The building project has meanwhile been expanded by a 400-bed clinic, a hotel, and apartments to create Al-Shefa'a Medical City. The UKE developed the business plan. The contract with the investor stipulates the development of a building and operational concept, as well as the transfer of the management of the project to the UCM.

Currently, Kuwait University has the following faculties:

- College of Allied Health Sciences (separated from College of Medicine in June 1982)
- College of Arts (separated on October 1967)
- College of Business Administration (est. as College of Economics and Political Science in April 1967) (Accredited by the AACSB)
- College of Dentistry (est. May 1996)
- College of Education (est. May 1980)
- College of Engineering and Petroleum (est. December 1974)—approved by ABET
- College of Law (est. April 1967)
- College of Medicine (est. July 1973)
- College of Pharmacy (est. February 1996)
- College of Sciences (separated on October 1967)
- College of Shari'a and Islamic Studies (est. 16 August, 1977)

Faculty of Medicine

After several years of intense study and careful planning, the Faculty of Medicine was formed with the objectives of producing high quality health care professionals and medical scientists and playing a major role in the development and upgrading of the country's health care system.

Since its establishment in 1973, the Faculty of Medicine has developed into an internationally recognized medical school, serving Kuwait and the Gulf region. The number of students enrolled in the program has increased from 48 in 1976 to the present 90 students per year. The total number of students enrolled in the seven year medical program is currently 600.

1339 students have completed the seven year program and received the B.M., B.Ch. degree since the first batch of students graduated in 1983. The Faculty employs 350 academic, technical and administrative staff.

The departments that make up the body of the Faculty of Medicine include Anatomy, Biochemistry, Community Medicine and Behavioural Science, Medicine, Microbiology, Nuclear Medicine, Obstetrics and Gynaecology, Paediatrics, Pathology, Pharmacology and Toxicology, Physiology, Primary Care, Psychiatry, Radiology and Surgery. The Faculty has moved into a system based case-triggered integrated curriculum from academic year 2006-07. As a prelude to this, the curriculum of the Health Sciences Centre common year has been revised incorporating medically-oriented basic courses, to be taught by the Health Sciences Centre staff.

Seven departments are currently running graduate programs, Anatomy, Biochemistry, Microbiology, Pathology, Physiology, Pharmacology and Nuclear Medicine. Since the programs began in 1983, more than 100 students have graduated. The Departments of Microbiology and Physiology are running both M.Sc. and Ph.D. programs. The Department of Pathology is approved to admit their first batch of Ph.D. students during the 2007-08 academic year. In addition to Mubarak Al-Kabeer hospital, other facilities utilized for teaching purposes are Al-Amiri, Al-Adan, Maternity, Farwania, Jahra, Ahmadi, Sabah, Chest, Al-Razi, Psychiatric and Ibn Sina hospitals, as well as several polyclinics throughout Kuwait. Teaching facilities housed inside the modern five storey medical school building include four lecture theatres, an auditorium, eight seminar rooms, seven multi-discipline laboratories, as well as a number of demonstration, seminar and conference rooms in the departments.

In addition, facilities at the newly commissioned Health Sciences Centre building are available to the use of the Faculty. A distance learning centre connecting two lecture theatres, Anatomy Dissecting room, a consultation room at the Faculty and an operation theatre at Mubarak Al-Kabeer hospital has already been commissioned. A virtual hospital (clinical skills lab) will be established shortly.

The technical facilities available to academic staff and students for research and teaching compare to those of older and more established institutions elsewhere in the world. As part of its increasing commitment to research and dedication to academic excellence, the Faculty maintains an equipment inventory in excess of 6 million Kuwaiti Dinars and includes three Jeol electron microscopes (one scanning and two transmissions), a General Electric gamma camera with an associated Star Computer, and a Siemens angiography unit. There are also several ultra centrifuges, gamma and beta counters, amino acid analyser in addition to numerous other sophisticated scientific and medical instruments. The Faculty maintains a full complement of highly qualified biomedical engineers to maintain and repair most scientific equipment.

In addition to the professional services provided by the clinical academic staff serving the teaching hospital and the specialized units in other hospitals, each department in the Faculty of Medicine provides special services for the Ministry of Health including consultation services in various hospitals, sophisticated diagnostic tests, and a variety of highly specialized procedures including Therapeutic Drug Monitoring and Toxicological Screening, as well as conducting seminars and workshops to the medical community. In addition to the teaching of medical students, the Faculty of Medicine also offers various courses of studies for the students of the Faculties of Allied Health Sciences, Pharmacy and Dentistry.

Health Care in Bahrain

Health care in Bahrain is as promising as its economy, which is the fastest growing in the Arab world. Bahraini government puts a high importance on its people's health in cognizance of the fact that they are the movers behind the nation's growth. This structure hinges on highly skilled, world-class medical practitioners and advancements in medical research, state-of-the-art facilities and newly discovered diagnostic techniques that all work together to provide the highest quality of health care to citizens and expatriates.

At present, the country's existing health care landscape consists of three full service private hospitals manned by Bahraini and expatriate medical professionals trained abroad, four government hospitals, 19 health centres, five government maternity hospitals and various private practitioners with varied specializations from neurosurgery to dentistry.

Medical care is afforded to every resident of the country through public medical services that are often free. Although hospitals are equipped with both human and technical resources to provide first-rate care to its patients, the health sector is adopting the US and Western Europe patterns of extending assistance to those in need by providing private medical services in the form of health insurance, which are more needed by Bahrainis. The evolution of the Bahraini health care sector has a lot to do with early American Mission hospitals, which offered free medical care to those who couldn't afford it. Today, the organization no longer offers free services. However, its legacy continues in the government's existing health care structure that extends free or affordable health care to both citizens and expatriates.

The government itself is actively pursuing the development of the medical sector by inviting new players who can positively contribute to its growing health care industry. Investors are required to coordinate with the Ministry of Health which oversees all health-related affairs and issues of government, including pharmaceuticals and licensing. Pharmaceutical companies seeking to enter the Bahraini market will also need authorization from the Ministry of Commerce and Industry Investments and Environmental Affairs. This friendliness towards foreigners is another reflection of Bahrainis' openness to foreign influence aside from an obvious affinity for expats.

This type of scenario is particularly beneficial to foreigners who have come to Bahrain as expats. As the nation appears to be a bustling, productive yet concerned metropolis, it is mostly viewed as an ideal place for migrants, especially those who are coming with their kids. Due to the country's relatively small population, it is never a problem getting a medical professional to take a look at a sick person's condition. Doctors who are manning the hospitals have come from medical schools offshore where they acquired more advanced and specialized techniques for whatever specialization they have. Couple that with the most advanced medical equipment and the highest possible quality of care is offered to all Bahraini residents, locals or expats.

Faisal al-Hamer said the national health bill will jump to more than 550 million dinars ($1.45 billion) a year by 2025, leaving the government no option but to privatise the health care system, the local Gulf Daily News reported on Tuesday.

"The health care cost is escalating so rapidly that no government, irrespective of its wealth, can continue to provide free health care," Hamer was quoted as saying at a conference in Bahrain. "We are finding it increasingly difficult to meet the costs of providing free health care to the people and have no option but to go on to compulsory health insurance to offset some of the costs." Bahrain is a small island in the Persian Gulf and has a number of renowned hospitals to take care of the citizens who need medical attention.

Some of the important hospitals of Bahrain are as follows:

American Mission Hospital

The American Mission Hospital started its operations in the year 1893 under the leadership of missionaries. It is a private non-profit body and provides all kinds of medical services at an affordable price. Many kinds of donations are granted to the hospital from capable institutions. Some of the various departments are as follows:

- Surgery and Anesthesia
- General Practice
- Pediatrics
- Orthopedics
- Dentistry
- Dermatology
- Ophthalmology

Some of the clinics which offer special services are women clinic, baby clinic, anti smoking clinic, chest clinic and diabetes clinic.

Bahrain Specialist Hospital

The Bahrain Specialist Hospital was inaugurated on Wednesday 26 th of February, 2003 and provides adequate medical facilities under a committed group of doctors and nursing stuff. There are 83 patient rooms, 12 patient day surgery units, 4 VIP suites, 6 premiere suits, private deluxe rooms, semi private deluxe rooms, 12 day surgery beds and ICU rooms. Some of the medical services are cardiology centre, neurology, urology, pulmonary medicine.

International Hospital of Bahrain

International Hospital of Bahrain, WLL is the first private medical centre of Bahrain and started to function in the year 1978. The hospital offers state of the art medical services and some of them come in the form of general surgery, geriatrics, neurology, neurosurgery and orthopedic surgery.

A burgeoning medical sector; medical city, Bahrain

King Abdullah bin Abdulaziz of Saudi Arabia donated 2 billion Saudi Riyal (BD100 million) for the construction of a medical city in Bahrain. Earlier, the Saudi king arrived in Bahrain for his first two-day visit to the kingdom. The medical city will be affiliated with Arabian Gulf University (AGU), one of the best medical institutions in the region. The Saudi king said the medical city will be a gift from the people of Saudi Arabia to the people of Bahrain and the GCC.

Commenting on the medical city plan, AGU President Dr, Khalid Al Ohali said his institution was honoured by the gesture, adding that the city will be named King Abdullah bin Abdulaziz Medical City to express appreciation to the Saudi king.

His Majesty King Hamad bin Isa Al Khalifa returned the gesture by donating Imam Turki bin Abdullah Al Saud's historic sword to the Saudi king. The sword has remained with Bahrain for about 140 years since it was entrusted by the late Imam Saud bin Faisal Al Saud to Shaikh Isa bin Ali Al Khalifa. King Hamad said the sword has remained a symbol of unity between both countries over the years. He also expressed delight while bestowing the Shaikh Isa bin Salman Al Khalifa Medal First Class on King Abdullah for his contributions to Arab and Islamic nations.

While no official details have been released about the medical city, the investment from Saudi Arabia is an indication of how much the sector is growing in the region. According to research, the health care sector in the UAE alone is expected to grow at an annual rate of more than 13 percent to 2012.

The general level of health care in Bahrain is good. Of course many expatriates prefer private hospitals to the public hospitals, but in a real emergency you are advised to go to the country's largest government-run hospital, Salmaniya, which has all the services you would expect of a top hospital. Your problem as a non-Arabic speaker will be getting yourself understood in an emergency, although most hospital staff speak English. Private hospitals used most often by expatriates are Awali Hospital, International Hospital of Bahrain, American Mission Hospital (AMH), the Bahrain Defence Force Hospital (BDF) or Bahrain Specialist Hospital. They all have GP services that expats can use.

The public hospitals can be used by expatriates and locals alike, but you must make sure that you have your CPR card with you. Although public hospitals should treat you immediately, there have been stories of delays when expatriates did not have their CPR cards with them. You should, as an expatriate, try to take out personal medical insurance. Your employer may provide this, but it is by no means standard in Bahrain. Having medical insurance enables you to have treatment at the hospital of your choice, but should also allow you to be treated outside the country if your condition is serious. There are many international companies you can get cover from, as well as well-respected local companies.

There are many pharmacies that open 24 hours a day. Some work on a rota system, with those open on any particular day listed in the GDN, while some others are also open 24 hours a day, every day, and are also listed in the GDN. Most pharmacies can give you basic medicines for colds, etc. If you go to a hospital to visit a GP, which is normal for expatriates here, the hospital usually has its own pharmacy, making it easier for you to reclaim your expenses if you are covered by insurance.

In an emergency, call 999 for an ambulance. You need to decide which hospital to go to. Often you are best served by going to the hospital you are used to, but remember some of the smaller private hospitals have a very restricted services during the night, if your condition is serious you should probably go to Salmaniya Hospital in Manama.

MEDICAL UNIVERSITY OF BAHRAIN (MUB)

This is the new medical university; The Premier and Mr Ahern unveil a plaque to mark the opening of the MUB

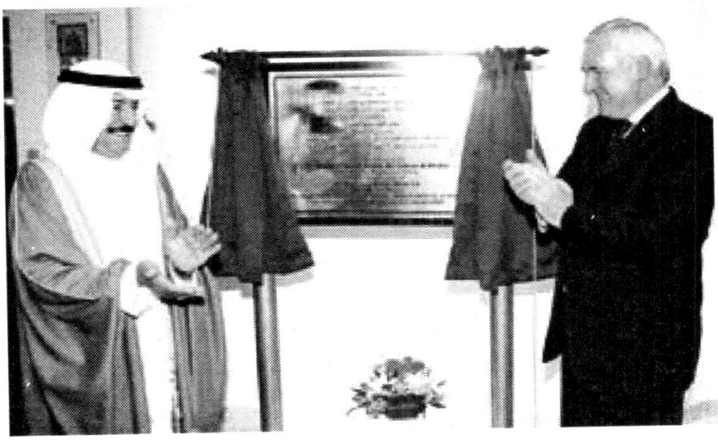

Bahrain made history with the opening of a globally-recognized medical school. The Medical University of Bahrain is affiliated to the Royal College of Surgeons in Ireland (RCSI). It is the first complete university to be established outside Ireland by the RCSI. It shows Bahrain's drive to attract foreign investment in higher education is paying off, said Prime Minister Shaikh Khalifa bin Salman Al Khalifa.

The MUB is the latest in the series of world-class centres of higher learning being developed in the kingdom, he said. "This educational pillar mirrors the government's success in attracting foreign investment in the field of higher education," said the Prime Minister. "The MUB also reflects the government's commitment to ensuring quality educational services. "The programmes at MUB will be delivered to the highest international standards, with qualifications that will be recognized worldwide." "The project was born out of the vision of the Prime Minister and Ireland is proud to join Bahrain in this great journey of co-operation in health care," he said. RCSI-MUB Board chairman Dr, Faisal Al Moosawi said more such universities were needed in Bahrain due to the rapid growth of the health care sector.

"The university has facilities to teach 2,000 students in its new Muharraq campus. It will offer admissions to Bahrainis, GCC citizens and students from other nationalities," he told a Press conference at the RCSI-MUB.

He said 90 per cent of the students in the university's nursing school and 40pc in its medical school were Bahrainis. "This will further help meet the demand for medical professionals in the country, with more Bahrainis willing to enter the field," said Dr, Al Mousawi. RCSI-MUB president Kevin O'Malley said the first batch of doctors and nurses to serve in Bahrain hospitals would be graduating by June, 2010. "During their study, they are trained at the BDF Hospital as well as Health Ministry hospitals along with the King Hamad General Hospital, which is under construction," he said. RCSI-MUB nursing and midwifery school director, Batool Al Mohandis said the university offers students similar programmes offered in Ireland.

"We have the same curriculum as in Ireland. Our goal is to provide high quality education without the need for Bahrainis to leave their country and spend a fortune," she said. Ms Al Mohandis said the university fees was 50 pc less than their main campus based in Dublin, Ireland. "Here, a student has to spend BD13,000 per year to obtain a bachelors degree from the medical school and to complete the programme a student needs six years," she said. The new campus is part of the King Hamad Medical City, which will feature the Bahrain Health Oasis and the King Hamad General Hospital.

Lebanon health care

With a highly Trained and professional Lebanese staff, is present in University Hospitals in Lebanon. With state of the art technology and over thirteen years of experience, Home Care Middle East (HCME) provides

Complete Health care Services at Home such as:

- Nursing Care
- Elderly Care
- Baby and Mother Care (New services added)
- Travel assistance
- Electronic Remote Patient Monitoring (NEW)
- Therapeutic Services
  - o Physical Therapy
  - o Speech Therapy
  - o Oxygen Therapy
- Lab Exams
- Medical Supplies and Equipments

They serve: Syria (Damascus and Aleppo), Jordan (Amman), Saudi Arabia (Jeddah, Ryad, Dammam), Oman (Muscat), Qatar (Doha), UAE (Dubai, Abu Dhabi), Kuwait (Kuwait City), Bahrain (Manama) and other arab cities.

Health Care in Oman

Oman offers high quality health care equal to that of Western Europe and the United States, except with regards to highly specialized treatments. Since Oman has a high ratio of medical facilities (both public and private) to residents, it is generally very easy to obtain care. However, for rare and extremely specialized procedures people sometimes need to travel outside of Oman. Wealthy Omanis often seek minor care abroad as well, traveling to hospitals in London or the United States. Interestingly, many Omani doctors and nurses are actually foreigners who have come to Oman to take advantage of the high salaries.

American Mission Hospitals, which used to operate on a part-private (for those who could afford treatment), part-free (for those who couldn't) basis, played an important part in the development of medical services. They can still be found today, though they no longer offer free treatment.

Oman now has a public health service providing free or very low cost health care for its nationals. These facilities are also available to foreigners. Tourists visiting Oman should have travel insurance that includes cover for private medical treatment, though they will have emergency access to state medical facilities regardless of whether or not they are insured.

Common expatriate health problems include alcoholism (particularly among bachelors, who frequently suffer from loneliness and depression) and respiratory problems caused by sand and dust in the air. The dust problem is aggravated by the construction projects that are common throughout Oman.

Hard work and long hours in the country's extreme heat take a toll on the human immune system, and manual labourers can suffer sunstroke and sunburn. Your employer should excuse you if the temperature reaches

50°C (122°F), though since these conditions are common (especially in summer), you may find him ignoring them instead. Summer humidity causes added discomfort and leads to common eye infections. Dehydration is a potentially lethal threat that can affect anyone spending time outdoors, including doctors. Make sure to have plenty of water on hand if you will be spending time outdoors.

Iraq Health care; Baghdad Medical City

Baghdad Medical City formerly known as Saddam Medical City is a complex of several teaching hospitals in Bab Al-Moatham, Baghdad, Iraq The Medical City includes the Baghdad University College of Medicine. The largest hospital in the complex is the Surgical Specialties Hospital built in 1980. The second largest is the Baghdad Teaching Hospital, built in the early 1970s, which contains the out patient clinics and the emergency department. The complex has over a thousand beds for patients, collectively it is run by Baghdad Medical City.

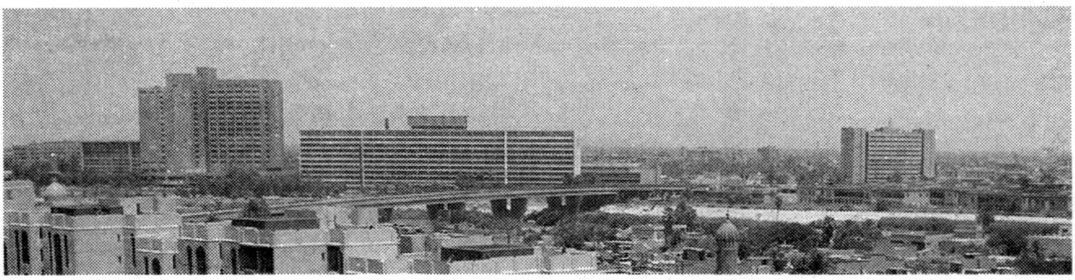

Baghdad's Medical City

The Biggest Hospital has Become Sick. Not even the elevators work now at Baghdad Medical City, built once as the centre for best medical care. One of the ten elevators still does, and the priority for this is patients who have lost their legs—and there are many of them. The rest, the doctors, patients and students at the four specialized teaching hospitals within the building complex, just take the stairs, sometimes to the 18th floor.

This is in a city that had been given dreams of great development some years back. Much of the corporate-led media in the U.S. and Europe still insists that the situation in Baghdad has "improved". As with Baghdad Medical City, so with Baghdad, and so with Iraq. The elevators are just another reminder of a country that's not working.

It's a hard day's work for Razak when he is operating the elevator. "The smell of my sweat mixes with the smell of at least 20 other people who crowd into the lift." It gets less sweaty to the extent there are more wheelchairs. Razak has been doing his job for the last ten years, the first five of them quite happy ones. "We used to have a special elevator just for doctors and professors," he says. "But by now most have left, and some have been killed."

"There is no air-conditioning in the building, when temperatures can be 48C, almost no qualified staff to serve patients, no antibiotics, and sometimes not even basic material for intravenous treatment," says Dr. Samir Abdul Zahra, who treats patients while also doing his medical studies. There are no senior doctors around. "Most of them left because of the situation in the city, the lack of security," Dr. Zahra says. And that affects teaching as much as treatment. "We are educating ourselves now. This means also that young doctors are taking on complex cases they are simply not qualified to deal with."

This dilemma is particularly acute at Baghdad Medical City because it is the largest medical complex in Iraq, and the most serious cases are usually taken to this hospital.

At this complex now, it is not even safe to drink tap water any more. Sometimes doctors cannot find water even to wash their hands. Equipment is often not sterilized. And the prescriptions they write can mean little. "Most of the medicines we have here are out of date, and we lack almost all basic antibiotics," says Dr. Saad Abu Al-Noor, a pharmacist at the supply warehouse at Baghdad Medical City. "We cannot get medicines from the stores because of lack of security, and because there is just too much corruption all over."

Patients in need or their family members are sent out to the shops to buy catheters, disposable syringes and essential medicines, Dr. Noor said. "If the patient is lucky, he can find the items in the black market. And then the question is if they can afford these things. The price is ten to 20 times higher than it should be." And finally, when all is at hand for the very few, and a doctor of some kind is available, electricity is often lacking for serious treatment. The hospital gets about two hours of electricity a day. It has some generators, but these have to be cut out frequently.

The Medical City, located in central Baghdad, includes the Baghdad University College of Medicine. The largest hospital in the complex is the Surgical Specialties Hospital built in 1980. The second largest is the Baghdad Teaching Hospital, built in the early 1970s, which contains the out patient clinics and the emergency department. The complex had over a thousand beds for patients. Now some patients just stray in hopelessly, with nobody to care.

Appendix to Chapter 3 (at the end of the book).

4

Dubai Health Care City (DHCC): Oases for Health Tourism

The Health Care City is very unique, because it is a city within a city, where both the pharmaceutical industry and health care are under one roof. The developers and the owners are the Dubai Holding. This project will cost $1.8 billion. The following institutions will be housed here:

- research and rehabilitation centres,
- medically training institutes,
- private hospitals and clinics,
- pharmaceutical offices and spas.

This project has been devised for promoting medical tourism. For this reason there are also some flats, residential villa's and five star hotels, which are surrounded by an artificial lake. The Health Care City in Dubai is situated on the Old Metha road, beside the creek and nearby Al Wasl hospital and Wafi City. By early 2010 it is likely to have its own Dubai Metro station on the Green Line.

The hospitals which are under construction can be categorized as follows:

- General Hospital I—Cardiology
- General Hospital II—Obstetrics
- General Hospital III (150 beds)
- Long-Term Care Facility (100 beds)
- Nursing Home (50 beds)
- Orthopaedic Hospital (20 beds)
- Plastic Surgery Hospital I (25 beds)
- Plastic Surgery Hospital II (25 beds)

- Rehabilitation Hospital (300 beds)
- Sports Medicine Hospital (100 beds)
- Long-Term Care Facility (100 beds)
- Urology Hospital (30 beds)
- University Hospital (400 beds)

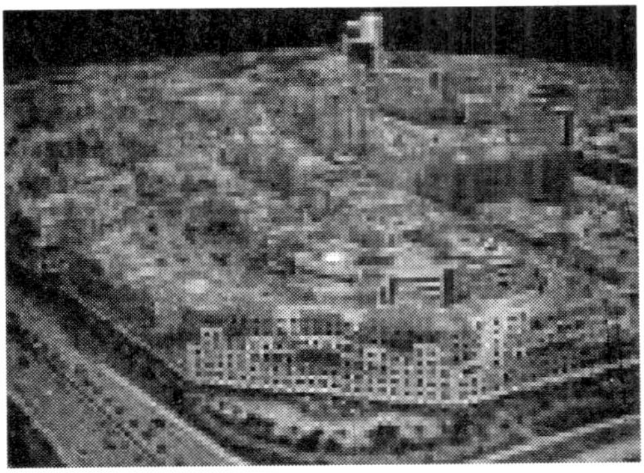

At present, candidates for the postgraduate training program are sent to Boston (USA). But the final goal is to set-up a teaching hospital and a postgraduate medical training centre, which will be associated with the Harvard Medical School. This academic centre promises the most exhaustive medical reference search in the country, by having a research centre of the sciences of living and the Al Maktoum Medical Library. The research centre of the sciences of living is an auditorium with 300 seats. Therefore it is a large project with also a nursing school in the expectancy, which will accommodate 200 students, offering basic and masters level training.

At present the Health Care City of Dubai functions partially. There are approximately 760 staff members, of which 130 doctors. According to the expectations phase 1 and 2 will be fully operational by 2010. Up till now the next list of private hospitals and offices has been announced:

- American Academy of Cosmetic Surgery Hospital
- American University of Beirut Medical Centre
- Dr. Sulaiman Al Habib Medical Centre
- Eleva Women's Hospital
- London Great Ormonde Street Hospital Dubai Office
- Mayo Clinic Middle East
- The City Hospital (Welcare, Varkey Group)
- The Creek Hospital Dubai (Welcare, Varkey Group)
- University Hospital
- Universitatsklinikum Hamburg-Eppendorf

The following pharmaceutical companies are already operational with offices and laboratories in Dubai Health Care City:

- AstraZeneca
- Johnson and Johnson
- Novo Nordisk
- Wyeth Pharmaceuticals

The City of Dubai

It is the second largest emirate in the United Arab Emirates (UAE). Its year-round sunshine, coupled with an unprecedented level of investment and a luxurious lifestyle, has not only turned it into a popular tourist destination, but also an essential health care location. Dubai offers an unparalleled quality of life in a virtually crime-free, tolerant society; world-class hotels and entertainment; enviable sports and leisure facilities; and excellent value shopping—all of which combine to make living and working in Dubai a pleasure. Dubai is one of the safest cities for tourists. Safety is not the only USP of Dubai. Right from the fleet of Bentleys that dot its roads to its spick and span environs, world's best luxury hotels as well as fashion brands. The only reminder that one is in an Islamic nation is the sight of many lovely women silhouetted in burqas as also the religious fervor that marks the observance of holy month of Ramzan. Another pointer is the safe distance between members of the opposite Sex. The city has a seductive charm, more so in the night when taxis zip past offering a glimpse of Burj Dubai (818 metres), which is a skyscraper in the Business Bay district of Dubai and the tallest man-made structure ever built. In recent times both Burj Dubai and Burj Al Arab, a super luxury hotel, have not only eclipsed the city's skyline but also become its biggest tourist attractions. The stinking rich soak in the luxury of the 1053-feet high awe-inspiring hotel while others gape at this modern-day architectural marvel resembling the sail of a dhow, an Arabian vessel. Though the dazzling night vision of luminous skyscrapers kissing each other establishes Dubai as a 21st century city, yet the place has on old-world charm too. The dhow cruise on Dubai creek is a passage through both modernity and tradition. On one side neon lights blaze and on the other dim-lit facade of some of its original buildings can be seen. Ski Dubai at Mall of Emirates shopping mall brings you even snow skiing and claims to be the largest indoor ski resort in the world. The natural beauty of this man-made wonder casts a spell. The human enterprising endeavor further extends to Palm Jumeriah, an artificial fantasy island created by land reclamation. The Jumeriah beach park overlooking the Arabian Gulf, too, presents an alluring picture with its sparkling clean water, picnic tables, washing areas, pebbled pathways and much more. The desert safari brings the magic of sand dunes. Available at 200 dirhams, (average Rs. 2,600), its worth every penny; the skilled native drivers maneuver their way up and down the sand dunes. As the vehicles stand ramrod straight atop the dune, the adrenalin rush brings a heady mix of exhilaration and fear. The camp offers the typical tourist paraphernalia: henna tattoos for hands, getting pictures clicked in traditional Arabic costumes. But piece de resistance is the belly dance. The soaring temperatures are not much of a dampener as the air conditioning finds its best use in the UAE—in the shopping malls, in dwelling places, even inside the bus stations. Light woolens are a must at night, irrespective of the time of the year one is visiting Dubai. During the return journey, the Dubai airport offers an out of the world shopping experience—just four hours away from Delhi.

Good health care is assured

With over 93% people well employed, good attention to health care is assured. Dubai is well known as the city of choice that offers a strategic location and a reputation for successfully developing innovative projects like DHCC. With a total number of 19,523 health care professionals in Dubai in both the private and public sectors including 6,064 doctors, Dubai is the perfect platform for Dubai Health Care City to emerge as the leading health care services centre in the region.

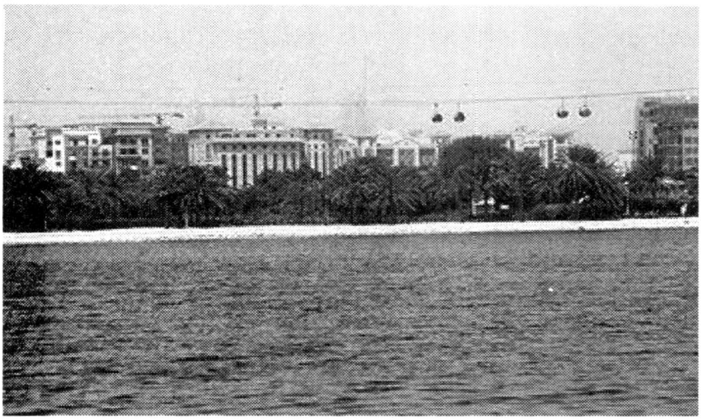

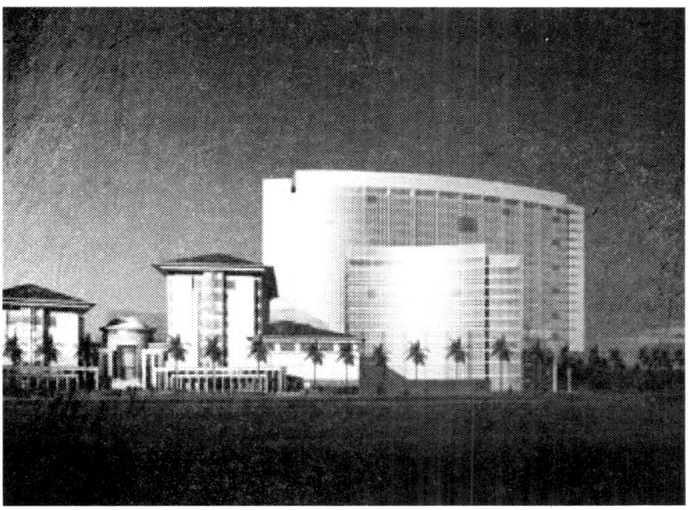

Dubai Health Care City (DHCC)

Located strategically between Europe and South East Asia, DHCC is a pioneering project that is poised to fill the gap that exists within the health care industry in the region. Due to the nature and scale of this project, patients, health care providers, professionals as well as the region as a whole will reap the benefits of the region's first integrated health care cluster. The mission of DHCC is to create a platform for the provision of health care, education and research services within an informed regulatory framework. We are at the forefront of health care delivery by continuously responding to emerging health care needs to improve the lives of people and by introducing initiatives such as continuing medical education programs for health care professionals. We are committed to scientific research through identifying and funding research needs in the region.

Dubai Health Care City (DHCC) was created by the Government of Dubai, with the objective of becoming, a globally acknowledged location of choice for health care and a centre of excellence for specialist medical services, medical education, and life science research. Dubai is investing in the infrastructure development of First phase called medical community, approximately four million square feet of space to establish regional medical care, including academic tertiary care and specialty referral hospitals, primary and secondary care centres, educational facilities, basic and clinical research facilities, and commercial biotechnology research and development facilities. Harvard Medical International (HMI), as DHCC's key strategic collaborator, has been working with DHCC to develop DHCC's capabilities and service offerings in the areas of medical education, health care delivery, and research. HMI has created a Dubai-based team to help carry out the terms of the partnership and ensure that objectives are met.

"Dubai Health Care City was launched in 2002 in cooperation with Harvard Medical School. The aim of the project is to build a world-class health care and training facility for residents of the Persian Gulf. Dubai Health Care City officials estimate that Persian Gulf residents spent $25 billion annually traveling abroad for medical treatment. That means a cool $25 billion of medical tourism lost. Since most of the Gulf residents go to Singapore, Malaysia and the United States for treatment, guess who's going to gain in the long run? It is reckoned that Dubai will be a major destination for medical tourists, especially Muslims. Maybe they'll offer discounts in the duty free shops to anyone who gets a facelift. DHCC will treat the region to a host of medical services grouped in a highly convenient setting. Physician offices, ambulatory surgery centres, general hospitals, specialty hospitals, rehabilitation and long-term care facilities, hospice, and diagnostic laboratories are brought together to deliver diagnostic and treatment services to an international standard. DHCC is the prime location for ultra-modern outpatient facilities, health care commercial offices and retail services. The Ibn Sina building houses clinics and laboratories featuring the latest in radiology and MRI technology. The Al Razi Medical Complex features outpatient surgical clinics complete with state-of-the-art analytical and diagnostic laboratories, and surgical suites. In line with

DHCC's innovative strategy, the Dubai Medical Suites offers day clinics and surgical suites for short-term lease to allow world-renowned visiting doctors to serve the region's specialized health care requirements. This arrangement is the first of its kind in the region.

Harvard Medical School Dubai Centre (HMSDC)

The Medical Community is home to medical, dental, nursing and allied health schools. These schools offer Continuous Medical Education (CME) courses and postgraduate education. A key member of this community is the Harvard Medical School Dubai Centre (HMSDC) for Postgraduate Medical Education and Research, which offers fellowship and observership programs. The community also aims to build a world-class research infrastructure. One of the pioneers in this field is the Dubai Harvard Foundation for Medical Research (DHFMR) which aims to lead the creation of regionally-relevant basic science research.

Complementing the conventional medical services are a vast array of diagnostic laboratories, pharmacies, medical equipment companies, health care recruitment firms, health care consulting firms and pharmaceutical companies.

Complementary Services

The Medical Community delivers an impressive portfolio of complementary support services. Most notably, DHCC offers a one-stop shop for our customers' legal requirements such as visas and other government-related documentation. For the convenience of our customers and visitors, wide selections of retail and food and beverage outlets are available throughout the city. A five star hotel dedicated to patients' families, staff, visiting doctors and students is yet another example of comprehensive support services.

Conglomeration of hospitals

Overall, there are 17 hospitals planned for DHCC with a total of 780 beds. By specialty categorization, hospitals proposed/under construction include:

- Plastic Surgery Hospital I (25 beds)
- Plastic Surgery Hospital II (25 beds)
- Orthopedic Hospital (20 beds)
- Urology Hospital (30 beds)
- General Hospital I—Cardiology
- General Hospital II—Obstetrics
- General Hospital III (150 beds)
- University Hospital (400 beds)
- Sports Medicine Hospital (100 beds)
- Rehabilitation Hospital (300 beds)
- Long-Term Care Facility (100 beds)
- Nursing Home (50 beds)

The teaching hospital and postgraduate medical training centre is affiliated with Harvard Medical School. The academic centre will have a Life Sciences research centre, a 300-seat auditorium, and the Medical Library, which promises to have the most comprehensive medical reference collection in the country. Applicants for the postgraduate training programme are sent to Boston for the time being. The University Hospital is expected to be ready by the end of 2008. A nursing school will accommodate 200 students, offering basic and masters level training.

DHCC is currently partially functional, with a staff of 760+, including 130+ physicians. The following is a list of private hospitals/ offices that have been announced so far at DHCC:

- University Hospital
- Universitatsklinikum Hamburg-Eppendorf
- Mayo Clinic Middle East
- Dr. Sulaiman Al Habib Medical Centre
- The City Hospital (Welcare, Varkey Group)
- The Creek Hospital Dubai (Welcare, Varkey Group)
- American Academy of Cosmetic Surgery Hospital
- American University of Beirut Medical Centre
- Eleva Women's Hospital
- London Great Ormonde Street Hospital Dubai Office

Pharmaceutical companies that have established offices/labs in DHCC:

- AstraZeneca
- Novo Nordisk
- Johnson and Johnson
- Wyeth Pharmaceuticals

Medical Education

Among the partnership's most important developments is the design and launch of the Harvard Medical School Dubai Centre (HMSDC). The HMSDC, established in May 2004, will house the Institute for Postgraduate Education and Research, and be the centre of DHCC's education activities. Currently, through the HMSDC, HMI fosters the development of postgraduate and continuing medical education (CME) programs designed to train specialty physicians, nurses, and allied health professionals, and bring updated knowledge and practices to the entire region. Since the inception of the DHCC-HMI partnership, the partners have teamed to organize CME programs focused on diabetes, musculoskeletal health and sports medicine, respiratory medicine, gastro-entrology and large-scale, multidisciplinary programs on primary care issues of particular regional concern.

To ensure that patient care and education services provided by

DHCC meet international standards of excellence, HMI and DHCC have established the Centre for Health care Planning and Quality (CPQ). The overarching goal of the CPQ is to oversee health care quality and accreditation within DHCC—across all structures and processes including, facilities, education, and patient care, and aligned with international standards of excellence—and ensure that the services provided through DHCC are commensurate with regional demand. It is also committed to establishing itself as a centre for research and scientific discovery. To this end DHCC and HMI have joined to create the Dubai Harvard Foundation for Medical Research to support training and research programs through HMSDC, as well as collaborative research programs around the world. The Foundation will be the mechanism through which DHCC attracts philanthropy as well as private and governmental funding for developing leaders in science and medicine in the region.

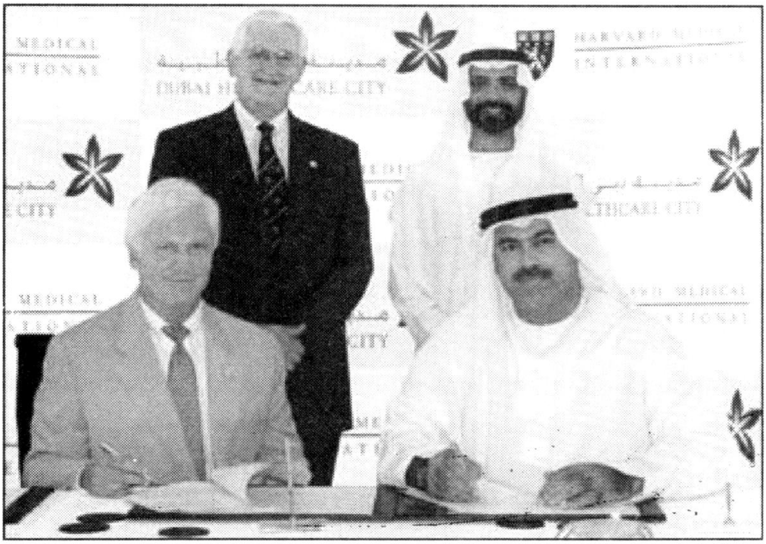

Centre for Health care Planning and Quality (CPQ)

The CPQ is a result of a committed long-term collaboration between DHCC and HMI throughout their partnership. The organization's charter covers a complexity of roles, from licensing health care providers to operate in Dubai Health Care City, to setting standards of high-quality care and providing quality training and performance evaluation. The overarching goal of the CPQ, however, is to support the ongoing development of Dubai Health Care City into a location of choice for health care delivery and ensure that the health care services provided at DHCC are comprehensive and aligned with regional demand. The council set-up by DHCC's Centre for Planning and Quality (CPQ) will be led by prominent alternative medicine practitioners, responsible for licensing CAM professionals under specific rules and regulations as well as its other regulatory functions.

The Centre for Health care Planning and Quality (CPQ), a joint initiative of Dubai Health Care City (DHCC) and Harvard Medical International (HMI) which oversees health care quality, clinical planning, education, project management, training, licensing and credentialing within DHCC has held a series of meetings with regional bodies to explore possibilities of collaboration. CPQ's consulting program has been asked to assist in the enhancement of health care services and education throughout the region.

Dr, Mariam Al Mazrouei, Medical Director of Dubai Health Care City said, 'The underlying goal of the CPQ is to support continuous improvement across every aspect of Dubai Health Care City and throughout the region. Moving forward, the CPQ also aims at offering its services in health systems development and educational development to organizations throughout the Gulf Region. In line with this the team from CPQ is holding a series of meetings with regional health care and medical education leaders.' Dr. Andrew Barrer, Acting Chief Executive Officer of CPQ and Executive Director of Harvard Medical International said that the CPQ team visited and held talks with medical organizations in Qatar, Egypt and Saudi Arabia to discuss possibilities of collaboration and to share the new systems created for Dubai with colleagues throughout the region.

Dr. Barrer elaborated, 'The first trip this year was to Doha to meet with members of the Qatar Foundation, Rand Corporation, Hamad Medical Corporation (HMC), Science and Technology Park and the Specialty Teaching Hospital on making alliances and exchanges on how CPQ can add value to their projects. We discussed developing quality standards for existing and new hospitals, public policy research, health care facility design standards and consulting and training in scientific research standards and processes.' 'In Cairo the CPQ team visited the President and Dean of the Misr University of Science and Technology (MUST) School of Medicine to talk about developing an education alliance and in providing services to help them develop their faculty and curriculum to bring it to international standards,' said Dr. Barrer.

'In Riaydh, Kingdom of Saudi Arabia, the CPQ team held meetings with King Faisal Specialist Hospital and Research Centre on how we could work together to improve medical education services and scope in the region through developing collaboration with Harvard Medical School Dubai Centre in developing the postgraduate education program to allow for training sites within DHCC,' said Dr. Andrew Barrer.

Alternative medicine therapy

Ahmad Sharaf, Senior Vice-President, Health care and Energy, Tatweer, said:

> 'In its endeavour to offer world-class health care services, DHCC has opened its doors to alternative medicine therapy, which is gaining wide acceptance worldwide. With this, DHCC further reiterates its

commitment to provide a balanced combination of traditional and modern medicine while catering to a larger segment of the community.' Dr. Muhadditha Al-Hashimi, CEO, Dubai Health Care City, said: 'The establishment of the Complementary and Alternative Medicine Council is our response to global trends, reflecting the growing popularity of alternative medicine and traditional practices. The council also demonstrates DHCC's efforts to operate on the global level as an efficient and leading market player.'

Dr. Ayesha Abdullah, Chief Executive Officer, Centre of Health care Planning and Quality, said: 'The use of these alternative therapies is growing. A survey by the National Centre for Complementary and Alternative Medicine, part of the National Institutes of Health in the United States, has stated that in 2002, more than 36% of the Americans used one form or the other of alternative therapy during the preceding 12 months, while nearly 50% had availed of these therapies at some point in their lifetime.'

The results of market survey conducted recently in Dubai generated almost identical numbers at 28% and 48% respectively in 2006. The same study concluded that 55% of the public prefer the implementation of formal regulations for CAM to increase public confidence and wider use. 'There is an obvious need to regulate this market to assure quality and safety. CPQ is proud to be the pioneer in developing CAM regulations with the establishment of the CAM Council, which is unique to this region,' added Dr, Abdullah.

Dr. Andrew Weil is one of America's leading practitioners in CAM. He is Director of Program in Integrative Medicine at the University of Arizona. He is also the founder of the 'Foundation for Integrative Medicine' and Editor-in-Chief of the journal Integrative Medicine. He has authored several books on the subject.

Teresa Hale is a nutritionist, and the Founder and Managing Director of the famous Hale Clinic in London. Dr. David Riley specializes in Homeopathy, and is a clinical associate professor at the University of New Mexico Medical School. He is also the Editor-in-Chief of EXPLORE, a journal of science and healing. Dr. Nishiti Joshi is a CAM specialist and the founder of the renowned Joshi Clinic in London, while Dr. Andrew Jeon is the Executive Vice-President and Chief Operating Officer of Harvard Medical International.

United States Medical Licensing Examination

Dubai Health Care City to Offer United States Medical Licensing Examination (USMLE) Step 3 Exams for the First Time outside the United States... DHCC is a highly regulated institution with a long-term vision for providing for high-quality health care, medical education and research in the region. The four entities involved in delivering DHCC's vision are:

- Dubai Health Care City Freezone (DHCC FZ)
- Centre for Health care Planning and Quality (CPQ)
- Harvard Medical School Dubai Centre (HMSDC)
- Dubai Harvard Foundation for Medical Research (DHFMR)

The leadership of DHCC is committed to the principle of accessibility for all, professional and academic development, and international recognition for quality of care as well as patient privacy, rights, and satisfaction.

Dubai Health Care City: Two Communities, One Destination

Dubai Health Care City, the world's first health care free zone, boasts two complementary communities, namely, the Medical Community and the Wellness Community. The Medical Community, occupying an area of 4.1 million square feet, focuses on clinical services for disease treatment and prevention, while the Wellness Community, 19 million square feet, completes DHCC's health care continuum by housing hospitals, outpatient clinics, luxury spa resorts, and the entire spectrum of wellness services. The wellness community will take some more time to see the light of the day.

The Mohammed Bin Rashid Al Maktoum Academic Medical Centre

The Mohammed Bin Rashid Al Maktoum Academic Medical Centre is at the core of the DHCC's clinical and educational structure. This central core comprises five components, namely, the University Hospital; the Harvard Medical School Dubai Centre Institute for Postgraduate Education and Research; the Dubai Harvard Foundation for Medical Research; the Al Maktoum Harvard Medical Library; and Boston University Dental Health Centre and Institute for Dental Research and Education—Dubai.

Listed below are some of the many features and benefits of Dubai Health Care City:

Free zone set-up:

- 100% tax-free
- 100% foreign ownership
- No corporate tax
- No income tax
- No customs duty
- No restrictions on capital, trade barriers or quotas
- Competitive pricing
- Clinic lease/purchase options

Commercial benefits:

- Low operating costs
- State-of-the-art facilities
- Flexible real estate designed to suit the industry (laboratories, pharmacies, etc.)

- Integrated health care community providing specialized quality medical care
- Access to a network of regional and global health care professionals

Business convenience:

- No bureaucracy or red tape
- One-stop shop for government services (visa service, permits, etc.)
- Business support services (hospitality, events, etc.)
- Fast-track company registration
- Simple company laws and legal framework
- Quick access to knowledge workers due to fast-track immigration process

Patients:

- Convenient location between Asia and Europe
- Quality health care services
- Wide selection of health care specialities and sub-specialities in one location
- Brand name operators
- Integrated health care e-network (HIRAS, Electronic Medical Records, Health Information System)
- Information on operators' outcomes and doctors' portfolios
- Patient confidentiality and rights—Patient centricity

Health Care Professionals:

- Establishment of the Mohammed Bin Rashid Al Maktoum Academic Medical Centre
- Provision of specialties and sub-specialties not available in the region
- Continuing Medical Education programs
- Integrated continuum of care
- Prime location
- Stringent regulatory environment

Health Care Investors:

- Ownership rights
- Patient referral network
- Stringent regulatory environment

- Integrated health care network
- DHCC brand
- Prime location

Complementary Facilities:

- Hotel and conference centres
- Telemedicine facilities
- Residential community
- Recreational facilities

Real Estate Investors:

- Prime location
- Proximity to different facilities
- Supporting infrastructure (FM, catering, etc.)

Educators and Students:

- Formation of the Mohammed Bin Rashid Al Maktoum Academic Medical Centre
- Internationally accredited education
- Prime location

Government:

- International licensing and quality standards
- Prime location
- Strategic partnerships with international health care providers
- Availability of in-house staff with health care knowledge
- Saving costs of patient traveling
- Attracting medical and health care service businesses to Dubai
- Attracting highly-educated professionals specialized in health care
- Increasing Dubai's city profile as the regional location of choice for quality health care services

Visitors and Families:

- Development of hotel and furnished apartment facilities for patients and families
- Transportation
- Proximity of retail area
- Education and support facilities

THE MEDICAL COMMUNITY

Through the Medical Community, DHCC will treat the region with a host of medical services grouped in a highly convenient setting. Physician offices, ambulatory surgery centres, general hospitals, specialty hospitals, rehabilitation and long-term care facilities, hospices, and diagnostic laboratories are brought together to deliver diagnostic and treatment services of international standards.

DHCC is the prime location for modern outpatient facilities, health care commercial offices and retail services. The Ibn Sina building houses clinics and laboratories featuring the latest in radiology and MRI technology. The Al Razi Medical Complex features outpatient surgical clinics complete with state-of-the-art analytical and diagnostic laboratories, and surgical suites.

The Medical Community is home to medical, dental, nursing and allied health schools. These schools offer Continuing Medical Education (CME) courses and postgraduate education to health care professionals. A key member of this community is the Harvard Medical School Dubai Centre (HMSDC) for Postgraduate Medical Education and Research, which offers fellowship and observership programs. The community also aims to build a world-class research infrastructure. One of the pioneers in this field is the Dubai Harvard Foundation for Medical Research (DHFMR) which aims to lead the creation of regionally-relevant basic scientific research.

Health Care Commercial Services

Complementing the conventional medical services at DHCC, there are a vast array of diagnostic laboratories, pharmacies, medical equipment companies, health care recruitment firms, health care consulting firms and pharmaceutical companies.

As an alternative setting to medical office buildings, a cluster of villas is devoted to conventional and alternative medicine outpatient clinics. A number of these villas will be dedicated to day surgery and cosmetic procedure clinics operated by internationally-renowned plastic surgeons. This cluster is beautifully landscaped and is located immediately adjacent to a large medical wellness resort.

Multidisciplinary Health Care Hub

True to DHCC's identity as a completely integrated health care hub, the Wellness Community will house representatives from each health care-related service, such as medical equipment companies, insurance firms, pharmaceutical companies, health care consultants, and complementary and alternative medicine suppliers.

Spa Resorts

One of the key features of the Wellness Community is the number of luxury spa resorts, two seven-star hotels, villas, marina, and retail which are located alongside the creek. Managed by globally-renowned specialist spa resort operators, these resorts will render every guest a soothing and memorable recovery time.

Hotels

One luxury five-star hotel and one affordable boutique hotel will cater to visiting patients, their families and rotational health care providers. The hotels will have medical floors to serve visiting patients who may require more recovery time before traveling safely. The hotels will also serve as ideal venues for health care conferences.

Residential

For the long-term accommodation needs of DHCC's health care providers, the Wellness Community offers residential properties for lease and for purchase. As an added convenience, these residential buildings also feature a long list of retail and food and beverage outlets.

Structure

The organization is built around an informed regulatory framework and close affiliations with leading academia from around the world in order to provide clinical and wellness services, medical education and research in health care.

The health care regulatory framework, known as the Centre for Health care Planning and Quality (CPQ) is jointly established by Partners Harvard Medical International to ensure that the health care providers at DHCC implement rigorous, high quality clinical standards and therefore excellence in quality of patient care.

In addition to the regulatory body, DHCC has also partnered with Harvard University to create the Harvard Medical School Dubai Centre (HMSDC), the first Harvard Medical School facility of its kind to be established outside the United States, HMSDC is currently addressing the need for professional development in the region, across all therapeutic areas through Continuing Medical Education (CME).

The Dubai Harvard Foundation for Medical Research (DHFMR) will support a partnership between DHCC and Harvard Medical School in USA to create and sustain a regional community of leaders in medicine and life sciences to advance scientific knowledge for the benefit of humankind.

Lastly, The Maktoum Harvard Medical Library (MHML) will include a unique patient and family education centre and an extensive library of resources for health care professionals, including state-of-the-art facilities for obtaining digital and print educational and reference materials.

Partners Harvard Medical International and DHCC have jointly established the Centre for Health care Planning and Quality (CPQ), as a regulatory body implementing rigorous quality clinical standards to ensure patient safety and quality patient care. CPQ also plays a major role in planning to ensure an appropriate balance between clinical services within DHCC in order to meet patient needs, demands, and expectations.

CPQ's aim is to become a regular centre for clinical regulation and accreditation through creating an environment of care that ensures quality patient care and safety, in line with international best practices via development of:

- Licensing of health care professionals and facilities.
- Quality standards for health care practice.
- Assessment of clinical practice as a tool for quality improvement.
- Rules and regulations governing clinical practice.
- Complementary and Alternative Medicine (CAM) regulations.
- Public Health and Health Safety rules and regulations governing non-clinical facilities.
- Health, Safety, and Environment standards.
- Patient care and patient safety initiatives to drive continuous quality improvement.
- Planning health care activities in DHCC to create an integrated health network.
- Health Information Reporting and Analysis System (HIRAS).
- Guidelines for health care facility design review and fit-out.

Harvard affiliation

The organization now known as Partners Harvard Medical International (PHMI) was founded originally as Harvard Medical International (HMI), a self-supporting subsidiary of Harvard University and Harvard Medical School (HMS). HMI was created to extend internationally the Medical School's tradition of excellence in clinical medicine, medical education, and biomedical research.

Through numerous collaborations with health care delivery organizations, academic medical institutions, and other key stakeholders, PHMI has played a major role in the development of health and education infrastructures globally. Through more than 50 programs developed in over 30 countries, they have provided training and education for hundreds of health care professionals, leaders, and students around the world, and helped their clients to achieve measurable progress, as well as national and regional recognition.

HMI became PHMI in the spring of 2008 under the terms of a new agreement between Harvard University and Partners Health Care, a major academic health care network that includes two of the flagship teaching hospitals of Harvard Medical School. PHMI's governance structure includes representation from Harvard University and Harvard Medical School, as well as Partners Health Care. Its services and programs continue to draw upon the expertise of faculty and staff across Harvard University, at the Medical School, and at all of the Medical School's affiliated teaching hospitals and institutes.

In 2003, HMI entered into a long-term collaboration with DHCC. As

DHCC's key strategic collaborator, PHMI has played a significant role in the development of the Health Care City and other major initiatives of the Government of Dubai. It teamed up with DHCC to develop the regulatory and governance structure for the Health Care City, as well as entities to support education and research: the Harvard Medical School Dubai Centre (HMSDC) and the Dubai Harvard Foundation for Medical Research (DHFMR). PHMI continues to provide significant input in the development of DHCC and the Maktoum Academic Medical Centre, including playing a lead role in the planning, design, and construction oversight of the University Hospital.

As DHCC's key strategic collaborator, HMI has been working with DHCC to develop DHCC's capabilities and service offerings in the areas of medical education, health care delivery, and research. HMI has created a Dubai-based team to help carry out the terms of the partnership and ensure that objectives are met.

To learn more about our Harvard-related initiatives, namely HMSDC, DHFMR, and MHML, browse through the sections herein.

Khalid Al Malik—CEO Tatweer, Dubai. Khalid Al Malik is the Chief Executive Officer (CEO) of Tatweer, a post he has held since January 2007. His impressive experience spans 18 years in both the governmental and private sectors.

Al Malik's tenure at Tatweer began in 2003 when he joined the Dubai Development and Investment Authority, Tatweer's predecessor, as the Director of Operations. During this time, he spearheaded several key initiatives, such as the Quality, Health, Safety and Environment (QHSE) committee, the Dubai Government Excellence Program, and the company's culture vehicle Al Ruwad.

He was then promoted to the CEO of Dubai Industrial City, one of Tatweer's entities with the vision of catalyzing the growth and expansion of the industrial sector in Dubai. He was then appointed as the Senior Vice-President of Industry and Knowledge to lead the development of both Dubai Industrial City and Moutamarat, the first pan-Arab initiative for creating business knowledge, before taking the reigns as the CEO of Tatweer.

Al Malik took the first step of his career in 1990, when he joined the IT division of the prestigious UAE Armed Forces, and he holds a Master's degree in Business Administration (MBA), with a concentration in e-commerce.

A keen sportsman, he was elected to be the General Manager of the Emirates Motor Sports Federation to revive and promote the motor sport culture in the UAE. In just two years' time, he increased the Federation's membership by 100%, in addition to revamping the Federation's marketing activities.

Al Malik embodies Tatweer's values and is focused, passionate, and dynamic. He has a personal and professional commitment to excellence, and has infused Tatweer with his own brand of energetic leadership, vision and spirit.

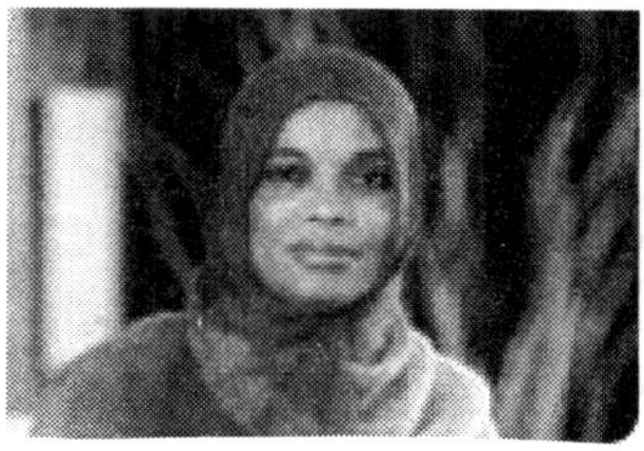

Dr, Ayesha Mohammed Abdullah—Senior Vice-President of DHCC. Ayesha Mohammed Abdullah is Senior Vice-President of Dubai Health Care City (DHCC). Ayesha is an 18-year veteran of the health care and engineering industries.

Dr. Ayesha Abdullah plays a key role in realising DHCC's strategic objectives. She is responsible for strategic planning and operations, development of education and research vision, development of new businesses, and managing strategic partners such as Harvard Medical International (HMI), Harvard Medical School (HMS), and Moorefield's among others.

In her previous position as Chief Officer at the Centre for Health care Planning and Quality (CPQ), she was instrumental in building CPQ into a premier quality regulatory body.

Ayesha's core competencies include strategic health care planning, project management, managing multi-disciplinary teams, strong technical competency, project design, and customer service.

Ayesha holds a Bachelors of Science, Biomedical and Electrical Engineering degree from USA, an MBA with a Finance focus and a Ph.D., M.Phil. in Strategy Management/Planning Studies from UK.

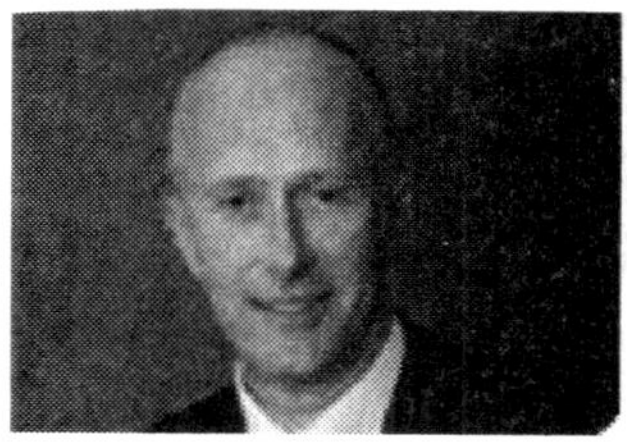

Kenneth Bruce MacPherson—Vice-President of Operations. As the VP of Operations of Dubai Health Care City (DHCC), Kenneth Macpherson is responsible for finance, information technology, and project development, as well as legal, administrative and procurement aspects of the world's only integrated health care free zone.

A British national, Macpherson brings with him a wealth of industry experience to DHCC. With an association of more than 23 years in finance and general management gained through a results-oriented career graph, he has held several key positions in high profile companies in the UAE and the UK.

Prior to joining DHCC, Macpherson was Executive Finance Director at Combined Diving and Inspection Services in Sharjah for over four years.

Earlier, as Group General Manager and Group Finance Advisor of Al Nabooda General Enterprises for more than seven years, he offered his industry expertise to one of the oldest family organizations in Dubai.

Macpherson has also served as Financial Controller in the Sub-Sea Group of Companies, a division of the US Energy conglomerate MW Kellog in the UK and Sharjah.

Holder of the Higher National Diploma in Accounting from Aberdeen College in Scotland, he is an Associate Member and a Fellow of the Association of Chartered Certified Accountants (ACCA), UK.

Dubai Health Care City has partnered with the Dubai Bone and Joint Centre (DBAJ) and Boston University (BU) in an ongoing initiative to provide the region with diverse health care practices.

DBAJ is the first comprehensive centre in the region dedicated to musculoskeletal diseases, delivering high quality medicine, comparable with western standards, providing the latest innovative treatments as well as evidence-based medicine according to international protocols.

BU Dental Health Centre and Institute for Dental Research and Education provides the latest in dental practice, and education and research to the Gulf region.

Across the world, musculoskeletal conditions affect hundreds of millions of people, at a huge cost to society. In the Middle East alone, there are thousands of people who are afflicted with some form of musculoskeletal ailment.

Up until now, patients requiring specialized musculoskeletal care have had to travel to Europe or America for treatment. The launch of the Dubai Bone and Joint Centre (DBAJ) will change all that. It is closer, more economical and offers world-class treatment and facilities. DBAJ offers a solid clinical practice coupled with tangible research. It will be the first comprehensive centre in the region dedicated to musculoskeletal diseases, delivering high quality medical care, comparable with western standards, providing the latest innovative treatments as well as evidence-based medicine according to international protocols.

DBAJ physicians treat a wide variety of disorders affecting the musculoskeletal system, including the care of fractures and injuries to tendons, ligaments, joints, bone and muscles. On staff are specialists in joint replacement, surgical spine care and rheumatology. Our goal is simple: to return patients to normal function as quickly and safely as possible. To reach this goal, the medical professionals at the DBAJ enlist a comprehensive, cutting-edge approach to the prevention, assessment, and treatment of musculoskeletal injuries. By combining extensive clinical expertise with a compassionate, caring treatment philosophy, we have created an environment known for its quality care.

Boston University Institute for Dental Research and Education, Dubai

Boston University Institute for Dental Research and Education Dubai at DHCC is a unique development in the Gulf Region. Boston University is the first to bring education in dental specialties to the region using United States standards. The institute will offer the Certificate of Advanced Graduate Study (CAGS) and Master of Science in Dentistry (MSD) by a team of specialized faculty trained from the US. The programs will combine a balance of extensive clinical experience with a strong academic program with an emphasis on original research. All of the faculty are specialists in their field and have trained in their specialty in the United States, many of them at Boston University. Additionally, the faculty members have joint appointments at Boston University School of Dental Medicine. In addition to the full-time faculty, senior faculty members from Boston University, generally departmental Chairs and program directors, will visit the Institute periodically to lecture and give clinical demonstrations.

The institute is complemented by the Boston University Dental Health Centre, Dubai. The centre, a 20,000 sq. feet state-of-the-art facility, has globally renowned dental professionals providing comprehensive care to patients utilizing modern techniques and equipment, as well as a strong continuing dental education (CDE) program. Emerging as the regional hub for medical excellence in education, research and patient care, the centre's mandate entails raising the standards of dental care in the region through endorsing the vision of one of the world's oldest private research and teaching institutions.

Joining the DHCC community is easy. The Client Relations team is a one-stop-shop committed to providing administrative and business support needs to any company interested in setting up operations at DHCC. This comprehensive offering includes complete licensing and governmental services. These services are made available to both individuals and multi-national companies setting up operations in DHCC.

The centralized services are designed to streamline a company's operations by providing clear, transparent, and systematic processes and a single point of contact for activities. Moreover, timely responses and fast and efficient implementation will relieve companies from the hassle and inertia of bureaucratic red tape. Assistance in locating key resources and the Centre for Information resources make this unit particularly valuable to companies doing business in DHCC. All activities are customer-oriented with a view to optimizing utility to our client companies and maximizing the efficiency of their operations.

To help assist you and save your time, we have provided all of the necessary list of regulations and forms for your convenience in the following sections.

How to apply for Commercial License and Registration?

Once you have completed all formalities with the Sales Department and Centre for Health care Planning and Quality (CPQ), you can then proceed to Government Services to begin the process of Commercial Licensing and Registration. The following links clearly lay out the documentation required and sample templates to begin processing.

There are 3 types of applications for licensing and registration for DHCC.

- Application for a FZ LLC where shareholder is an individual person(s)
- Application for a FZ LLC where shareholder is a corporate client (company)
- Application for a Branch of a UAE or Foreign Established Company

1. Application for a FZ LLC where shareholder is an individual person(s):

Please complete the following forms:

- DHCC License Requirements
- Application For License DHCC FZ
- Board Resolution FZ LLC individual Shareholder 1, Shareholder A
- Board Resolution FZ LLC for more than one Shareholder
- Specimen Signature
- Personnel Sponsorship Agreement
- Certificate of Authorization
- Articles of Association
- Memorandum of Association
- Government Services Tariff

Please refer to the checklist provided to ensure that you have completed all of the documents needed.

Once your documentation has been submitted in full along with the License and Incorporation fees, the application will be forwarded to Dubai Holding (DH) for approval. Once we receive approval, we shall then be in a position to issue a letter addressed to a bank of your choice in the UAE. This letter will enable you to open an account in the new company's name. You will deposit your capital shares into this account and obtain a Proof of Capital from the bank.

This letter should be presented to DHCC whereupon your License and Incorporation certificate will be issued.

2. Application for a FZ LLC where shareholder is a corporate client (company):

- DHCC License Requirements
- Application For License DHCC FZ
- Board Resolution FZ LLC for more than one Shareholder
- Board Resolution FZ LLC individual Shareholder
- Specimen Signature
- Personnel Sponsorship Agreement
- Certificate of Authorization
- Articles of Association
- Memorandum of Association
- Government Services Tariff

Please refer to the checklist provided to ensure that you have completed all of the documents needed.

Once your documentation has been submitted in full along with the License and Incorporation fees, the application will be forwarded to Dubai Holding (DH) for approval. Once we receive approval, we shall then be in a position to issue a letter addressed to a bank of your choice in the UAE. This letter will enable you to open an account in the new company's name.

You will deposit your Capital shares into this account and obtain a Proof of Capital from the bank.

This letter should be presented to DHCC whereupon your License and Incorporation certificate will be issued.

3. Application for a Branch of a UAE or Foreign Established Company:

- DHCC Check List Legal Documents required for a Branch of a Foreign Company
- Application For License DHCC FZ
- Board Resolution To Establish a Branch Tabbed
- Specimen Signature
- Personnel Sponsorship Agreement
- Certificate of Authorization
- Government Services Tariff

Please refer to the checklist provided to ensure that you have completed all of the documents needed.

Once your documentation has been submitted in full along with the License fee, the application will be forwarded to Dubai Holding (DH) for approval. Once we receive approval, we shall then be in a position to issue your Commercial License.

Legal Requirements

Please note that in each of the above application sets, the following documents must be signed in the presence of a DHCC representative:

- Board of Resolution
- Articles of Association
- Memorandum of Association

In the event that this arrangement cannot be met, then the documents must be Notarized and Legalized. Documents consisting of more than one page must be sealed.

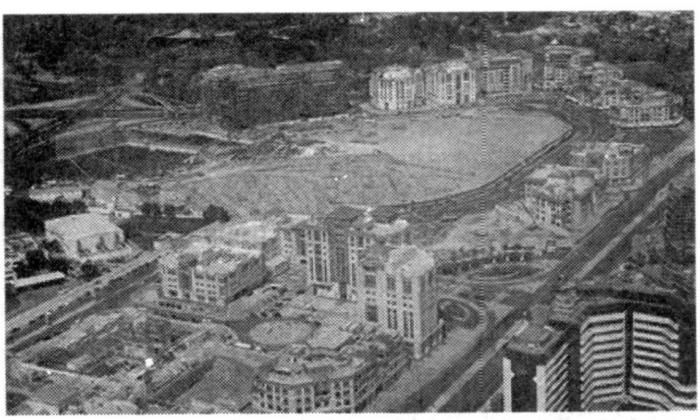

DM Health Care Group

From one clinic in 1987 his company, DM Health care Group, now has one of the largest health care networks in the GCC. By 2015 it plans to have 300 establishments and 10,000 staff across the Middle East and India. Not bad for someone who says they didn't have a long-term goal. "I always believe in destiny and that you have to work hard," he says. Both appear to have paid-off as the week before we met he had just returned from India where he received the 'Pravasi Bhartiya Samman'—a top award given by the President of India for achievements by Indians overseas.

The firm's slogan is 'Health care for All' and Moopen firmly believes that employers and the UAE government must continue to fund health care for their employees. "I feel that somebody has to spend. I do not know whether it has to be the government or the employer, but definitely not the employee. "For the population who are natives of this country it is the responsibility of the government to take care of them. For expatriates it is the responsibility of the employer to make sure they have coverage through insurance to make sure their health care is taken care of when they are here. "I strongly feel it has to be included as part of the cost for the employer. If someone can pay AED10,000 to stamp the visa of an employee I think they can add another AED1000 to provide health care," he says. The large number of expatriates, which make up nearly three quarters of the UAE population aged fifteen to 64 years old, has a direct impact on health care requirements in the country. Figures from industry researchers RNCOS show that the UAE has one of the lowest hospital bed ratios by international standards and in 2007 it was less than two beds per 1000 of the population, around half what it is in most developed economies.

However, Moopen defends this by saying the demographics mean that the region generally has a lower health care requirement than other developed nations. For example, in the UAE figures show that those aged 65 years old only make up 0.9 percent of the population, compared to maturing populations such as Germany, where the age group accounts for 20.3 percent.

There are also two other important factors says Moopen: expatriates are generally within the healthy age group of 25 to 55 years old, and they have a tendency to return home to their own countries if they require long-term care. "That is important for us when planning as we have to look more at acute illnesses, rather than chronic illnesses, because immediate care is usually given here. The primary care in the UAE is as good as in any other country as it has to be taken care of immediately," he points out.

However, no matter how healthy a population is, he believes health care is something they cannot cut back on, even in a recession. "We have found that even in the very bad, supposedly recession-hit years, in 2009 we had grown by increasing our establishments and increasing our employees. "Health care still has a supply-demand gap... It is something that is essential. It will be one of the last areas to be affected by recession," says Moopen. In fact, the RNCOS research backs this up and has forecast that the health care sector in the UAE alone will grow at an annual rate of more than thirteen percent until 2012. As part of their 'Vision 2015' plan, Moopen plans to see the group increase its facilities to 300 within the next five years. It plans to have 175 pharmacies and 75 clinics, of which they currently have 50 and 25 respectively.

"It is easier to increase the number of pharmacies as we do most of it through acquisitions," he says. At present, up to 75 percent of the company's revenue comes from Dubai, therefore much of its expansion plans are outside the emirate and the UAE, with Saudi Arabia being its main focus. "One major country we have not covered so far is Saudi Arabia —a huge country with a big population. Once you enter there and start establishing the business, the numbers will be easily achieved."

"When you look at health care one of the most important things is manpower. Getting qualified people and good people is an issue, especially in health care. It is a challenge which we have to live with." Previously, a lot of the doctors and nurses were recruited from India. However, the growth in the Indian economy has meant that the differentiation between wages in India and the GCC has now changed and it is harder to persuade Indian staff to uproot and move to the Middle East. There is also the issue of retention of staff when they arrive in the UAE as nurses often leave the private sector and move to the government sector, where wages are generally higher. Moopen also believes the government could do more to speed up the licensing process for staff. "I find sometimes it is extremely difficult. It is important that their qualities are looked at—but there are certain situations where you have people who have been qualified for many years—they come here and can't get a license. "I think the authorities should look at it much closer and help the private sector to come into health care," he adds.

Two other areas that Moopen believes the region's government should loosen up its regulations are: in-vitro fertilization (IVF) and organ transplants.

At present, IVF treatment is only offered in government operated hospitals.

"They want to have more controls on that. They don't want people to play around," Moopen added. UN research has found that fertility in the UAE is already a big issue and over the last three decades the UAE fertility rate has dropped from 5.7 children per woman to less than two. Moopen believes "it is time for the authorities to look at providing such avenues for the private sector". "The government should look at the individual organizations and establishments and those who have accreditation and good reputation—the government should allow such establishments to take care of these areas," he says. In terms of worldwide organ transplants, he says, "it is something that needs to be looked at in detail, from a cultural, religious as well as a social angle."

All of DM Health care Group's facilities are private operations but Moopen has not ruled out private-public partnerships with the UAE government and is looking into opportunities to manage government-run hospitals. The group's headquarters are currently in Dubai Health Care City (DHC) and while Moopen says the health care sector has not been impacted by the credit crunch he believes it has been impacted by the downturn in the real estate sector. He says the DHC development "has not matured yet" and still requires a lot of investment. Many projects have been put on hold in Dubai, including some in DHC. The group currently has no clinics in DHC, only administrative offices. Therefore, the only impact that Moopen is hoping they will see in DHC is that their rent may come down.

Samsung Medical centre opens its shop in DHCC

The centre is the first of its kind for Samsung Medical Centre outside Korea and the decision was made based on the agreement signed last October between Index Holding and Samsung Medical Centre. The two parties are confident that Dubai in the United Arab Emirates is the ideal venue to host such an international medical centre. Samsung Medical Centre in Collaboration with Index Holding will provide advanced medical services for Emaratis and residents in Dubai, UAE, GGC countries, Middle-East and North Africa region. The centre occupies an area of more than 10.000 square feet in Dubai Health Care City.

Samsung Medical Centre in Collaboration with Index Holding comprises of a team of Medical, Nursing and Allied Health Professionals in addition to the medical visits by specialists from Samsung Medical Centres and hospitals in Korea. Samsung Medical Centre in Collaboration with Index Holding provides specialized medical services in Cancer, Cardiology, Nephrology, Urology, Gastroenterology, Women Health and Family Medicine.

"Opening Samsung Medical Centre in Collaboration with Index Holding is a new medical achievement added to the continuous achievements of Dubai. We are pleased that a world-class centre like Samsung Medical Centre has decided to open its first medical centre in the world in Dubai. The decision reflects the investors' trust in Dubai, the United Arab Emirates and in the vision of its wise leadership represented by His Highness Sheikh Mohammed Bin Rashid Al Maktoum, Vice-President and Prime Minister of UAE Ruler of Dubai and the continuous support of His Highness Sheikh Hamdan Bin Rashid Al Maktoum, Deputy Ruler of Dubai Minister of Finance and Industry, President of Dubai Health Authority," said His Excellency Qahdi Al Mroushid, Director General, Dubai Health Authority.

"This project that was initiated by Index Holding under the patronage of Dubai Health Authority is a new achievement added to the ongoing success in the medical sector in Dubai and the United Arab Emirates," he added.

Samsung Medical Centre in Collaboration with Index Holding aims to attract medical tourism to the region and to exchange knowledge and experiences. "After an extended research and study of this project and its importance to the medical sector in the region on the long-term, we decided to invest in it. We will continue working in collaboration with Samsung Medical Centre to enhance the health of Emarati and non-Emarati residents in UAE. We would like to thank Dubai Government and all its institutions for their unremitting support to the medical and private sectors which we consider as major incentives that attract international leading institutions to Dubai and encourage us to achieve the best," said Abdul Salam Al Madani, President of Index Holding.

"We have decided to open the first Samsung Medical Centre, the first of its kind outside Korea, in Collaboration with Index Holding in Dubai, United Arab Emirates due to the trust we have in this city and its capabilities in providing all the requirements for establishing such project. The Dubai Emirate offers world class facilities and infrastructures that compete with those in the largest developed countries around the world. Dubai under its wise leadership represented by His Highness Sheikh Mohammed Bin Rashid Al Maktoum has a worldwide outstanding reputation and the two countries enjoy a steady friendship and business relations'. In addition, UAE's leadership vision and its continuous support to the medical sector is an incentive to us to invest in this project, as we will be able to provide advanced medical services for patients in the Middle East, GCC countries and North Africa," he added.

Dr. Ayesha Abdullah, Senior Vice-President of Dubai Health Care City said, "Dubai Health Care City is delighted to welcome Samsung Medical Centre—a major international brand—who shares our commitment to delivering high-quality, patient-focused care. Though its collaboration with Index Holding, I am confident that the Samsung Medical Centre will further contribute to making DHCC the leading location for health care but more importantly, to improving the health of the community."

Samsung Medical Centre was established in Korea in 1995 and currently includes 3 specialized hospitals in Seoul and other provinces. The hospital ranks the first for eight years successively and is known to be the best specialized hospital in Korea. Samsung Medical Centre hosts more than 40 centres and specialized units in all medical specialties and employs more than 10,000 employees including 5,000 specialized medical staff and is considered as one of the largest advanced medical complexes in Korea. Also as a designated teaching hospital for Sungkyunkwan University School of Medicine, Samsung Medical Centre produces outstanding future leaders in health care.

Moorefield Eye Hospital, Dubai

This is the first eye hospital from Moorfield UK, outside the country. It organized a CME programme for the eye doctors of the region. The first session took place December 21 and covered the management of pediatric ocular anomalies both from a medical and surgical perspective, and a review of contact lenses for children and teens. The session took place as Moorfields revealed the findings of its school Vision Programme in the UAE, which covered around 1,000 pupils. Keith Wilken, Senior Orthopist at

Moorfields, gave a presentation titled Vision Screening in Pre School and School Aged Children. According to Keith, of the 982 children covered by the recent UAE School Vision Programme organised by Moorfields, 167 pupils (pupils) 'failed' or required a referral to a professional. "The rate of vision-related problems picked up by the programme was about the same as we see elsewhere around the world. The top three problems picked up by the programme were bilateral visual acuity, unilateral visual acuity, and strabismus (squint). The need for, and benefits of, vision screening for schoolchildren are clear and the professional programme we are running in partnership with The Vision Care Institute complements this extremely effectively."

In addition to considering the typical pediatric ocular anomalies, the pediatric eye care program also reviewed the use of contact lenses by children and teens, drawing on the substantial experience of Johnson and Johnson.

Dr. Razmig Knajian, Senior Manager of Professional and Medical Affairs for Johnson and Johnson Vision Care in the Middle East and Africa, commented, "Contact lenses provide self-esteem benefits to children beyond simply correcting vision. They also improve their perception regarding physical appearance, social acceptance among friends, ability to play sports, confidence in academics (due to low spectacle satisfaction)."

Johnson and Johnson Vision Care opened The Vision Care Institute—a professional education centre for eye care specialists—in Dubai Health Care City in June 2008, so that eye care professionals from across the Middle East could learn more about the latest developments in the field under the leadership of top eye care professionals from within, as well as from outside, the region. The aim of The Vision Care Institute is to enhance patient satisfaction through innovative education and training programs.

Dr, Chris Canning, CEO and Medical Director of Moorfields Eye Hospital Dubai, commented, "Training and the sharing of our extensive medical experience and knowledge with the regional professional eye care community is an important part of Moorfields' role in the Middle East. We are very pleased to be working with Johnson and Johnson on this pediatric eye care programme at their excellent training facility at The Vision Care Institute in Dubai and believe that this training initiative will help make an important contribution to the development of professionals within the industry."

Royal Ayurveda Clinic in DHCC

Dr. Ayesha Abdullah, Managing Director, Sciences Cluster and Executive Director for DHCC, Tecom Investments Business Parks, opened the clinic in the presence of His Excellency Wasantha Senanayake, Consul-General of Sri Lanka in Dubai, and Hiroki Matsumoto, Managing Director, Japan External Trade Organization (JETRO), Dubai and MENA.

Royal Ayurveda is dedicated to providing high quality patient care with an unrelenting attention to clinical excellence and patient safety in disease management, positive health promotion, as well as relaxation and vitalizing therapy. Patients will have access to full-fledged and systematic Ayurvedic consultations, body constitution (dosha) determination, pancha karma or other disease-specific treatments with herbal medicines, oil massage treatments, cleansing and detoxifying therapies, as well as nutritional and lifestyle counselling.

The 5,000-year-old Ayurveda or 'Science of Life' aims at treating the sick as well as the healthy. It cures the disease and also rejuvenates and tones the body by strengthening the immune system.

Dr, Ayesha Abdullah, said:

> "We welcome Royal Ayurveda, the first of its kind in the region, to Dubai Health Care City. Royal Ayurveda joins a strong list of complementary and alternative medicine providers (CAM) at DHCC. Dubai Health Care City is pleased to be a pioneer in further developing its base of integrated medicine services as a response to global trends that reflects the growing popularity of alternative medicine and traditional practices."

Royal Ayurveda adopts the Rasayana Treatment (Ayurvedic anti-aging) approach to enhance the human body's healing power and immunity. The unique and powerful treatment in Ayurveda is particularly known for the better management of contemporary disease conditions.

Masao Tsuji, Managing Director of Royal Ayurveda Anti-Aging Clinic said, "Ayurveda is widely accepted as a tested and proven health care practice across the world and is now making strong inroads into the Middle East region. Dubai Health Care City offers us the perfect platform to reach out to a wider clientele, and helps position us in the premier league of Ayurveda providers in the region."

Royal Ayurveda's concept and structure is developed from the collaboration of well established and highly experienced institutions from Sri Lanka, Japan and the UK. The Sri Lankan counterpart provides the authentic and traditional Ayurvedic practices, therapies and herbal medicinal prescriptions that have been used over more than 5,000 years and enriched by the Indian and Sri Lankan culture and heritage. The Japanese counterpart is a pharmaceutical company that brings with it over 100 years experience in manufacturing high quality herbal medicines. The UK counterpart contributes to the renowned academic and research input for developing high professional standards.

Dr. Palitha Serasinghe, Consultant Ayurvedic Medical Practitioner, Director and Clinic Manager said, "Ayurveda integrates the elements of nature in its treatment, thus ensuring mind-body harmony. In today's stressed and fast-paced life, our therapies for rejuvenation, wellness and anti-aging will add to personal efficiency, overall good health and well-being. Royal Ayurveda offers effective anti-aging treatment to slow down the process of wear and tear and degeneration. Our patients can look forward to receiving premier treatment from our highly qualified team of practitioners."

Dubai Health Care City provides CAM treatments in 12 areas: Homeopathy, Ayurveda, Traditional Chinese Medicine, Unani Medicine, Osteopathy, Therapeutic Massage, Naturopathy, Guided Imagery, Thai Chi, Pilates, Chiropractic, and Yoga. Patients can have the confidence that these practices are regulated by a strict governance structure and DHCC is the first health care institution outside the USA to implement CAM codes using ABC Coding Solutions.

Complementary and Alternative Medicine (CAM) is a diverse group of medical and health care therapies and systems that may be separate from or integrated with conventional medical therapies. A common factor shared with all CAM therapies is a holistic and individualistic approach to health and healing, and an appreciation of the physical, emotional, mental and spiritual dimensions of the human being.

Latest news at DHCC

- The American academy of cosmetic surgery hospital at Dubai Health Care City receives jci accreditation.
- Boston university institute for dental research and education organizes cme program in dentistry.
- Dubai Health Care City celebrates arab health success.
- Samsung medical centre to open 6,800 square foot facility in Dubai Health Care City.
- Dubai Health Care City and dubiotech share stand at Arab Health 2010.
- Oman insurance to offer cover for all 12 complementary and alternative medicine treatments at Dubai Health Care City.
- World leading eye experts to lead unique 'retinal master class' in Abu Dhabi for regional eye care surgeons.
- Postgraduate medical education symposium calls for developing unified international standards for health care reform.
- Boston university institute for dental research and education Dubai holds dental awareness and screening sessions.
- Dubai's community supports the first health festival at DHCC.

Smart cell storage centre at DHCC

In the United States, stem cell storage has become so commonplace, it is now no more unusual than buying a cot or stocking up on nappies, claims Darryn Keast, founder and director of Dubai Health Care City's MedCells, the regional distributor for UK firm CellsLife. And while Keast may be guilty of slight exaggeration, it is true that the storage of so-called naive cells is soaring in popularity. It is easy to see why, Stem cells are currently involved in the treatment of very few conditions, but they have the potential to make a life-saving difference and are at the forefront of medical research. The idea is to preserve a baby's umbilical cord blood at birth by freezing the cells in liquid nitrogen. This allows parents to preserve the stem cells for many years, ready for use at any time in the future should you need them.

The cells can be manipulated at a later date to transform into other cells. Some stem cells are more "plastic" than others—that is they are able to make more types of cells. It is these transformational properties that have led to the creating of the stem cell storage industry, explains Keast.

"The fact that the umbilical cord is a rich source of stem cells has prompted private companies to offer frozen storage of these cells from umbilical cord blood collected at birth," he says. "Created during the earliest phases of development they have the potential, given the right stimuli, to become specialized cells such as red or white blood cells".

Albeit a fairly new aspect of medicine, stem cell storage is popular in Dubai and the rest of the United Arab Emirates. Keast believes the country is taking the right steps to make sure it is well placed for any further breakthroughs. "The formation of stem cells for storage and use in the treatment of children with these diseases," he says. "There are now specialised stem cell storage centres all around the country." But stem cells are not an overnight sensation. Since the first stem cell transplant in 1988, much attention has been focused on stem cell storage and potential stem cell therapy applications. Currently, they are primarily used as the basis of bone marrow transplants, a technique used to treat diseases such as leukaemia. But funding for stem cell research has increased dramatically recently, as confidence in the potential clinical benefits of stem cell therapy grows.

To date more than 75 medical conditions can be treated with stem cells, and more than 20,000 cord blood transplants have been successfully recorded worldwide. Here are just some of the areas where cord blood stem cells are being used to where cells are missing or have deteriorated:

Dubai Health Care City (DHCC): Oases for Health Tourism:

- o Diabetes
- o Multiple Sclerosis
- o Recovery from stroke
- o Neural regeneration
- o Retinal regeneration
- o Tissue and organ engineering
- o Heart disease
- o Alzheimer's disease

While stem cell storage certainly advantages, it is important that the parents are reliably informed about its capabilities may be growing in popularity in but there is still a lack of informatics there, says De Wiest.

Some remarkable successes using stem cell treatment in the region, the main advantage of storing a child's cord blood is the potential to cultivate a bone marrow transplant in the case of leukaemia. De Wiest claims the advantages of using stem cells for this treatment are undisputed. "It is superior because you have them at your disposal and you know they will work," she says. "For bone marrow you need a perfect match and this way you don't need to rely on one of your siblings being able to provide a donor. The chances are much greater—also the quality of life after a cord blood treatment transfer is much better."

The topic of stem cells is not without controversy, though. Cord blood storage is one thing, but some scientists have been pushing for the study of embryonic stem cell research, which gives rise to debate over the rights and status of the embryo *versus* the life-saving potential of such research.

This controversy should not be confused with cord blood banking, says Keast. "Embryonic stem cell research has ethical and moral considerations but umbilical cord blood is not controversial as it is sourced from a live human without adverse effect," he says. "Cord blood procurement is free from the negative associations of embryonic research."

ARAB HEALTH CONGRESS 2010

The Arab Health Exhibition and Congress, Dubai, UAE, was once again the focus for the word's health care sector in January. Now in its 35th year, the show achieved an estimated 20 per cent increase in visitor numbers. Highlighting the increasingly important role played by the Middle East health care industry, health care authorities, medical device manufacturers, medical supply distributors and health care professionals from across the region and the globe convened in Dubai for Arab Health 2010.

Highlights of 2010 Arab Health Congress

The Arab Health Congress 2010, with over 5,500 delegates, is by far the most extensive scientific and educational platform for health care professionals in the world. Regional health care pioneers honoured Health Care pioneers in the United Arab Emirates, the Kingdom of Saudi Arabia and Jordan have been honoured for their contributions towards regional innovation and development in the annual Arab Health Achievement and Innovation Awards,. Middle East 'centre of world' for health care companies.

The Middle East is becoming the "centre of the world" for specialised health care companies seeking a share of the region's new hospital construction market, according to a leading industry player. HRH Princess Haya urges medical community to invest in prevention.

Her Royal Highness Princess Haya Bint Al Hussein, wife of HH Sheikh Mohammed Bin Rashid Al Maktoum, Vice-President and Prime Minister of the United Arab Emirates and Ruler of Dubai, today urged the medical community to invest in prevention in a keynote speech at Leaders in Health care, the flagship gathering at the Arab Health Exhibition and Congress.

GCC health care spending: robust growth seen in 2010

The health care sector in the Arabian Gulf will continue to enjoy high growth in 2010, despite the global slowdown, led by government investment in infrastructure improvement, according to leading industry observers.

Arab Health 2010—the main event for the Health Care Industry

The Arab Health Exhibition and Congress is, by far, the largest health care exhibition in the Middle East, and the second largest in the world. Arab Health is viewed as a must-attend global event in the health care calendar. Established 35 years ago, it provides a platform for the world's leading manufacturers, wholesalers and distributors to meet the medical and scientific community in the Middle East and beyond.

At the 2009 event 2205 exhibitors from 59 countries showcased their products and services. Over 56,000 professionals from 145 countries—comprising 70% decision makers and 85% visitors directly involved in purchasing products and services attended Arab Health last year. With the addition of extra halls this number of exhibitors and visitors will grow in 2010.

Arab Health also features the world's largest and most comprehensive conferences programme—Arab Health Congress. The 2010 Congress will feature 17 internationally accredited conferences, addressed by 400 eminent and internationally acclaimed speakers and hosting more than 5,500 delegates and conference attendees.

With its line up of innovative educational activities, such as free accredited education and strategic tie ups with regional institutes, Arab Health leads the way in delivering the best interactive opportunities to the show participants and an ideal B2B environment to the audiences.

The Arab Health exhibition delivers to exhibitors the right balance between dealers and distributors, senior decision makers and end users. Arab Health is the business destination of choice for the Middle East Market estimated to be close to $80 billion per year. Due to the huge increase in the expatriate population it is also one of the fastest growing regions with an estimated annual growth of 16%.

The Arab Health Exhibition and Congress, Dubai, UAE, was once again the focus for the world's health care sector in January. Now in its 35th year, the show achieved an estimated 20 per cent increase in visitor numbers. Highlighting the increasingly important role played by the Middle East health care industry, health care authorities, medical device manufacturers, medical supply distributors and health care professionals from across the region and the globe convened in Dubai for Arab Health 2010. Held at the Dubai International Convention and Exhibition Centre from 25-28 January, the organiser, IIR Middle East, was delighted with the success of the 2010 show.

"We are thrilled that the region's health care industry, once again, chose Arab Health as a platform for seeking regional and international partners in this burgeoning sector," said Simon Page, Director of the Life Sciences Division of IIR Middle East. "Demand for health care is growing driven by aging populations and lifestyle related diseases such as diabetes, particularly in the UAE and Gulf Region. Governments are being forced to tackle this issue head on which ultimately means a lot more investment in the health care infrastructure in these countries.

"In spite of significant project delays in other non-health care industry sectors, the pipeline of health care projects in the region remains remarkably robust, particularly for Saudi Arabia and the United Arab Emirates. This has been reflected in the growth in the exhibitor, visitor and delegate numbers for this year's Arab Health.

"With the additional four new halls to the Dubai International Convention and Exhibition Centre, Arab Health 2010 had, for the first time in several years, the opportunity to grow and become an even bigger event. It meant that many existing clients had the opportunity to expand their stands, whilst new companies, not previously able to participate at the event, were be able to join us in Dubai for this year's event."

"With the opening of the new Sheikh Saeed halls providing a further 20,000 m^2, as estimated, Arab Health 2010 grew by more than 20 per cent in size from last year," Page added. "Arab Health touches all aspects of the health care industry in the Middle East. Tens of thousands of medical professionals, government officials, wholesalers, dealers and distributors converged on the Dubai International Exhibition Centre for the region's main event for the health care industry."

For many visitors, this was their first experience at Arab Health. For others, they return to the event year-on-year to network with distributors and manufacturers from across the globe.

"This was my first time at the Arab Health Exhibition and I was very impressed with the exhibition. I have made contact with many valuable distributors which was excellent in terms of building business relationships," said G. Sudhakar, from the Haji Pharmacy in Dubai.

Another visitor, Anil Grover from Al Mansouryah General Trading, who has attended the event in the past commented, "Arab Health is a very good show and it has grown significantly over the years. Based on this year's showing, I now feel it is one of the biggest and the best."

Research into the health care market in the Middle East indicates positive growth and we can expect further expansion on all levels.

Dubai-based research firm Proleads has released the latest figures on current investment in both the public and private health care sectors in Saudi Arabia, which is leading regional growth. The Proleads figures show government investment in health care-related projects in Saudi Arabia is currently running at more than US $5 billion, compared with around US $1 billion of private sector investment.

Another report by Alpen Capital also forecasts the GCC may need in excess of 25,000 additional beds by 2020 to address growing demand for in-patient treatments. The largest share of demand is accounted for by Saudi Arabia followed by the UAE.

Exhibitors at Arab Health 2010 were in agreement that the health care industry in the region was set to grow even further. Pleased with the turnout, many exhibitors and show sponsors were keen to re-book and expand their presence for next year.

Maher El Hassan, Marketing Director MENA, Karl Storz, and Platinum Sponsors for this year's event, said: "Arab Health continues to be the 'Exhibition of the Year' for Karl Storz and we intend to participate in 2011 with a larger presence that reflects our image and our commitments to our customers and partners in the region."

As Gold Sponsors, Carestream Health were enthusiastic about this year's visitor numbers and especially the high concentration of decision-makers who attended the event and visited their stand.

"At Arab Health 2010 we were able to showcase our latest medical imaging and IT solutions to a large number of executive-level decision-makers from all over the region," said Mirna Bassil, Marketing Manager for Emerging Markets, Carestream Health. "We were extremely pleased with the high-caliber of delegates and visitors at this year's event. We look forward to our participation at Arab Health 2011."

For Shigadrywithearth Co, a Japanese infection control company that sponsored the Arab Health Infection Control Program, Arab Health 2010 was a fantastic platform for knowledge transfer and business enhancement.

"As a premier health care event we were pleased to have participated at Arab Health 2010," said Chaminda Serasinha, Shigadrywithearth Co. "It was indeed great to have witnessed one of the largest gatherings of health care professionals from around the world. Unlike standard exhibitions, this attraction of health care professionals allows the exhibitors to target their branding purposefully. As first time exhibitors we felt that the exposure and visibility we got for our products was commendable with many an inquiry left for constructive follow-up. Our presence was also helpful in understanding immediate and eminent market needs which will be valuable for on going product development. As a whole we are happy to have invested at Arab Health 2010, especially as a sponsor."

Many exhibiting companies use Arab Health as a platform to conduct business and conclude successful business deals. Although most of the deals were kept under wraps during the event, Siemens Health care were at liberty to announce the biggest single order contract in Middle East, signed during Arab Health 2010.

Siemens Health care announced a contract win of US $69 million to supply diagnostic imaging equipment to all Ministry of Health hospitals across Iraq. The recently signed contract will provide the Iraqi Ministry of Health with unrivalled diagnostic imaging equipment, fully serviced over a period of 5 years.

Maurice Faber, Vice-President Siemens Health care Sector Middle East said, "We are very proud to announce this agreement as it means we are playing an active role in the helping to rebuild health care services in Iraq. One major result of this contract will be improved health care for all Iraqi people, and advanced breast cancer screening facilities for women in Iraq."

The Minister of Health, Iraq, His Excellency Ali Saleh Al Hasnawi, comments, "We have been a regular customer of Siemens for more than 30 years and are confident of the quality of their products, innovative solutions and excellent service history."

This year's event also saw an array of leading health care experts and dignitaries attend the exhibition and conferences.

The event was inaugurated by HH Sheikh Mohammed bin Rashid Al Maktoum, Vice-President and Prime Minister of the United Arab Emirates and Ruler of Dubai. Along with other government dignitaries, the UK business Ambassador Lord Ara Darzi, a leading figure responsible for health care innovation and reform across the UK, attended Arab Health 2010 to promote excellence in British health care manufacture, services, technology and innovation. Lord Darzi attended the opening ceremony, gave a keynote address to senior surgeons and clinicians and unveiled the first portable home haemodialysis machine designed by a UK company.

There were a number of country pavilions at the event demonstrating the power of the event to attract marketing investment from around the globe.

Exhibition Director, Terri D'Elia, from IIR Middle East explains: "The health care industry is one of the few that is still showing buoyancy in these critical economic times. This year our showcase featured 30 national country pavilions and in excess of 70 exhibiting countries including France, Germany, United Kingdom, China, India, Korea, the USA, Brazil and Canada, to name a few. The largest country pavilion was Germany while the largest private exhibitor was Getinge Group."

The Swiss Pavilion, organised by Osec in close co-operation with the Swiss Business Hub GCC, saw 25 Swiss companies showcasing a range of their health care products and services.

Mr. Pascal Blanc, Head of Trade affairs for Osec was extremely pleased with the decision to bring together a national stand for Switzerland.

"The economic development in the oil-rich Gulf States in combination with a fast growing health care industry is creating unprecedented business opportunities for anybody involved in health care," he said. "Our visibility in Hall 7 was fantastic and we were happy with our location in the exhibition.

"The Swiss Ambassador to the UAE visited our stand on the opening day and was pleased with the image that this health care show has created for Swiss companies hoping to expand into the Middle East."

The Arab Health Congress 2010, with over 5,500 delegates, is by far the most extensive scientific and educational platform for health care professionals not just in the world.

"For many, the Congress represents significant financial and time saving as, until recently, only limited CME courses were available in the region forcing many to travel abroad," said Simon Page, Director of the Life Sciences division of IIR Middle East.

"The 2010 Arab Health Congress featured 18 conferences addressed by 500 internationally acclaimed speakers. Sponsored by the Cleveland Clinic Centre for Continuing Education, 15 conferences provided professionals with high-level CME accreditation approved as American Medical Association Physician's Recognition Award (AMA PRA) Category One credit."

For the Arab Health Congress, IIR Middle East collaborated with the Cleveland Clinic, a not-for-profit academic medical centre that integrates clinical and hospital care with research and education, to expand medical education activities.

Dr, William Carey, Director of the Cleveland Clinic Centre for Continuing Education, said collaboration with Arab Health allowed broader quality continuing medical education activities "benefiting the local medical community as well as the region and beyond. Providing AMA PRA Category One credit at Arab Health 2010 significantly expanded accredited postgraduate education in the Middle East."

This year, the Leaders in Health care Conference featured topics on sustainable and green health care that will not only be environmentally friendly and cost-effective but will contribute to the overall quality of patient care and a higher quality of life for all people.

Discussion centred on the definition of sustainable health care and whether or not it works in engaging the most successful and cost-effective medical therapies that include treatment and prevention to ensure a healthier population. Leaders in the health care field spoke about preventive approaches, operational efficiency and increased profitability which are all components of sustainable health care.

"The Leaders in Health care Conference, in its sixth year, has become the must attend event for the Arab Health Congress. This year's theme "Sustainable Health care Systems" provided timely information from industry experts on issues that affect every health care organisation. The 500 participants voted on the Leaders in Health care Business Forum Outcome Statements and will have the opportunity to offer their solutions to these issues which will be presented in a follow up forum next year. We hope we will see everyone back again next year to hear what the audience has to say about how to make health care systems sustainable and if the next year brings about any working solutions," said Pam Page, Conference Producer.

The 2010 edition of the Medial Imaging and Diagnostics Conference was the tenth anniversary edition of this extremely popular conference which saw more than 1000 delegates attended this event. Once again, oncology marked the Molecular Imaging and Nuclear Medicine Conference for 2010 highlighting key areas for cancer management in metabolic imaging and nuclear medicine.

Another popular conference for 2010 was the sold-out Middle East Laboratory Management and Medicine Congress (MEDLAB, 2010). An impressive panel of regional and international experts presented new ideas, updates and insights on diagnostics test to the 1500-strong audience.

Many other conference streams, such as the 3rd Middle East Urology Update, also experienced a steady increased in delegate numbers compared to last year.

"The 3rd Middle East Urology Update gathering grows annually and this year, more than 100 core specialist urologists attended. This steady increase in delegate numbers adds to the credibility of the conference programme highlighting the outstanding calibre of our speakers," said Raza Chevel, Conference Producer.

Undoubtedly a testament to the growth and development of the health care sector in the region, Arab Health remains a global player in the field of medical innovation, health care education and health care sustainability and development. Poised to attract more foreign direct investments this year the Middle East growth will be driven by the favourable regulatory environment, increasing private sector participation and the introduction of compulsory medical insurance schemes together with the expected completion of the Dubai Health Care City this year. The success of Arab Health 2010 has paved the way for an even bigger and better show in 2011.

Regional health care pioneers honoured

Excellence singled out at Arab Health Achievement and Innovation Awards. Health care pioneers in the United Arab Emirates, the Kingdom of Saudi Arabia and Jordan have been honoured for their contributions towards regional innovation and development in the annual Arab Health Achievement and Innovation Awards. The awards were made in front of more than 700 of the region's leading health care professionals at a gala dinner on 26 January 2010 at the Grand Hyatt Hotel, Dubai.

Abu Dhabi Health Services Company (Seha) was the diamond sponsor of this year's Arab Health Awards. The gold sponsors were Roche, Miele, Cerner, dothealth, Microsoft Health Vault and Microsoft Amalga. The Excellence in Imaging and Diagnostics Award went to Tawam Hospital, Al Ain, UAE, with the judges describing the hospital's mammography screening programme as a "brilliant exposition of implementation of global standards in a difficult and controversial area." Mafraq Hospital, Abu Dhabi, UAE, received the Excellence in Surgery Services Award with the judges recording "excellent assimilation of a new technology and very good results."

The award for Excellence in Laboratory Services went to the King Hussein Cancer Centre Department of Pathology and Laboratory Medicine, Jordan, described by the judges as a pioneer in the region.

The award for Excellence in Patient Centreed Care was made to Al Corniche Hospital, UAE, which the judges said was providing an additional dimension in improving health care in Abu Dhabi.

The Rashid Hospital Trauma Centre in Dubai received the Excellence in Hospital Emergency Department Award and was described as "an exciting and interesting project" achieving excellent results.

Ambulatory Health care Services of the Abu Dhabi Health Services company (Seha 2) received the Human Resource Development Award. The judges said work being carried out by Seha 2 is "innovative and groundbreaking considering the tremendous human resources challenges that health care organisations are currently facing."

For its successes in many clinical and technical areas, the judges gave the Excellence in Electronic Health Records Award to the National Guard Health Affairs of Saudi Arabia.

For an "excellent ongoing project," the Excellence in Patient Safety Award went to Lifeline Hospital, Abu Dhabi, UAE.

An Outstanding Contribution of an Individual to the Middle East Health care Industry Award went to Dr, Azad Moopen, Chairman of the Dr, Moopen Group, Dubai.

The Arab Health Exhibition and Congress—the biggest health care event in the Middle East—at Dubai World Trade Centre closes tomorrow (28 January 2010) and has seen 20% year-on-year growth with the opening of new halls adding a further 20,000 square metres of exhibition space.

Arab Health is the flagship event of IIR Middle East's Life Science Division and the region's premier event for the health care sector. A total of 2700 exhibiting companies from 70 countries are taking part.

Middle East 'centre of world' for health care companies

Two full-scale operating theatres to be erected on biggest company stand at Arab Health Exhibition and Congress.

The Middle East is becoming the "centre of the world" for specialized health care companies seeking a share of the region's new hospital construction market, according to a leading industry player.

"The trend is particularly true for operating theatres," said Salah Malek, Middle East Managing Director of Maquet, the world's leading specialist in surgical workplaces and medical technology. "In the developed world the market is more about upgrading facilities but here the number of hospitals keeps on mushrooming and new operating theatres are on a steep growth curve."

Maquet, part of Sweden's Gettinge Group, will be part of the biggest single company stand measuring more than 800 square metres next month at the Arab Health Exhibition and Congress—the biggest health care exhibition in the Middle East which is set be even larger in 2010.

With the addition of four new halls at the Dubai International Convention and Exhibition Centre, the Arab Health Exhibition running from 25-28 January 2010 has been expanded by 20,000 square metres to accommodate more exhibitors, according to the organizer, IIR Middle East.

Maquet will be erecting two full-scale and fully-equipped 35 square metre examples of their operating theatres on the stand. When the exhibition closes for the first day, Maquet will, overnight, convert the two theatres into one 70-square metre hybrid theatre equipped with medical imaging technology ready for day two.

More than 2,000 of the modular Variop operating theatres have been constructed around the world and Maquet have installed almost 60 of them, along with three intensive care units, in the Middle East. "The health care market in the Gulf Co-operation Council countries is expected to grow at about 9% annually to reach $47 billion to $55 billion by 2020, according to a recent report by Alpen Capital," said Dave Panther, Sponsorship Director of the event. "Maquet are a good example of a major international company recognising the continued growth in health care in the region and the opportunities this affords, which is reflected in the increase in the size of Arab Health in 2010 by around 20%."

The Arab Health Exhibition and Congress is the flagship event of IIR Middle East's Life Science Division. In January this year, more than 2205 exhibitors from 59 countries showcased products and services with well over 50,000 professionals from 145 countries attending. There are expected to be around 2,500 exhibitors at the 2010 event, many taking bigger stands than in previous years.

Arab Health features the world's largest multi-track medical congress at which health care professionals can earn continuing medical education (CME) credits. The 2010 conferences will be addressed by around 500 speakers and host more than 5,500 attendees. Sponsored by the Cleveland Clinic Centre for Continuing Education, 15 of the 18 conferences provide CME credits.

The Arab Health Achievement and Innovation Awards, recognising individuals, hospitals, departments, teams or organisations contributing to the growth and development of the industry, will also be presented as part of the event. The winners will be announced during a gala dinner on 26 January 2010 at the Grand Hyatt Hotel for more than 700 of the region's leading health care professionals.

HRH Princess Haya urges medical community to invest in prevention

Princess Haya gives keynote speech at Leaders in Health care—flagship event of 2010 Arab Health Exhibition and Congress. Her Royal Highness Princess Haya Bint Al Hussein, wife of HH Sheikh Mohammed Bin Rashid Al Maktoum, Vice-President and Prime Minister of the United Arab Emirates and Ruler of Dubai, today urged the medical community to invest in prevention in a keynote speech at Leaders in Health care, the flagship gathering at the Arab Health Exhibition and Congress.

"If we want to see sustainable development in the health sector, we as members of the medical community must also be personally involved and take responsibility for the choices we make," said Princess Haya. "Unless we have long-term vision, unless we invest in prevention, we will soon be overwhelmed by the level of diabetes, heart disease and other non-communicable diseases."

The focus of this year's Leaders in Health care was sustainable and green health care that would not only be environmentally friendly and cost-effective but also contribute to the overall quality of patient care and a higher quality of life for all people. Princess Haya, who delivered the keynote address, highlighted the need for sustainable health care systems, stressing that hospitals are one of the largest consumers of energy in the world today.

"They use twice as much energy per square foot as office buildings and generate millions and millions of tons of waste per year," She said. "If the earth's ecosystem is to continue to support us, we need to preserve public health and provide health care in ways that will sustain our environment."

Topics of discussion also included principles of sustainable health care, preventive approaches to health care, operational efficiency and increased profitability as well as the meaning of 'going green' and why it's good for business.

Among other high-level speakers who took part in Leaders in Health care were: Brian De Francesca, Executive Vice-President, TBS Group and Senior Partner, Capitol Health, USA; Heinrich Von Wulfen, CEO, EMEA and CRM, Siemens Health care Sector, Erlangen, Germany; G. Steven Burrill, Chief Executive, Burrill & Co., USA; Dr. Walid Fitahi, CEO, International Medical Centre, Jeddah, Saudi Arabia; Professor Elias Mossialos, Centre Director, London School of Economics Health, UK; Dr, Mark Parrish, Director of Health Solutions Group Asia Pacific and Middle East, Microsoft, Australia.

The Arab Health Exhibition and Congress, organized by IIR Middle East, closed today at the Dubai World Trade Centre, featured more than 2700 exhibiting companies from 70 countries. Attended by in excess of 50,000 visitors it was the largest gathering ever of health care professionals in the Middle East.

GCC health care spending: robust growth seen in 2010

The health care sector in the Arabian Gulf will continue to enjoy high growth in 2010, despite the global slowdown, led by government investment in infrastructure improvement, according to leading industry observers.

"In spite of significant project delays in other non-infrastructure sectors, the pipeline of health care projects in the region remains remarkably robust, particularly for Saudi Arabia and the United Arab Emirates," said Simon Page, Director of the Life Science Division of IIR Middle East, organisers of this month's Arab Health Exhibition and Congress.

Arab Health—the biggest health care event in the Middle East—takes place at the Dubai International Convention and Exhibition Centre from 25-28 January 2010. With the opening of new halls providing a further 20,000 square metres, Arab Health will grow by more than 20% in 2010, Page added.

Page was speaking as Dubai-based research firm Proleads released the latest figures on current investment in both the public and private health care sectors in Saudi Arabia, which is leading regional demand growth.

The Proleads figures show government investment in health care-related projects in Saudi Arabia is currently running at more than $5 billion, compared with around $1 billion of private sector investment.

In addition, per capita health care spending in the Gulf Co-operation Council (GCC) countries is expected to continue growing faster than the global average, according to a recent report from Alpen Capital.

"Growth in income levels as well as an increase in health insurance coverage will boost demand for health care services," the report said. "Moreover, per capita health care requirements and spending will also increase as the GCC population ages and the disease mix changes."

The Alpen Capital report also forecasts the GCC may need in excess of 25,000 additional beds by 2020 to address growing demand for in-patient treatments. The largest share of demand is accounted for by Saudi Arabia followed by the UAE.

The Arab Health Exhibition and Congress is the flagship event of IIR Middle East's Life Science Division and the region's premier event for the health care sector. At the 2009 event, 2205 exhibitors from 59 countries showcased products and services with more than 55,000 professionals from 145 countries attending. There are expected to be around 2,600 exhibitors at the 2010 event.

Arab Health features the world's largest multi-track medical congress at which health care professionals can earn continuing medical education (CME) credits. The 2010 conferences will be addressed by around 500 speakers and host more than 5,500 attendees. Sponsored by the Cleveland Clinic Centre for Continuing Education, 15 of the 18 conferences provide CME credits.

The Arab Health Achievement and Innovation Awards, recognising individuals, hospitals, departments, teams or organisations contributing to the growth and development of the industry, will also be presented as part of the event. The winners will be announced during a gala dinner on 26 January 2010 at the Grand Hyatt Hotel for more than 700 of the region's leading health care professionals.

The Arab Health Exhibition and Congress is supported by the UAE Ministry of Health, Dubai Health Authority and the Health Authority Abu Dhabi.

Haret Hreik care centre leading the way for health reform

The Primary Health Care Centre (PHCC) that was inaugurated in Haret Hreik in January could be a first step toward a thorough reform of Lebanon's public health care system, Dr. Luigi Triggiano, a member of the Italian municipality of Arezzo told *The Daily Star* in an interview.

"The centre is intended as the starting point of a new process," Triggiano, who acts as scientific coordinator for the project, said. "It is only a small step, but we hope that it lead to many innovations in public health care."

The centre in Haret Hreik is the first of three centres funded by the UNDP's ART GOLD program.

In addition to the funding, ART GOLD brings together municipalities from Europe with their counterparts in target countries to supply them with technical expertise and counseling. As a result of this approach, the municipality of Arezzo is supporting the centres in Beirut's southern suburbs with training and equipment.

Triggiano has been involved in this project from its beginnings in 2007, when a field trip to Lebanon brought him together with the mayors of the southern suburbs. In several working groups hosted by ART GOLD, it was established that a top goal for the development of the suburbs would be the establishment of a primary health care centre.

"We found that it would not be efficient to simply provide health services to the poor, or combat only certain diseases," Triggiano explained. "A PHCC provides health care with a long-term view, not just day-to-day treatment."

To this effect, the health dispensaries in the southern suburbs are being transformed into health care centres, staffed by a team of experts that cover a wide range of fields.

A primary health care centre brings together experts from different disciplines, such as family doctors, pediatricians, gynecologists, obstetricians, professional nurses and also social workers.

"The PHCC makes sure that a patient gets the most suitable cure," the doctor stressed. "It acts as filter, referring patients to the right place, and for very little money, they are sure to get a high quality of care."

"The staff can address health issues with a new approach—at the same time medical, biological, social and psychological. As an example, I was told by a gynecologist that she was very relieved to be working next door to colleagues from other fields. Where before, she didn't have the time and the knowledge to help her patients with the many other problems they complained to her about, she can now refer them to someone in the centre who can."

For Triggiano, the centre presents a real opportunity for reform. "The ministries concerned with public health, meaning the ministries of the interior, of health and of social affairs, could use this experience to deepen their understanding of public health," he estimated. "We hope that an intensive dialogue between the administration, the municipalities and the centres will take place," he added.

The doctor sees one of his main tasks in encouraging that dialogue. "The system relies on good relationships between all actors, on their communication and cooperation," he emphasised. "It should be any government's duty to ensure everybody's right to good health."

In order to achieve this goal, integration between the concerned bodies is needed, Triggiano argued. To him, unity between all national and international actors is essential.

"I hope that this small project can push us towards more unity. If we work together, we can overcome individual limitations."

The doctor admitted that this viewpoint was somewhat idealistic. At the same time, he affirmed his belief in the importance of an efficient public health care system. As he put it: "A population's health is its most important asset."

Source: *The Daily Star.*

List of hospitals in the United Arab Emirates

They are categorized by emirate and whether they are federal government, local government or private hospitals.

Abu Dhabi Emirate

Abu Dhabi City

- Shaikh Khalifa Medical City (SEHA—Abu Dhabi Health Services Company, managed by Cleveland Clinic)
- Dar Al Shifaa (Private)
- Al Noor Hospital (Private)
- New Medical Centre (Private)
- Ahalia Hospital (Private)
- Franco-Emirien Hospital (Private)
- Al Reef International Hospital (private) 02-6328000
- Al Mafraq Hospital (SEHA—Abu Dhabi Health Services Company, managed by Bumrungrad International Ltd.)
- Al Rahba Hospital (SEHA, managed by Johns Hopkins International)
- Al Corniche Hospital (SEHA, managed by Johns Hopkins International) 02-6724900
- Zayed Military Hospital 02-4448
- Silkor Laser Hair Removal www.silkor.com (Private)

Al Ain

- Oasis Hospital, Al Ain (Private)
- Tawam Hospital, Al Ain (SEHA, managed by Johns Hopkins International)
- Al Ain Hospital, Al Ain (SEHA)
- Al Jimi Hospital, Al Ain (Ministry of Health)
- Madinat Zayed Hospital (HAAD—Health Authority Abu Dhabi)
- Marfa Hospital (HAAD)

Western Regions

- Al Mafraq Hospital (Al Mafraq) 58-23100
- Delma Island Hospital (Delma) 87-81888
- Ghayathi Hospital (Ghayathi) 87-41666
- Madinat Zayed Hospital (Madinat Zayed) 88-46888
- Ruwais Hospital (Ruwais) 02-6022350

Dubai

Hospitals and Clinics under Department of Health (Dohms) Authority

- Dubai Hospital (Dubai Government DOHMS)
- Rashid Hospital (Dubai Government DOHMS)
- Al Baraha Hospital (Ministry of Health)
- Al Amal Hospital (Ministry of Health)
- Al Maktoum Hospital (Dubai Government DOHMS)
- Al Wasl Hospital (Dubai Government DOHMS)
- Zulekha Hospital Dubai (Private)
- Jebel Ali Hospital (Private)
- American Hospital Dubai (Private)
- Welcare Hospital (Private)
- Emirates International Hospital (Private)
- Iranian Hospital (Private)
- Neuro-Spinal Hospital (Private)
- Belhoul Speciality Hospital [1] (Private)
- Belhoul European Hospital [2] (Private)
- Medcare Hospital (Private)
- Silkor Laser Hair Removal www.silkor.com (Private)
- Canadian Specialist Hospitals Dubai

Hospitals and Clinics under Dubai Health Care City (DHCC) Authority

- Harvard Medical School University Hospital
- Medical Group Practice FZ LLC—UGRS International (www.the-european-institute-ugrs.com)
- Universitatsklinikum Hamburg-Eppendorf
- Mayo Clinic Middle East
- Dr. Sulaiman Al Habib Medical Centre
- The City Hospital (Welcare, Varkey Group)
- The Creek Hospital Dubai (Welcare, Varkey Group)
- American Academy of Cosmetic Surgery Hospital
- American University of Beirut Medical Centre
- Eleva Women's Hospital
- London's Great Ormond Street Hospital—Dubai Office
- Isis—The French Pediatric Clinic

- Biolite Skin Clinic UK dubai branch—www.biolitedubai.com
- Physiocare FZ LLC—http://www.physiocare.ae
- German Clinic—http://www.germanclinic-dubai.com

Sharjah

- Sharjah Teaching Hospital (Private)
- Al Qassimi Hospital (Ministry of Health)
- Kuwaiti Hospital (Ministry of Health)
- *Zulekha Hospital Sharjah (Private)
- Al Zahra Private Hospital (Private)
- Royal Hospital (Private)
- Central Private Hospital (Private) [3]
- Khorfakkan Hospital

Ajman

- Khalifa Bin Zayed Hospital (Ministry of Health)
- Ajman Medical Complex (Ministry of Health)
- GMC Hospital (06-7463333 Private)

Ras Al Khaimah

- Saqr Hospital (Ministry of Health)
- Saif bin Ghubash Hospital (Ministry of Health)
- RAK Hospital (Private Hospital)

Fujairah

- Al Fujairah Hospital (Ministry of Health)
- Dibba Hospital at Dibba Al-Fujairah (Ministry of Health)

Umm Al Quwain

- Umm Al Quwain (Ministry of Health)

Dr. Sulaiman Habib Medical Centre, Dubai Health Care Centre

Habib Medical Centre, Dubai Health Care Centre is forecasted to be commissioned for operation by the end of year 2006 (HMC at DHCC). HMC at DHCC will be equipped with the state of the art of medical equipments in all departments. Its main goal is to provide excellent medical services to patients and to become a referral centre for the entire Middle East region. HMC at DHCC will be able to provide treatment for 800 patients per day and will adhere to international standards from initiating the construction of the building to provision of all phases of medical services to patients.

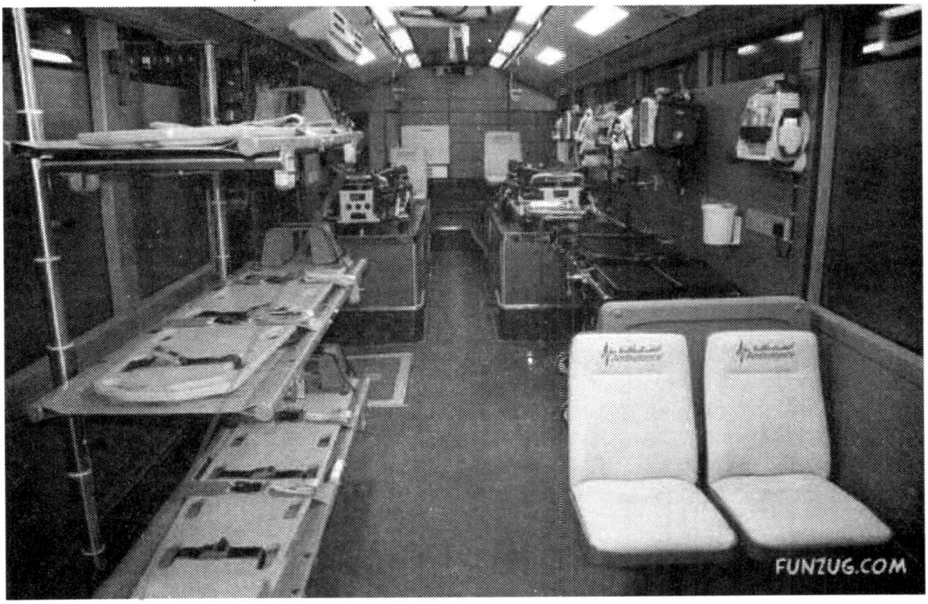

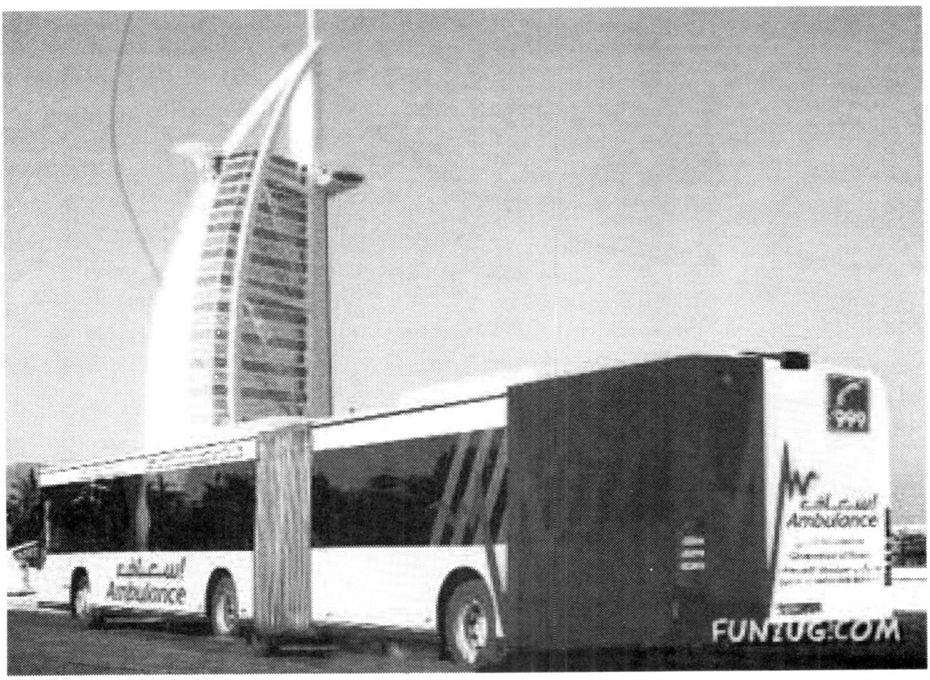

The car is longer than 20 meters to accommodate more than 45 injured at one time and includes two operating rooms and intensive care room and family medical as well as medium-sized stretchers and seats for minor injuries.

City Hospital in DHCC

Indeed, many of the world's most prestigious hospitals have been essentially exclusive for years, with the world's top specialists and surgeons tending to and saving some of the world's most powerful people. But the difference now is that patients expect more than just a top-rate clinical service—they want the customer service to match as well. At The City Hospital in DHCC, for instance, patients have the option of 'topping up' their treatment package to make the most of its luxury facilities. "The VIP service provided at their facility comprises of the same quality of health care that is offered to all patients, however it includes a number of elements that add an extra significance to the comfort that results from the stay at the facility," explains Rania Roxana Akkela, marketing and communication officer at The City Hospital. "These kind of services are currently provided only for the in-patient department and consists of extra constituents such as larger and different style rooms, wider variety of foods, flower arrangements, decorations, complimentary beverages and snacks, as well as a full entertainment system." Bigger rooms and free food may be a step up from the norm, but aren't exactly mind-blowing. But the VIP health care service also incorporates some of the best elements of Dubai's numerous health spas. "Furthermore, the guests of the VIP floor get access to the health club and spa floor which includes, two Jacuzzis, a swimming pool, sauna and steam room as well as a fully equipped gym and two beauty enhancing rooms where the patients can get facials and massages." VIP health care might make for good marketing, but it can be a tricky strategy for a hospital to promote. After all, the concept of VIP services is that they are exclusive. The idea of hospitals, after all, is that they are there to treat the sick and needy. That is why, explains Akkela, the facility is so keen to emphasize the lack of difference in a patient's clinical experience—whether they are VIP or not. "The City Hospital clinical outcomes are benchmarked internationally with the APACHE score for ICU ([intensive care units], Vermont Oxford Network for NICU [neonatal intensive care unit] and Medi-Clinic International for cardiothoracic data—we are proud to provide these services combined with VIP hospitality for those who like to experience these services," she says.

Indeed, Akkela maintains that despite high-end services, the goal of the facility is to provide high quality patient care. "At The City Hospital, our main focus lies on the provision of state of the art health care revolving around the patient care.

Regardless of whether or not The City Hospital wants to develop its VIP services or not, it has been an extremely tough year for the economy. Not exactly the best time, would have thought, to be launching high-end services. But Akkela insists that the interest in VIP services have not tailed. "Despite the global economic crisis, we have not experienced any decrease in the demand of VIP services as a result of the economical downturn," she said. "The UAE market has a definite demand for this category of services. It seems that VIP people are becoming more and more educated towards health care, and the demand for add value services is escalating."

In fact, The City Hospital is planning development of its services to also include the out-patient department in the near future.

American Academy of Cosmetic surgery hospital. (AACSH) decision to set-up a hospital at DHCC is a step in that direction. Dubai's reputation as a luxury holiday destination is providing a boost to VIP health care services in the region, whic is why the AACSH decided to set-up in the free zone. But does VIP health care benefit anyone other than the well-off or the hospital's bank balance? "Research shows that the way you treat a person before and after any type of medical procedure defines the pace of the healing process. And this is so true—if a person gets his surgery done in a well organized place where even small details are taken care of, that brings a feeling of safety and helps the patient relax. This will lead to less post operative complications and a quick and smooth recovery to normal lifestyle." "Any hospital today regardless what kind of services it provides is trying to promote its customer service," admits Qadir. AACSH, it seems, is no different. "VIP health care. requires unique medical customer service as patients who come to a high quality facility understandably have higher expectations and demands when it comes to quality of any services provided."

Delivering against the promises of VIP health care is no easy task—and as The City Hospital has shown, it is crucial that clinical services are first standardized across the facility. But if a patient can afford to pay for more comfortable or more attentive treatment, there is no reason why hospitals shouldn't be encouraged to offer the service. Although in health care, unlike retail, patients will have to remember—or at least hope—that the consultant is always right.

5

Sheikh Khalifa Medical City (SKMC), Abu Dhabi

The Sheikh Khalifa Medical City is located in Abu Dhabi, the capital city of the United Arab Emirates. The health care facilities that comprise SKMC are situated on an island about five miles wide and nine miles long. Architecturally, Abu Dhabi is an intriguing city where the domes and minarets of traditional mosques are surrounded by ultramodern skyscrapers, tree-lined boulevards, gleaming fountains and parks. The Sheikh Khalifa Medical City operates under the management and direction of the General Authority for Health Services for the Emirate of Abu Dhabi and is managed by Cleveland clinic USA. The Medical City has several 'Centres of Excellence' and aspires to practice contemporary medicine comparable to the best hospitals and medical centres in the world. SKMC provides comprehensive health care services in all of the disciplines

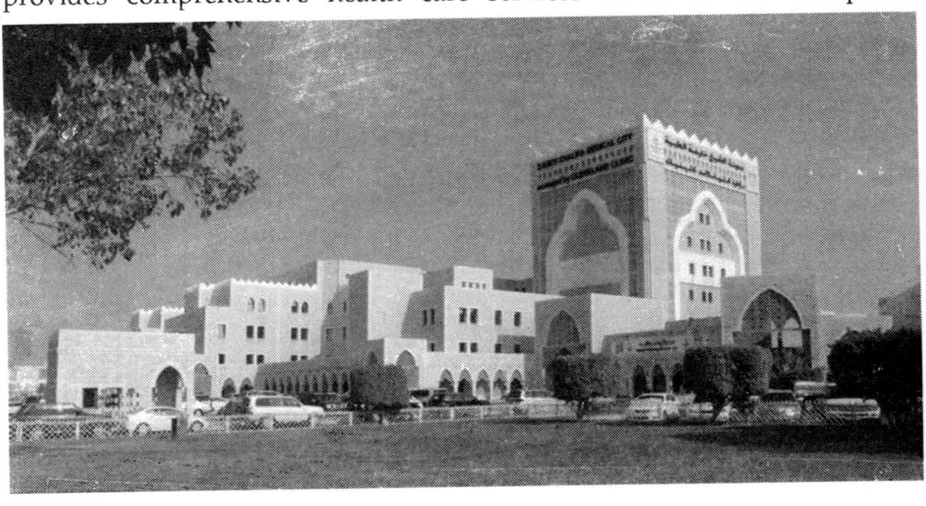

relevant to the needs and priorities of the community and promotes a work ethos sensitive to the social and cultural values of the Community to attain the highest levels of patient satisfaction SKMC aspire to be the health care provider of choice by offering a diverse and integrated set of medical services based on World Class quality compliant with the highest standards. SKMC is committed to the development of the health sector in Abu Dhabi by creating a compassionate and diverse culture that promotes medical education and research.

Link with Cleveland USA

Sheikh Khalifa Medical City (SKMC) operates under the management of Cleveland Clinic, consistently named by U.S. News and World Report as one of the nation's best hospitals in its annual "America's Best Hospitals" survey. SKMC is owned by SEHA, the Abu Dhabi Health Services Company, recently established to oversee operations of all public hospitals in the Emirate. SKMC is the flagship institution for the public health system in Abu Dhabi and has several 'Centres of Excellence', and aspires to practice contemporary medicine comparable to the best hospitals and medical centres in the world. SKMC provides comprehensive health care services in all of the disciplines relevant to the needs and priorities of the community to attain the highest levels of patient satisfaction. SKMC consists of 568-bed Tertiary Hospital, 14 outpatient specialty clinics and Abu Dhabi Blood Bank, all of which are accredited by the Joint Commission International (JCI). SKMC is also accredited as a Cycle III Chest Pain Centre with Primary Angioplasty Intervention. In addition, SKMC manages a 125-bed Behavioural Sciences Pavilion, 6 Family Medicine Clinics, 2 Walk-in Clinics, 2 Dental Centres, and an Urgent Care Centre distributed over the city of Abu Dhabi. For further information, please contact us at marketing@skmc.gov.ae or call +971508128892. About Abu Dhabi Health Services Company—SEHA SEHA is health in Arabic. The Abu Dhabi Health Services Company—whose corporate identity is SEHA—is an independent, public joint stock company created to manage and develop the curative activities of the public hospitals and clinics of the Emirate of Abu Dhabi. SEHA is committed to providing quality, cost effective health care on par with international standards measured through accessibility, affordability, choice and satisfaction. SEHA owns and operates 12 hospitals, 2,644 licensed beds, 62 Ambulatory, Primary Health and ancillary care clinics and 2 Blood Banks. SEHA employs more than 15,500 doctors, nurses and other clinical staff and administration.

The Cleveland Clinic

Cleveland Clinic, located in Cleveland, Ohio, is a not-for-profit multispecialty academic medical centre that integrates clinical and hospital care with research and education. Cleveland Clinic was founded in 1921 by four renowned physicians with a vision of providing outstanding patient care based upon the principles of cooperation, compassion and innovation.

U.S. News and World Report consistently names Cleveland Clinic as one of the nation's best hospitals in its annual "America's Best Hospitals" survey. About 2,000 full-time salaried physicians and researchers and 7,600 nurses at Cleveland Clinic represent more than 100 medical specialties and subspecialties. In addition to its main campus, Cleveland Clinic operates nine regional hospitals in Northeast Ohio, Cleveland Clinic, Florida, Sheikh Khalifa Medical City in Abu Dhabi, the Lou Ruvo Centre for Brain Health in Las Vegas and Cleveland Clinic, Canada. In 2008, there were more than 4.2 million visits throughout the Cleveland Clinic health system and 165,000 hospital admissions. Patients came for treatment from every state and from more than 80 countries. Visit Cleveland Clinic at clevelandclinic.org.

The Sheikh Khalifa Medical City is comprised of the following facilities:

Acute Care Facilities:

- Sheikh Khalifa Medical Pavilion (Previously known as the Sheikh Khalifa Medical Centre)
- Al Jazeira Pavilion (Previously known as Al Jazeira Hospital)
- Central Pavilion (Previously known as the Central Hospital)

Behaviour Science Facilities:

- Behavioural Sciences Pavilion (Previously known as the Psychiatric Hospital)
- National Rehabilitation Centre

Additional Facilities:

- Abu Dhabi Dental Centre
- Central Blood Bank
- Preventive Medicine
- Diabetes Centre

"Practices"

P— Professionalism
R— Respect
A— Accountability
C— Compassion
T— Teamwork
I— Integrity
C— Community
E— Education
S— Safety

GAHS Future Expansion Plans for Sheikh Khalifa Medical City

The General Authority for Health Services for the Emirate of Abu Dhabi has set forth as part of its overall strategy to develop health care services for the Emirate of Abu Dhabi a plan for the continued expansion of the sheikh Khalifa Medical City In addition to the renovation plans of the Al Jazeira Pavilion, the new Nephrology Clinic, expansion project of the Emergency Department at the Sheikh Khalifa Pavilion and New Primary Health Care Centres Plan; the projects in the final planning stages for the Sheikh Khalifa Medical City. There are plans for a new Administration Building that will utilize the ground floor for a Rehabilitation Centre, the first floor for Administration Offices and a Second floor dedicated to Education Services for the SKMC. Furthermore, an additional 10-12 operating theaters, a new helipad and also a free standing Laboratory Facility that will be built on the SKMC Campus and will provide laboratory services for the entire UAE. Additional parking and a landscaping development project of the campus are also in the final stages of planning. The expansion of the Sheikh Khalifa Medical City and other GAHS projects demonstrates the commitment of the General Authority to improve the delivery ofhealth care and provide medical treatment, services and technology that are at the highest standards available around the world.

Primary Health Care (PHC) Facilities:

- Zafra PHC Centre
- Ettehad PHC Centre
- Rowda PHC Centre

Centres of Excellence

It is the flagship institution for the public health system in Abu Dhabi and has several 'Centres of Excellence,' and aspires to practice contemporary medicine comparable to the best hospitals and medical centres in the world. SKMC provides comprehensive health care services in all of the disciplines relevant to the needs and priorities of the community to attain the highest levels of patient satisfaction. SKMC operates under the management of Cleveland Clinic, named among the top hospitals in the USA. SKMC is owned by SEHA, the Abu Dhabi Health Services Company, established to oversee operations of all public hospitals in the Emirate. It consists of a 550-bed Acute Care Hospital and 14 specialized outpatient clinics accredited by the Joint Commission International (JCI). In addition, SKMC manages a 120-bed Behaviour Sciences Pavilion, a 90-bed Rehabilitation Centre, 9 primary health care centres and 2 dental centres distributed over the city of Abu Dhabi.

The Khalidiyah Urgent Care Centre is a modern Urgent Care Centre that receives patients for urgent problems, such as abdominal pains, coughs/colds/flu, earache/sore throat, eye problems, mild-moderate asthma, minor cut wounds, sprains and minor broken bones, sudden back pain, sudden rashes, urine problems, and vomiting and diarrhea in adults. It consists of 19 modern treatment rooms and a pharmacy. X-rays and some blood tests are performed at the Centre, which is located in Al Khalidiyah Area, first right after Al Khalidiyah Mall. The Centre is open 24/7 and can be reached at telephone number +971 2 6653475. The overall strategy of the Sheikh Khalifa Medical City is to improve the current status of health care delivery by expanding its services and technology, upgrading and improving the physical condition of its existing facilities, combining its health care resources for a more efficient model of health care delivery, increasing its current bed capacity to accommodate the needs of its patients, and create a system for health care professionals to work as one team under the guidance of the Health Authority, Abu Dhabi. The Sheikh Khalifa Medical City employs approximately 4000 staff from different nationalities.

Shaikh Khalifa Medical City (SKMC)

It is a modern, acute care institution that opened in late February 2000. Services are provided through an inpatient facility and a large outpatient specialty clinic. The facility's mandate is to provide secondary and tertiary care to the citizens of the United Arab Emirates, (the UAE). SKMC is under the direction of the Office of His Excellency Sheikh Hamed Bin Zayed Al Nahyan who oversees a body established by the government of the Emirate of Abu Dhabi to guide improvement in health services within the Emirate. In the recent past, citizens of the UAE often travelled out of country to the UK or USA for health care. However, with the opening of SKMC, more services and complex care can be provided within the country.

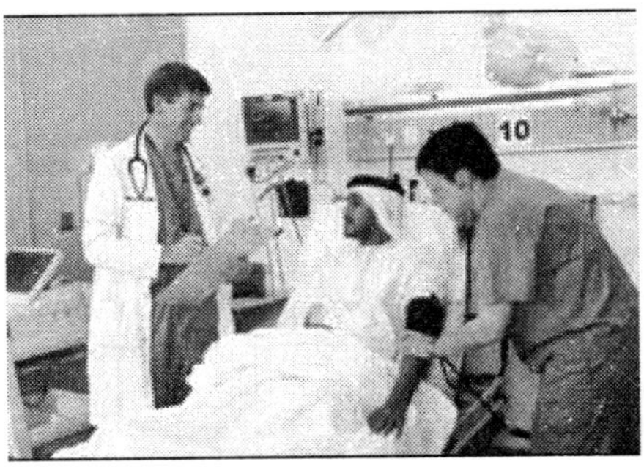
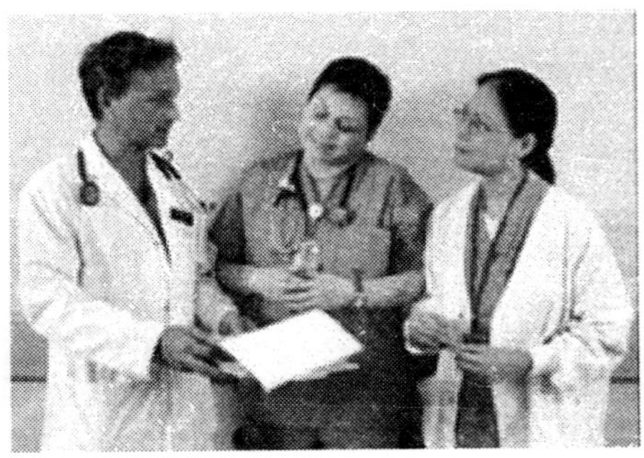

Staff members are recruited locally and internationally. SKMC's vision is to be a City of Excellence within the United Arab Emirates and to provide within its walls, medical care comparable to that available in recognized Medical Centres in North America and elsewhere.

In January 2002, SKMC underwent a process of hospital accreditation. The Canadian Council on Health Services Accreditation (CCHSA) provided the survey. The standards to measure the care provided within SKMC are the same as those used by the CCHSA to accredit similar Canadian hospitals. SKMC received a three year accreditation award—the highest award given to hospitals. SKMC's mission is to provide those services that are relevant to the needs and priorities of the communities we serve and to foster academic activity and scientific research.

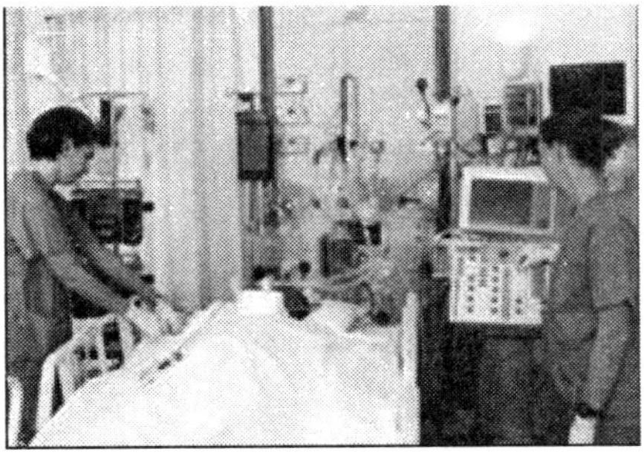

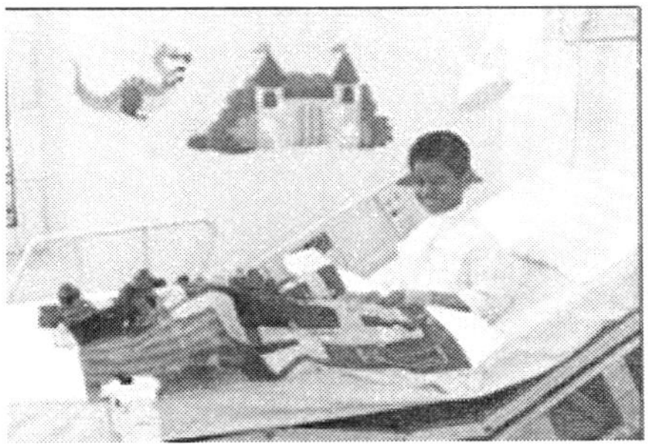

SKMC is an acute care hospital with 700 beds. Next door to the inpatient facility is a large, multi-disciplinary outpatient clinic, with a primary purpose to provide specialist consultations on a referral basis and to allow ongoing care. Emergency services are provided through a busy department, efficiently designed and staffed by consultants in Emergency Medicine. The equipment is modern and up-to-date and comparable to that of most North American facilities. SKMC is striving to provide new services. Recently, the Primary Care (i.e. family practice) and Home Care Programmes were introduced.

The Major Departments at SKMC include:

- Admissions/Registration
- Anaesthesia
- Cardio-Respiratory
- Clinical Dietetics
- Communications
- Central Sterile Supply
- Education Services
- Emergency Medicine
- Environmental Health
- Facilities Management
- Finance
- Housekeeping
- Human Resources
- Intensive Care
- Information Technology
- Internal Audit
- Laboratory Medicine
- Materials Management
- Medical Records
- Medicine (and its subspecialties)

- Outpatient Clinic
- Nursing
- Paediatrics
- Pharmacy
- Public Relations
- Purchasing
- Radiology
- Rehabilitation
- Security
- Surgery (and its sub-specialties)

One of the first things to consider about SKMC is that it is a relatively new organization. While it is no longer in a 'start up' mode, SKMC continues to undergo a great deal of growth and change. It is a dynamic atmosphere and for people who come here from very well established organizations, this work environment can be challenging.

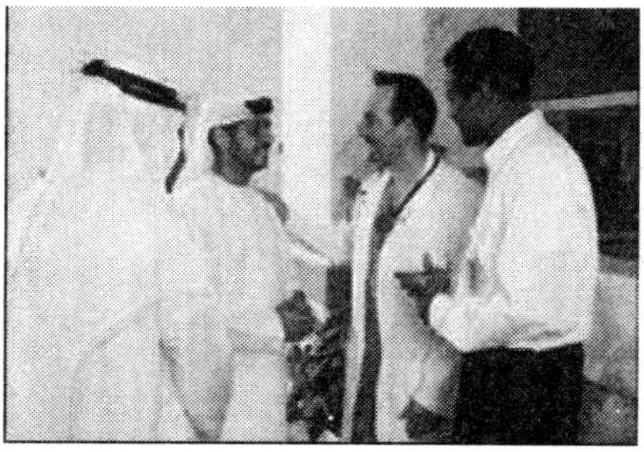

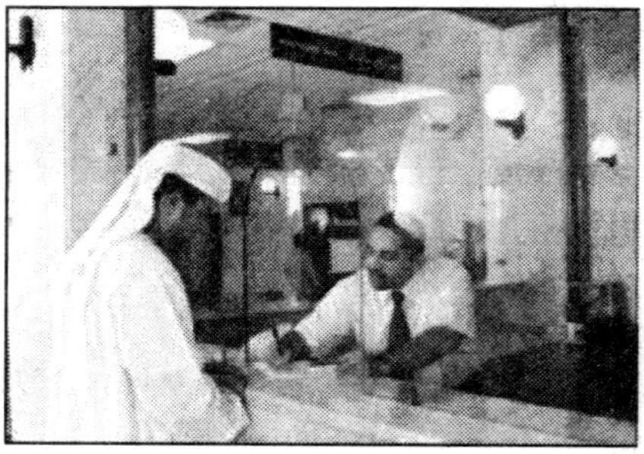

The island city of Abu Dhabi is a lush, modern metropolis, complete with tree- lined streets, futuristic skyscrapers, huge shopping malls and international luxury hotels. The city is surrounded by the sparkling waters of the Arabian Gulf which offer a striking contrast to the large parks and green boulevards spread across the island. Built on a grid system running from a central 'T', the city is easy to navigate. The 'T' is formed by the corniche, which runs along the end of the island furthest from the mainland, and Airport Road which runs the length of the island. Roads parallel to the corniche have odd numbers and roads running vertically have even numbers.

SKMC has a large, multi-cultural workforce with varying levels of responsibility and therefore, varying levels of compensation for positions within the organization. This multi-level staffing system, where compensation is based on one's country of origin is not uncommon in the Middle East. Staff members try to foster harmony in the workplace, among and between the different cultures and backgrounds of SKMC employees. SEHA owns and operates 12 hospital facilities, 2,644 licensed beds, and more than 40 ambulatory and primary health care clinics with more than 16,500 doctors, nurses and other clinical and administrative staff, making it one of the largest employers in the Middle East.

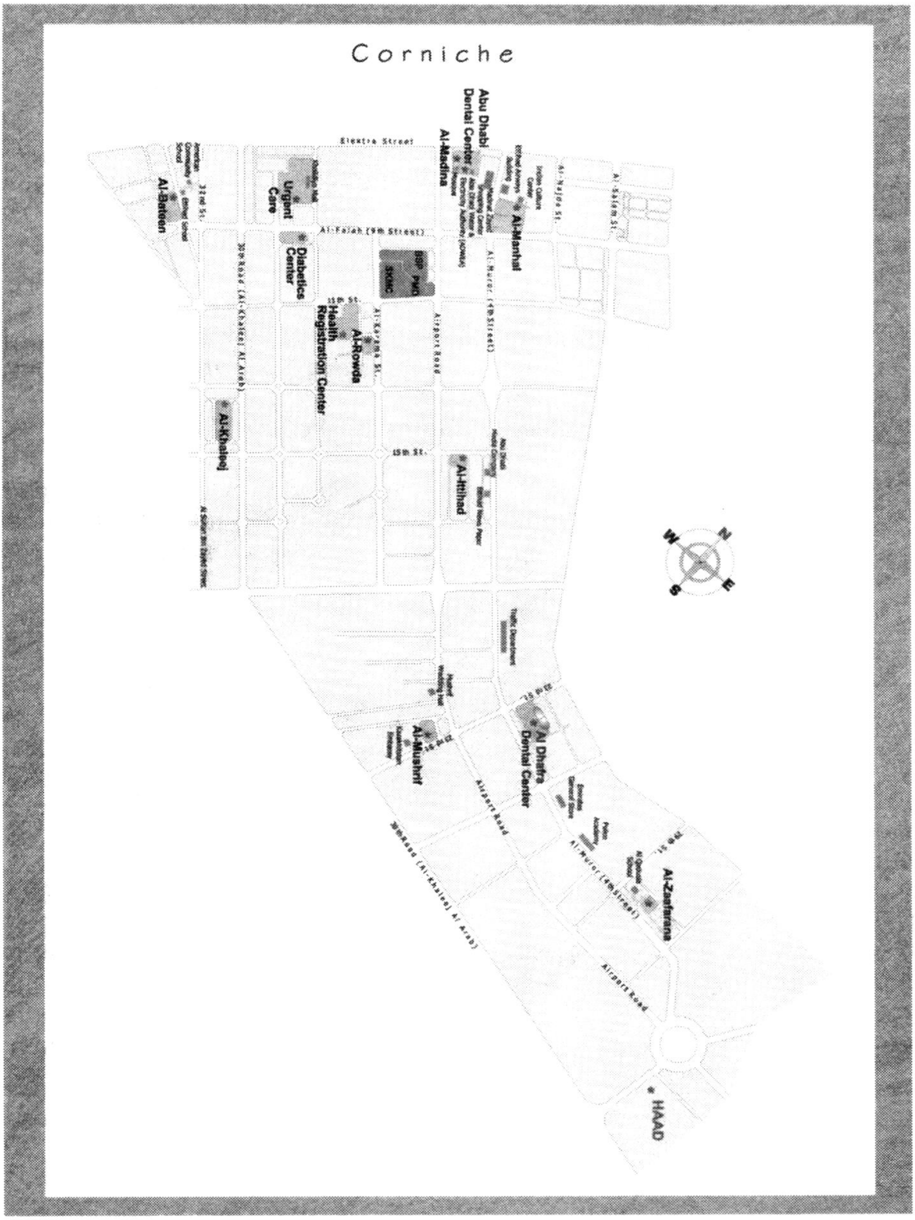

Primary Health Care

Primary health care is the individual's first contact with the health care system. It serves as the connector between the hospital and the community. On the island of Abu Dhabi, there are 9 primary health centres that have integrated services with Sheikh Khalifa Medical and Surgical Pavilions and form part of Sheikh Khalifa Medical City.

The primary health centres provide a variety of services. These include diagnosis of acute illness, chronic disease management, appropriate screening, well baby visit and child and adult immunizations. Nutrition services are provided and specialized medical services, such as a minor surgery and allergy testing, is provided by our Family Medicine consultants. Dental services are also provided and will be centralized in Zafra Clinic.

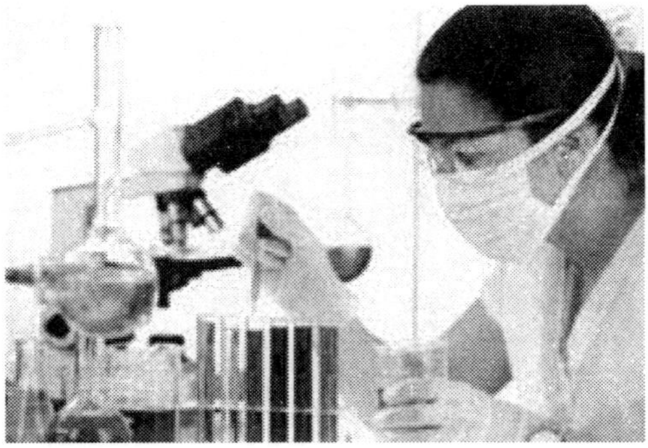

The aim of the primary health care system is to provide people with quality health care. To deliver a high quality of care, the individual should have suitable access to care, continuity of care and care should be patient focused. It should be provided by health care professionals who are continuous learners. To achieve this, only the best qualified individuals are hired at the Primary Health Care Clinics.

Family Medicine is the core around which primary care is organized. Men and women study additional years after their internship and must pass specialty examinations before they receive their specialty certification. General practitioners work along with family physicians in the primary health centres to provide medical care.

The clinics currently operated by Sheikh Khalifa Medical City are include:

- Ittihad
- Rodha
- Mushrif
- Manhal
- Bateen
- Khaleej
- Madina
- Zafranah
- Al Dhafra Dental Clinic

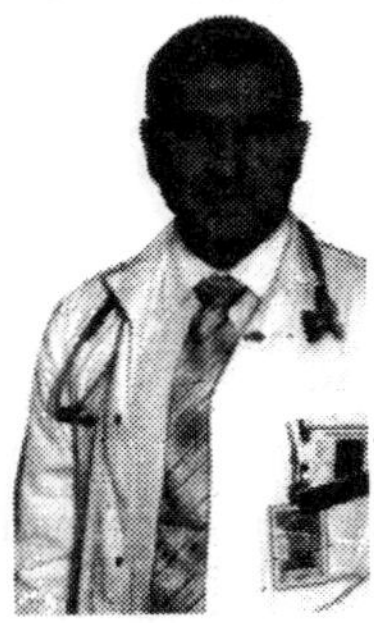

Dr. Ali Khalili, Chairman Family Medicine Department

Introducing Family Medicine to Abu Dhabi

For most of us in the health care industry, coming to Abu Dhabi is an eye opening experience. Here is a beautiful and modern metropolis that is establishing its identity in many areas, including health care. The health care industry has seen a great deal of resurgence and high tech makeovers in the last few years, however, it needed a proper foundation: namely, a primary health care system. Digging into the psyche of the populace reveals some lack of trust in the private and, to a lesser degree, public sector. Health care in Abu Dhabi is often viewed as substandard by its population.

That lack of trust translates into multiple visits to multiple physicians and often to multiple centres, as the patient tries to form a comfortable opinion of their condition. The department of Family Medicine was given the opportunity to improve and expand its services to the community. This shift in paradigm was planned in the last quarter of 2008 and early 2009, and began its tactical implementation in the second quarter of 2009. Many changes have taken place and will continue to take place ultimately benefiting the population at large, providing better accessibility and sustainability of primary care.

Family Physicians in Al Bateen FMC:

1. The development of a unified call centre, where any patient may call in to make an appointment in any of our family medicine clinics.
2. Structural upgrades, equipment upgrades and general renovations in all of our clinics. We have increased the number of utilizable rooms in each clinic to allow better flow of patients with less waiting times.
3. Change in the skill mix of each clinic resulting in improved registration services, better ratios of nurses to nursing assistants and most importantly the redistribution of the consultants and specialists to all clinics providing a definite improvement in the standards of care.
4. Implementation of CERNER in all clinics with the view of full EMR (Electronic Medical Record) by March of 2010.

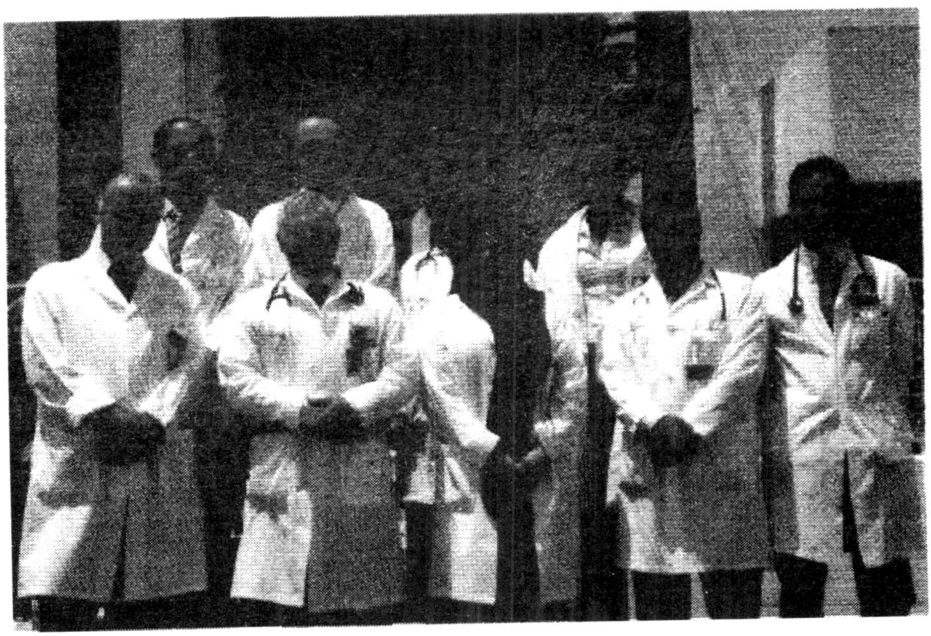

5. Provision of appropriate Family Medicine in the 6 newly designated* residential clinics and the availability of extended hours centres for the patient's needs, in the form of walk-in-based Urgent Care Centres.

Benefits of having your own Family Doctor

As Family Doctors, we need to encourage patients to stay with one family doctor by ensuring that they receive and appreciate the benefits of doing so. Although there is a myriad of reasons as to why having a family doctor could improve your health status, we believe the most important element is the relationship between the members of the family and their doctor. The trust developed between the patient and physician will help ensure the treatment of not only the medical but, more importantly, the psychological aspects which may cause or prolong many chronic illnesses. The breakdown of reluctance to share psychological or emotional issues can be better achieved by development of a satisfactory long-term relationship between the family and their physician.

Another extremely important and overtly lacking issue is that of advocacy. With the adoption of the family medicine model, the patients will have a qualified family physician advocating their needs within the health care maze and acting as a "champion" of their medical problems. This invariably lifts a huge burden off the patient's shoulders and further deepens the trust within their relationship further.

A third issue of significance is that family physicians are trained to consider multiple systems and diagnoses in their evaluation, and relate these to their previous knowledge of the patient. During explanation and discussion of findings and results, the patient's perspective may be explored so that appropriate management and follow-up will also take account of their preferences. This comprehensive and holistic nature of family medicine makes it a much more patient-centreed and friendly model of care. Every family medicine consultation is also an excellent occasion to practice Preventive Medicine. A brief counseling intervention, after dealing with the presenting problem, could cause a smoker to decide to enter our Cessation Program, or an obese patient to consider seeing our dietitian. A good doctor-patient relationship is likely to make these interventions more successful, whilst collaboration with our team of health care workers will lead to better outcomes.

Screening is also an important part of preventive medicine. We expect that the Electronic Medical Record (CERNER) will help to standardize and streamline our screening programs by prompting the physician to check that the appropriate screening has been offered to the patient at the appropriate time. Preventive medicine is also encouraged by community awareness programs whilst their effectiveness is augmented when the individual can discuss concepts and suitable action with their trusted physician. In short, trust is an honour and when that honour is bestowed upon a physician it is no longer mere a job, but a bond that inevitably leads to the patient's healing and comfort. Family physicians by virtue of their learning and training take on that honour and ultimately strengthen and transform it into a life long episode of care and devotion. We are by nature educators, comforters and inspirers of healthy living.

What does Family Medicine offer?

Our scope of practice is extremely wide and our physicians are well trained in all aspects of health care including appropriate referrals. The scope of practice includes all ages and all medical conditions. Psychiatric/ psychological counseling, post-operative follow-up care, minor procedures, patient education and minor emergencies, all add to the variety of the family physician's work.

Family Medicine Postgraduate Residency Program

Since our application and acceptance by the Arab Board almost 3 years ago, the family Medicine Postgraduate Residency Program has grown tremendously under the directorship of Dr. Fawaz Aboudi. Our vision of Emiratization has been successful due to the perseverance and dedication of our faculty including, Dr. Fayeza Nasser, Dr. Maha Al Fahim, Dr. Nassib Saba, Dr. Greta Shorey, Dr. Wameed Hassan and Dr. Ali Khalili.

We are proud to have one of the best regional programs with a total of 20 Residents in their 1st, 2nd and 3rd year.

Continuous Development in Family Medicine

Our patients can be assured that our family medicine physicians remain up-to-date in evidence-based medicine with excellent attendance at our weekly one-hour CME sessions at Al Bateen Clinic. The presentations are given by our own physicians or by guest consultants from other specialties. We are pleased that consultants from other specialities within SKMC give talks to the Family Medicine physicians to further improve our relationship and cooperation with hospital consultants, so that referrals we make to secondary or tertiary care will be appropriate and in the best interests of the patients.

Research and Quality in Family Medicine

The department produced its first review paper last year, which was accepted and published in the *Australian Family Physician Journal*. The article focused on the general review of Vitamin D deficiency and its association with many chronic diseases. This of course is a very important and widespread problem here in Abu Dhabi and in the Gulf region in general. The aim of the review was to bring to light the many important aspects of correcting and optimizing this very important component of our nutrition to all physicians at large.

Thanks to the enthusiastic research committee under the leadership of Drs. Valerie Stott and Mark Stroud, we are presently involved in at least 4 different research projects in areas of importance such as Type II Diabetes

Mellitus, Metabolic Syndrome, Hepatitis immunization and Vitamin D. 2009-10 should be very fruitful years indeed.

They are in the process of tackling the many facets of Quality Improvement under the leadership of Dr, Wameed Hassan. A multi-disciplinary committee involving members from all clinics and skill mixes is in the process of development, with the aim of standardization and improvement of the quality of care for the department, compliant with the JCIA standards by the end of 2011.

Dr. Mario Patricolo, Consultant Pediatric Surgeon and Urologist, recently introduced the details of the "Integrated Day Surgery Service" so that Family Physicians might spread the awareness of this service amongst our patients. The CME committee of the Family Medicine department also organized quarterly Primary Care Updates with recent topics including "Cardiac Failure", "Allergy in Primary Care" and "Ano-rectal disease." These half-day sessions allow for a more in-depth study and discussion of the latest advances which affect our practice.

SKMC Opens Family Medicine Call Centre in June—02 610 4000

The Call Centre was opened in June 2009 in support of the conversion of the Primary Health Clinics into the Family Medicine Clinics. The Family Medicine s to make appointments as opposed to walking into the Clinic. Patients can easily speak to a representative by calling 02 610 4000 and make an appointment with one of our qualified Family Physicians at Al Bateen, Al Khaleej, Al Manhal, Al Mushrif, and Al Zafaranah between the hours of 8:00 am to 5:00 pm. The Call Centre is staffed with a team of highly energetic individuals, trained in customer service. The feedback to date has been overwhelmingly positive and many patients have forged relationships with the call centre representatives. Weekly call volumes started out at around 700 calls a week and have recently surpassed 1,500. The friendliness and welcoming attitude of the staff has added an excellent service to the community and has helped everyone "add a doctor to their family." Please feel free to call in and make an appointment for you or your loved ones today.

The telephone rang!

"Would you please arrange a visit to see Baba; he is getting more and more noisy and upset!" The Home Care team sat discussing the day's cases and decided that Baba should be seen as soon as possible; so the driver was briefed, the car brought around and off we went. We eventually found the villa, an imposing structure in the Muroor District of Abu Dhabi, and introduced ourselves again. Baba is an aged gentleman, a real desert Bedouin from the Liwa Oasis, now suffering, as are many his age, from progressive Alzheimer's disease. His days of roaming the dunes are over; he is now virtually imprisoned in his room because of his old, worn joints and his disruptive behaviour now seriously aggravated by his advancing cognitive impairment.

The team examined him, took note of the large and supportive family in attendance and formulated a sensible plan for this frequently encountered and difficult psycho-geriatric problem. As leader of the Home Care team, I am most reluctant to prescribe strong sedatives or anti-psychotic medicines for such patients, especially since new data implies that the use of these drugs has been shown to shorten life. We suggested some calming measures, advised about focused distractions and arranged a follow-up visit in a week or two.

Before our next visit, a call was made to confirm the repeat visit; Baba's wife told us that we should be most welcome to come anytime, but that he was fine now and no longer upset. Naturally, we were intrigued by Baba's apparent change of fortune,—surely his wife must have been humoring us. Nevertheless, when we made our next trip to the big villa, we were all in for a big surprise! As we made our way through the traditionally darkened home, we found his bedroom 3A full of red Liwa-desert sand! There must have been at least 10 tons of it there. It had been retained in 2/3 of the floor space by rows of bricks, and his wife and extended family were sitting round chatting, drinking tea and coffee (which we were of course offered) and generally passing the time of day—in short they were continuing their desert family-life heritage.

Baba was content; even a cursory glance at his lined and weather-beaten face could see that! His bedding (a mat + comforter) had been laid on the pile of soft warm sand. Whenever he became agitated he would extend his fingers and feel the smooth grains sliding between them, and calm down. It could be said that he had returned from whence he came. It is said that life is a journey; Baba was born into the desert; he spent his life first playing then working in the sand. It is thus entirely appropriate that as he approached the last of his many years, he should again return to the sand, even if it was only the truck loads of it brought from the Empty Quarter and piled into his bedroom!

The whole Home Care Team was awed by the resourcefulness of this family and how their need to cradle their beloved Baba in his final time was so successful. We all thought how much we too would prefer such treatment when it is our turn to be old.

I relate this true story as an illustration of the way Home Care works in Abu Dhabi. I believe that medical narrative has distinct advantages when trying to convey an idea of which many are ignorant. I could describe to you how we cope with 380 patients, how we are expanding to help get the patients at home with their families, how we are adding paediatric IV therapy patients and more ventilator cases, but I thought that this story would be of more real human interest. Our patients are our clients; in Home Care they are also our friends and our Joy. (Dr, Martyn Thornington, MBBS, CCFP, FCFP).

SEHA

In March 2007, the government of Abu Dhabi created a new management model health care system. As a consequence, the Health

Authority-Abu Dhabi (HA-AD) was formed to regulate the standards of all hospitals in the emirate of Abu Dhabi with a mission to enforce, and subsequently monitor, the adoption of internationally recognized quality standards, while Abu Dhabi Health Services Company (SEHA) was formed to manage all public owned hospitals and clinics, working hand-in-hand to ensure the delivery of first-rate medical care to the residents of Abu Dhabi.

The Cardiac Sciences Institute

It is a modern, state-of-the-art centre of excellence providing superior cardiac services. The institute specializes in:

- Non-invasive cardiology
- Interventional cardiology

In addition, SKMC is home to the

- Electrophysiology, only cardiac rehabilitation service
- Cardiac surgery in the Emirate, facilitating a smooth and stress-free recovery for patients. It consists of seven divisions including:
  - Adult and Pediatric Cardiac Surgery
  - Adult and Pediatric Cardiology
  - Adult and Pediatric Cardiac Intensive Care
  - Cardiac Anesthesiology SKMC excels in the science and art of coronary angiography and interventions, and provides round-the-clock primary angioplasty procedures. Cardiac Surgery provides the entire spectrum of surgical treatment of cardiovascular disease from a newborn baby to the elderly. The Cardiac Sciences Institute at SKMC is the only facility in Abu Dhabi to offer certain cardiac procedures, including complex cardiac operations for congenital heart disease in combination with interventional procedures (hybrid procedures), as well as all electrophysiology studies and ablation. With more than 50 highly qualified physicians, this institute is the largest and most integrated in local and international medical research and clinical trials, intensive care units as well as unique programs including primary angioplasty and electrophysiology.

The Surgery Institute

It offers secondary and tertiary surgical services and aims to provide the highest quality of care, consistently exceeding international standards of practice. Individual subspecialty divisions include: general dentistry, general surgery, neurosurgery, ophthalmology, oral-maxillofacial surgery, orthopedic surgery, otolaryngology, pediatric surgery, plastic surgery, thoracic surgery, urological surgery, and vascular surgery.

Guided by the objective to offer specialized and minimally invasive techniques, the Surgery Institute developed and expanded its services in solid organ transplantation and hepato-biliary surgery as well as bariatric surgery.

With a philosophy based on team-work and cohesive collaboration, SKMC has the ability to deal with the most complex of clinical problems from the UAE and beyond. The ICU is a modern area equipped with the most advanced technologies, and staffed by highly qualified specialist physicians from around the world. The eight state-of-the-art operating rooms at SKMC can handle a wide variety of procedures simple or complex, minor or major. In addition, SKMC is committed to the development of postgraduate medical training in the UAE and has one of the best Surgery Residency Programs.

The Pediatric Institute

It offers secondary and tertiary care to infants, children and adolescents by top qualified pediatricians using the latest technology. Within the Pediatric wards, 80 inpatient beds are dedicated to pediatric acute care, 20 beds for pediatric critical care, including pediatric cardiac surgery, 11 beds for dedicated pediatric emergency cases and 10 beds for day services. The Institute also manages a large outpatient department for general pediatric care, as well as cardiology, endocrinology and diabetes, gastroenterology, hematology and oncology, hepatology and nutrition;, infectious diseases, nephrology, neurology and pulmonology, etc.

The delivery of pediatric care is not limited to the Pediatric Institute; the diagnosis and treatment of patients is a result of the collaborative work of several SKMC departments including Anesthesia, Emergency, Medicine, Surgery, Radiology and Urology. All departments that work with pediatric cases are skilled in treating infants and children, while all pediatric ICU patients have around-the-clock care from board-certified pediatric intensive care physicians and pediatric nurses. With 14 new single rooms, the number of pediatric beds will stand at around 140. Quality improvement, clinical research, and internship and resident training programs are additional strengths of the Pediatric Institute.

The Medicine Institute

It is the main provider of acute medical services for the residents of Abu Dhabi as well as many other residents of the UAE. In collaboration with the SKMC Quality Council, the Medicine Institute is committed to optimizing patient care through set quality improvement methods. Strong emphasis is placed upon postgraduate education, both for institute staff and in the residency training programs for UAE National graduates. The Medicine Institute admits patients through the Emergency Department, outpatient services, or by direct referral. Medical services are managed through subspecialty divisions, including dermatology, diabetes and endocrinology, gastroenterology, hematology, infectious disease, nephrology, neurology, oncology, pulmonology, respirology and rheumatology.

Emergency Department at SKMC

It is the main public emergency department and trauma centre within Abu Dhabi city. It is located on the ground floor of the Surgical Pavilion with a helipad for transport of critically ill patients, with easy and quick access to CT scanning and ultrasonography. In addition, consulting services are available across a wide range of medical and surgical disciplines, utilizing a 24-hour call system. SKMC's world-class physicians in the ED have significant experience and expertise in trauma care and, together with the Surgery Institute, have had a real impact on the improvement of trauma care and its medical education in the UAE. The ED also has extensive experience in pre-hospital care as well as undergraduate and postgraduate medical education.

SKMC promotes mutual cooperation between the general medicine and psychiatric units to offer patients the best care possible. The Rehabilitation Unit is considered the most advanced community unit in the Middle East, with both a day centre and half-day accommodation for the rehabilitation of patients. In addition, a community case management team (CCMT) is also available. It is made up of a psychiatrist, a psychologist, a social worker and a nurse, who make regular visits to patients at home.

The principles of good Medicine are based on the following:

- Comfort of the patient first and foremost throughout their experience in the clinic.
- Evidence-based Medicine—treatment based on assured diagnostics.
- *Professionalism*—appropriate professional conduct in order to create system is built. Family medicine physicians have specific patient confidence qualifications through postgraduate study examination.
- *Advancement*—continual training, allows them to work within the SKMC Family Medicine System. The knowledge development and self-importance of early diagnosis along with patient comfort and well-learning of physicians being are crucial aspects of Family Medicine care.
- *Patient Advocacy*—a commitment to strengthen and maintain patient trust.

  The aim of the SKMC Family Medicine Clinics is to provide throughout the patients' health care preventative and primary care for common medical complaints, and to undertake early diagnosis and referral when specialty treatment is required.
- *Holistic Health care*—a combined approach to treatment that recognizes world-class professionals who are dedicated to the continuous development of medicine and strive to be the best in their field.

SKMC believes that in order to deliver a high quality of care, individuals should have easy access to continual care. A call centre was recently established to facilitate appointments at the Family Medicine Clinics. Appointments are usually given on the same day as the patient request is made.

Home Care Program

SKMC also has its own Home Care Program caring for 420 patients discharged from hospital who are willing to accept care at home and have mobility problems. Patient age in the Home Care Program ranges from newborn children to those in the twilight of their lives. Service is provided by a Consultant Family immunization programs, women's health Physician, a Specialist Physician with specialization in Cardiology, care, child care, teen health care, a range of acute to chronic care, geriatric care, Technicians, Dieticians and Occupational Therapists. The Home Care Program team helps, for example, patients requiring tracheostomy care, enteral feeding advice, wound care, 'activities, surgeries, and family counseling.

Family Medicine Clinics are the core around which the entire health care rests.

Abu Dhabi Blood Bank

Abu Dhabi Blood Bank (ADBB), located in the Al Khalidiyah area, is managed by the Laboratory Medicine department of SKMC. Supplying blood 24 hours a day, the ADBB functions as the major blood source for SKMC and the majority of Abu Dhabi's hospitals. ADBB is open for donations from Sunday to Thursday 07:00 to 21:00 (irrespective of public holidays) and on Saturday 08:00 to 13:00. A staff member is on duty, seven days a week, to issue blood and blood products to hospitals on demand. ADBB adheres to the most stringent international standards in the handling of blood and blood products, thereby ensuring the highest levels of patient safety. Highly qualified physicians, nurses, medical technologists, phlebotomists and ancillary staff work tirelessly to make certain that the blood supply in Abu Dhabi is safe and meets the needs of the health care community.

I-Care Solution

SKMC started the implementation of the Cerner Health care Information System (internally branded as the iCare solution) in July 2008 which was launched as part of a SEHA wide initiative to introduce the Electronic Medical Record (EMR) System for all of its facilities. Cerner is a leading worldwide provider of health information systems and technologies. The first phase involved the introduction of systems in Registration, Medical Records, Pharmacy, and Radiology. The second phase will include Physician Order Entry—Medications and Medical .Tests, Nursing Documentation, Laboratory, Surgery department, and Emergency department.

"The EMR system will eventually link all SEHA hospitals and clinics in Abu Dhabi, as it have been successfully implemented in Tawam, Corniche, Al Rahba hospitals, some of AHS clinics and today we are witnessing the implementation of the second phase at SKMC", he added.

Mr. Basheer Al Muhairbi, Information Technology Manager, SEHA added, "We are truly proud of the successful implementation of the HIS and are delighted to see this project implemented after months of studies, planning and hard work".

"By creating a unified electronic medical record for our hospitals and clinics across the region, the patient can utilize the services of any SEHA facility. The EMR system will help ensure patient information is available when and wherever a SEHA provider needs it. This system will noticeably accelerate the creation and management of patient records. It will always be up-to-date and complete. It is state-of-the-art", he added.

Dr. Tej Maini, CEO of SKMC, said "SKMC adopted the iCare Health Information System since July 2008. We were proud of the improvements that the new system brought us during the first phase. These improvements allowed our clinicians to partially run tests, make diagnoses, place orders, fill medications, document care and remit bills using a single information system. The new phase which will start from 5 December 2009 will add more features to our clinicians making the health care process safer and more efficient for our patients here at SKMC and for the population of the Emirate of Abu Dhabi who use SEHA's network of facilities".

Mr. Sulaiman H. Sulaiman, Chief Information Officer of SKMC said, "The second phase of the iCare solution is the next step in our journey to transform patient charts from its current paper state to the Electronic Medical Record (EMR) format. Studies have shown the implementation and utilization of the EMR enhances patient care and improves patient safety. At SKMC, our physicians will be able to quickly and easily retrieve test results in the exam room and review them with our patients. Additionally, the complete installation of the Digital Radiology PACS System in 2009 allowed our physicians to review x-rays and other imaging studies with their patients anywhere within SKMC and the Family Medicine Clinics."

"Our clinical and technical teams have been diligently working together to ensure that the transition to the new electronic system will be as smooth a possible. A comprehensive infrastructure and computer upgrade was conducted throughout 2009 to provide our staff with the right tools and access to use with the new system. Over 2800 of our staff have gone through an intensive training program to educate them on the use and benefits of the system. With the introduction of the new clinical functionality, we anticipate our staff to go through a big adjustment and a learning stage. Our experience tells, as a result of this change, we anticipate some delays over the first few days as staff become more familiar with the new system. We respectfully request our patients to be patient with the staff during this initial period", Mr. Sulaiman stated.

A number of clinicians and staff agreed that the HIS solutions saved them time and helped reduce missing charts and inaccurate information during the past year. It improved communication between care providers and patients, which facilitated quicker and more effective patient treatment. The new added features including Physician Order Entry for Medications and Medical Tests, Nursing Documentation, Laboratory, Surgery department, and Emergency department will add more value to the system and enhance the process of prescribing medications, requesting x-rays and other procedures, ordering laboratory tests, viewing the procedure results and documenting health information such as allergies and past medical history.

"SKMC has embraced the technology knowing that it will advance the care to our patients. We would like to thank all of our clinicians and employees for their involvement, dedication, and tremendous efforts in getting this system started, thus improving patient care. Additionally, we would like to thank the project team members for their dedication and commitment in building the system, training the employees, and deploying both phases of the iCare Solution," Mr. Sulaiman avowed. "SKMC management would also like to thank our patients in advance for working with us as we refine our processes during the implementation of the new system. The iCare system will ultimately allow us to improve patient safety and enable our employees to provide the highest quality of care possible."

Capsule Endoscopy

The newly offered service is the Capsule Endoscopy and SKMC is the first hospital in the region to use its full array of capsules. SKMC is owned and operated by SEHA, the Abu Dhabi Health Services Company, which is responsible for the curative activities of all the public hospitals and clinics in the Emirate of Abu Dhabi.

The Capsule Endoscopy technique has been started at SKMC under the supervision of Dr. Nigel Umar Beejay, Lead Consultant in Capsule Endoscopy, who was involved in using the first public demonstration of the capsule in the world in 2001 in Canada and who teaches and lectures internationally on capsule endoscopy.

Capsule Endoscopy is an examination of the digestive tract by using a self-contained wireless imaging device capable of transmitting images of the tract to an external receiver. Essentially, this allows doctors not only to visualize the small bowel (an area previously difficult to visualize) but also the complete bowel from gullet to colon. Moreover, such a procedure comes as a real relief to patients who are not candidates for conventional endoscopy with a camera inserted via a flexible tube, or who find such procedures uncomfortable.

Dr. Beejay, stated: "We are proud to announce that three types of capsule are available at SKMC to examine the esophagus, to examine the small bowel, and to examine the colon. Although the capsules have been available in other parts of the world, their use in the Middle East has been limited. Therefore, it is remarkable to have SKMC as the first hospital in the

Middle East to offer the full service of all three types of capsules in the UAE."

Remarkably, capsule endoscopy comes to SKMC at a time where it may be a possibility to offer colon cancer screening by colon capsule endoscopy rather than by conventional colonoscopy. The colon capsule technique may be preferable to patients especially women who may desire a less invasive method when looking for colon cancer.

The small bowel and esophageal capsules are internationally approved for visualization of the esophageal and small bowel lining in adults and children aged 10 years or more.

The most common applications for the small bowel capsule includes evaluation for the obscure GI bleeding (negative upper and lower endoscopy), iron deficiency anemia, suspected Crohn's disease, suspected small intestinal tumors, surveillance in patients with polyposis syndromes, and suspected or refractory malabsorptive syndromes (e.g., celiac disease).

Dr. Tej Maini, CEO of SKMC said, "We are proud to introduce these new techniques to our patients. It illustrates our commitment to deliver state-of-the-art medical practices. Less invasive approaches such as capsule endoscopy have well positioned us as an institution that allows its physicians to advance the standard of care for their patients. Physicians hired at SKMC are of a very qualified caliber and are always supported to offer the best care possible to our patients." Dr. Atul Mehta, Chief Medical Officer of SKMC stated, "Our interventional endoscopy team performs an average of 1500 endoscopy procedures yearly. The team has already performed two cases and have several others lined up to use the new capsules this year. Patient feedback has so far been excellent. We expect that up to 5% of the total number of patients undergoing endoscopy procedures at SKMC could be good candidates for the new capsule endoscopy technique."

Heart of the Matter

In a renewed call to tackle heart diseases—the number one killer in the UAE—expert cardiologist Dr, Wael Abdurahman Almahmeed, the Chairman of the Emirates Cardiac Society, consultant cardiologist and deputy chief medical officer at the Shaikh Khalifa Medical City (SKMC), said people in the Gulf develop coronary artery disease at a much younger age than their western counterparts.

"We have a big problem in terms of risk factors for coronary artery disease here, we have patients developing coronary artery disease at a young age of 50, which is 10 to 15 years less than the age at which their western counterparts develop it. This is the trend in the Gulf," said Dr, Almahmeed.

Noting the lack of good statistics in the UAE, Dr, Almahmeed cited a study conducted in Saudi Arabia about four to five years ago which found that about six per cent of the population had coronary artery disease and maybe up to 50 per cent of them have high cholesterol, up to 23 per cent have diabetes, 26 per cent of them have high blood pressure and 12.8 per cent smoke.

"We expect that we have similar numbers if not higher here in the emirates. We know for sure that about 25 per cent of the emiratis have diabetes, so we don't expect to have different numbers," he stated.

Coronary artery disease (CAD), also called coronary heart disease, is a condition in which plaque—made up of fat, cholesterol, calcium and other substances found in the blood—builds up inside the coronary arteries, which supply oxygen-rich blood to the heart.

Symptoms of CAD include central chest pain that goes to the neck and arm, shortness of breath, dizziness and palpitation. Dr, Almahmeed noted that the majority of CAD patients here are men but he attributed this simply to the demographics of the region, in which there are more men than women.

He emphasised however, that when women develop coronary heart disease, the prognosis is more complicated primarily due to age—coronary disease affects women usually 10 years after menopause, around the age of 60, while men are generally in their 50s when the disease hits them—and mainly because they're diabetic.

Women also do not present with the classic symptoms that men do, they may present with dizziness, shortness of breath, palpitations and vague pain but not central pain, and thus, these are often ignored by physicians, leading to misdiagnosis or late diagnosis. "Coronary artery disease in women manifests itself in a different way, particularly if they are diabetic, because the nerves are affected and that's why they don't feel the pain," Dr, Almahmeed elaborated.

Patients in the Gulf also tend to seek medical treatment later or present their conditions to their physicians late.

"In the West, when patients suffer chest pain, they go to the emergency very quickly. Here patients may wait. The average wait time is six hours here in the Gulf (while) in the West, it's around three hours," said Dr, Almahmeed.

He ascribed this to the lack of patient awareness with regards to the dangers of chest pain. According to the cardiologist, the number one cause of death in the UAE is heart disease and this includes stroke and cardiac arrest.

Lifestyle and genes are factors that contribute to the disease, however, in the Arab world, it's primarily lifestyle—the change from a rural Bedouin lifestyle to an industrialized sedentary one—which, over the course of time, may have dire effects on health.

Fifty per cent of UAE nationals are obese, especially the women.

"If you are obese, you're prone to develop diabetes, hypertension, high cholesterol, so you are at risk of developing coronary artery disease. Obviously, risk develops over a period of time, over 10-20 years. So, if we don't treat these risk factors today, within 10-20 years, we will face a huge burden of cardiac disease in this country," Dr, Almahmeed stressed.

He added that the responsibility in reducing the risk factors does not lie only on the patients and physicians; it involves teamwork and co-operation with all the relevant authorities to develop a national plan to deal with coronary artery disease. This includes ban on smoking in public places, providing more parks and pavements, open areas for playing sports and availability of affordable sports and exercise venues.

Urging people to move towards a healthier lifestyle Dr, Almahmeed advised, "Don't smoke, exercise at least thrice a week for half an hour each time and have a healthy diet, avoid junk food, fast food and food containing high levels of cholesterol."

Continuous Medical Education (CME) Conference on heart care

H.E. Dr. Abdulla Al Khanbashi said in the opening remarks, on behalf of H.E. Sheikh Nahyan Bin Mubarak Al Nahyan, "Under the leadership of the president, His Highness Sheikh Khalifa bin Zayed Al Nahyan, and with the guidance and strong support of Sheikh Mohammed bin Zayed Al Nahyan, Crown Prince of Abu Dhabi and the Deputy Supreme Commander of the Armed Forces, Abu Dhabi has a world-class health care system, with a clear focus on diagnosis, treatment, and public education. Regarding the scourge of heart disease, Abu Dhabi is committed to having the most advanced technologies, to detecting the disease as early as possible, and to implementing the most effective treatments and cures. Both SKMC and Zayed Military Hospital have excellent medical facilities that deliver high quality medical services. This conference is also an important indication of the strength of Abu Dhabi's commitment to excellence in health care."

The conference, accredited for 14.75 hours of Continuous Medical Education (CME), was attended by more than 200 Internists, General Practitioners, Cardiologists and Neurologists and Pharmacists during the first day. The conference includes seven different sessions covering all essential topics in the field of cardiac and vascular diseases. The first day included discussions on the status of cardiac disease in Asia and the Middle East, the management of cardiovascular co-morbidities (diabetes, dyslipidemia, hypertension), prevention of cardiovascular disease including impact of smoking cessation and importance of patient and public education. The talks were given by national and international speaker focusing on relevant topics to the Middle East and to the physicians of the community.

The second day focuses on peripheral vascular disease including an introduction to the epidemic of vascular disease which is vastly under diagnosed in this region. The topics are pertinent to the patients seen by the internists, general practitioners, cardiologists and neurologists in the community such as strokes and the role of safe carotid stenting, diabetic feet and its treatment which is a common problem in the Middle East. There shall be talks on Deep Venous Thrombosis (DVT's), venous problems, renal disease as well as evaluation of quality of cardiovascular care delivery in our region.

The speakers are experts in their respective fields and include international speakers from the World Health Organization (WHO) and from hospitals in Qatar, Kuwait, India, Sweden and USA.

Kidney transplant centre started functioning!

The first successful kidney transplant on a child in the UAE was performed at the Sheikh Khalifa Medical City (SKMC). The patient, a Pakistani girl who was operated upon in the first quarter of 2010, had an uneventful hospital stay and the clinical outcome was judged excellent. She was discharged from SKMC 10 days after the surgery. The five-year-old received the organ from her uncle, 40. The renal transplantation programme was started in February 2007 and was created under the guidance of Abu Dhabi Health Services (Seha) and Cleveland Clinic. Saif Bader Al Qubaisi, Chairman of Seha, accompanied by top officials, visited the child and her mother 10 days after the surgery to check on her recovery and commented favourably on the importance of organ donation, and how special donors are saving lives.

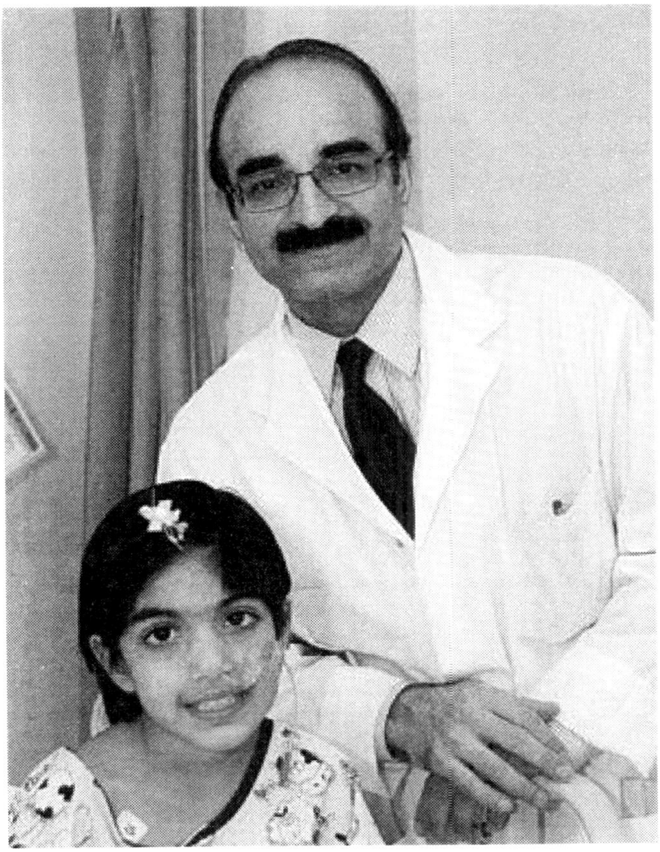

Dr. Abrar Khan with his patient

This historic surgery has had a tremendous impact on the life of this child—she will now live, play and enjoy her life just like any other child, the officials said. During his visit, Al Qubaisi praised the efforts of the surgeons and medical team of SKMC, saying: "The success is a source of great pride for Seha and SKMC."

World Thalassemia Day

Thalassemia Day on Thursday, 20 May 2010. The aim of World Thalassemia Day is to raise the awareness of the public on how to prevent thalassemia and that lives can be made more enjoyable and living with thalassemia can be made easier through education and appropriate care. SKMC is part of the SEHA Health System and is owned and operated by the Abu Dhabi Health Services Company (SEHA), which is responsible for the curative activities of all the public hospitals and clinics in the Emirate of Abu Dhabi.

To mark the World Thalassemia Day 2010, the Pediatric Hematology and Oncology Team at SKMC will organize several activities that are designed to bring the whole family together with others for the purpose of sharing information and raising the public awareness about Thalassemia. The group of activities organized target patients and their families as well as the public. For the children and families, a get-together will be organized on Thursday 20 May 2010 from 2:00 pm to 4:00 pm at SKMCs playground and will be attended by SKMC medical team, management members and patients families and visitors. Face painting, flower pot planting, arts and crafts will be arranged and gifts will be distributed amongst the children. Moreover, a group of 10 students from the Emirates College for Advanced Education will participate in this event. Coming to spread the joy amongst the children, they will visit some of the patients and spend valuable time with them. Furthermore, a booth at SKMC will be set-up during the day to provide information to staff and visitors and reinforce their knowledge about Thalassemia and the importance of pre-marital testing.

On the same evening, a booth will be set-up at Khalidiyah Mall (ground floor) from 06:00 pm until 9:00 pm targeting the public. Educational brochures and pamphlets on thalassemia and pre-marital testing in order to reach a UAE Free of Thalassemia will be distributed. Doctors and nurses will be available at the booth to help the public and educate them about the disease. Moreover, games and fun activities are arranged for children.

Dr. Atul Mehta, Chief Medical Officer at SKMC said, The Pediatric Hematology and Oncology division is determined to provide a wide array of services for hematology and oncology patients and supports public health education. We are committed to raising awareness of the public on pediatric hematology and oncology, and our booth during the thalassemia day, which will be set-up at Al Khalidiyah Mall, will serve this objective.

Dr. Ian Jefferson, Acting Chair of Pediatrics Institute at SKMC said, This event is the fifth participation of SKMC in the World Thalassemia Day.

We are objectively committed to raising awareness on Pediatric Hematology utilizing such international educational and health campaigns. Our Pediatrics Hematology division follows a multidisciplinary approach at SKMC where hematologists, pediatricians, cardiologists, endocrinologists, hepatoplogists, orthopedists, nurses, dentists, dietitians, social workers, physical therapists and psychologists in addition to other caregivers if needed link together in specialized care teams to look after each patients needs. SKMC Pediatric Institute is considered the largest and the most advanced in the UAE. It is our role to lead and take part in international health campaigns for children such as the two health campaigns we celebrated last quarter on Childhood Cancer and Hemophilia.

Dr. Azzam Al Zoebie, Senior Consultant and Head of the Pediatric Hematology and Oncology Division avowed that, SKMC is currently treating 66 children and 29 adults suffering from Thalassemia. The children with Thalassemia come to our Pediatric Short Stay Unit in the Surgical pavilion once every 3-4 weeks for blood transfusion as each blood infusion session would last 4-5 hours while the adults have their treatment and transfusion in the SKMC Infusion Centre. During their routine appointments, a physical exam is done by their physician to check their growth and development and tests to evaluate their organs function and iron status would be performed.

SKMC and Abu Dhabi Health Services Company (SEHA) are committed to providing the highest international standard of care for our patients and especially Thalassemia patients Dr. Al Zoebi added. We, at SKMC, are considered the first hospital, not only in the UAE but in the region, to offer the newly released oral iron chalator medication for our patients to use instead of the traditional injectable one and that has made a significant change in their lifestyle, compliance and outcome.

International Ambulatory Care Cay

The aim of celebrating the International Ambulatory Care Cay at SKMC is to gather nursing staff from all specialty clinics, introduce services provided at each specialty clinic at SKMC, and raise the awareness of the public and visitors about the role and duties of ambulatory care nurses.

During the day, nurses will be offering visitors free check-ups for the body mass index, blood pressure and blood glucose; and will distribute informational brochures about different health topics such as asthma, allergies, and promote positive habits as healthy eating and promote road safety and children safety. Baby car seats will also be displayed to new parents highlighting the importance of using car seats for children the minute they are discharged from the hospital after delivery.

Dr. Atul Mehta, Chief Medical Officer at SKMC said, "SKMC continuously participates in health campaigns, symposiums and activities. It is our mission to increase the awareness of the public about diseases prevention and healthy habits in addition to providing advanced surgical and medical services that meets internationally recognized standards of excellence to the residents of the UAE." Tarey Ray, Chief Nursing Officer commented, "SKMC employs almost 1600 nurses for inpatient and outpatient services. Amongst them, around 400 work at our 14 Outpatient Specialty Clinics and 6 Family Medicine Clinics, offering ambulatory care to our patients who do not require hospitalization. It is worth mentioning that in year 2009, we received 177,000 visits within the Outpatient Specialty Clinics and 321,000 visits in our Family Medicine Clinics." Mrs. Ray added, "Our Nursing Division is constantly evolving its practices to assure a high-level standard of quality and a focus on exceptional patient care and experience. We are very proud of our nurses who work in our clinics."

SKMC celebrates its tenth anniversary

Sheikh Khalifa Medical City (SKMC), managed by Cleveland Clinic, celebrated the tenth year anniversary of its Surgical Pavilion during the month of March 2010. SKMC is part of the SEHA Health System and is owned and operated by Abu Dhabi Health Services Company (SEHA), which is responsible for the curative activities of all the public hospitals and clinics in the Emirate of Abu Dhabi.

The chronicle begins with the establishment of the Central Hospital during the 1960s and then the establishment of Al Jazeera Hospital in the 1970s serving the whole population of Abu Dhabi under the management of the Ministry of Health. Numerous primary health care centres were opened during the same era in addition to the Abu Dhabi Blood Bank and a dental centre. During the 1990s, Behavioural Sciences Pavilion and Abu Dhabi Rehabilitation Centre were opened. This was followed by Sheikh Khalifa Medical Centre which was commissioned in the year 2000 to serve UAE Nationals offering a wide spectrum of medical and surgical services.

In January 2005, the Health Authority of Abu Dhabi announced the merger of Sheikh Khalifa Medical Centre, Al Jazeera Hospital, Central Hospital, Abu Dhabi Rehabilitation Centre, the 10 Primary Health care Clinics, Abu Dhabi Blood Bank, and a Dental Centre.

The new health care campus was renamed "Sheikh Khalifa Medical City (SKMC)", reflecting the true nature of the new organization. Following the merger, SKMC underwent a series of transformational events to take advantage of the new efficiencies realized from the unification. Both, the Sheikh Khalifa Medical Centre (currently re-branded as the Surgical Pavilion) and Al Jazeera Hospital buildings (currently re-branded as the Medical Pavilion) were connected to form the current 568-bed Main Hospital. Central Hospital was partially closed and scaled down to an emergency centre and an outpatient dialysis unit only.

Two years later and upon the signature of an official partnership between the Health Authority of Abu Dhabi and the Cleveland Clinic Foundation, the Cleveland Clinic which is heralded as one of the top hospitals in the USA took over the management of Sheikh Khalifa Medical City. During the same year, the Abu Dhabi Health Services Company, SEHA was formed. SEHA, a Public Joint Stock Company or PJSC, became the owner and operator of SKMC and SKMC became part of the SEHA HealthSystem as its Abu Dhabi flagship facility and largest hospital.

Under the management of Cleveland Clinic and the support of SEHA, numerous transformational projects were implemented. SKMC received the Joint Commission International Accreditation for its Main Hospital (Surgical and Medical Pavilions), Outpatient Specialty Clinics, Khalidiya Urgent Care Centre and Abu Dhabi Blood Bank. Abu Dhabi Central Hospital completely closed and all of its services were transferred to the main hospital in 2008 while a separate Urgent Care Centre located in Al Khalidiyah area under the management of the Emergency department was inaugurated to receive less urgent cases that are not life threatening.

In 2009, the Primary Health care Centres were transformed into six Family Medicine Clinics and two walk-in clinics. The two walk-in clinics will be transformed to Urgent Care Centres in 2010 similar to the centre located in Khalidiya area. Moreover, SKMC was accredited by the Society of Chest Pain Centres as a cycle III Chest Pain Centre, the only health care organization categorized under Cycle lll outside the USA and the 12th worldwide. SKMC also started new medical and surgical programs such the Renal Transplantation program and enforced education and research within all its divisions. A new electronic Health Information System (HIS) was also implemented at SKMC's facilities as part of SEHA's overall plan to introduce the Electronic Medical Records (EMR) in all its hospitals providing more functionality to improve the patient health care experience, greatly reducing the paper medical records, improving patient safety and enhancing patient confidentiality.

Commenting on this historic occasion, H.E. Saif Bader Al Qubaisi, Chairman of SEHA said, "The success we are witnessing at SKMC and in the health care sector in Abu Dhabi is the result of the continued support and wise leadership of our Rulers, and in keeping with SEHA mission to deliver world class health care to our patients and our vision to be compared with the best hospitals internationally. I want to congratulate the employees at SKMC whose hard work and dedication to excellence helped continuously achieve various accomplishments and successful patient's stories during the past ten years", he added.

Dr. Tej Maini, CEO of SKMC stated, "With SEHA's governance and Cleveland Clinic's leadership, the success and positive reputation of SKMC in the health care industry regionally would have been impossible without our multinational team of professional and well trained staff who make a difference by delivering high level of quality service to the community of Abu Dhabi and to our patients who come from all over the region. Since opening its doors exactly ten years ago and with all the mergers and changes that occurred, SKMC has succeeded in firmly establishing itself as one of the most prominent health care organizations in the United Arab of Emirates and the region."

Carl Stanifer, CEO of the SEHA Health System added, "I would like to add my congratulations as well to SKMC, its management team and professional staff. The residents of Abu Dhabi are indeed fortunate to have a hospital of the caliber of SKMC available to them. I have worked all over the world in 10 different countries including over some of the best hospitals in the United States and Asia and SKMC compares favourably with all of them. SKMC will continue to strive for greatness and we will continue to support its efforts to achieve result competitive with the best in class. The best is yet to come.

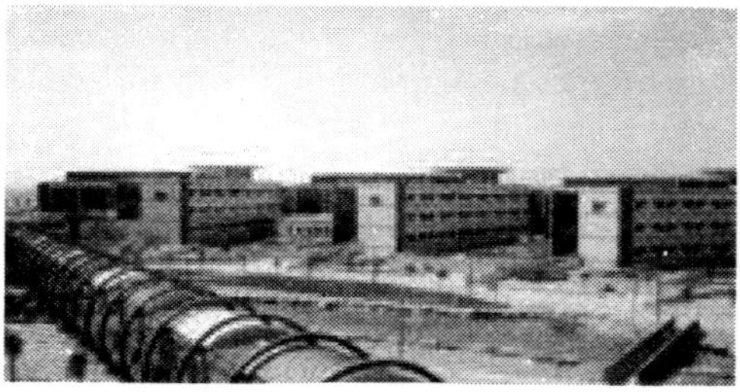

Zayed Medical Hospital

Zayed Military Hospital (ZMH) is located in Abu Dhabi, the capital city of the United Arab Emirates (UAE). ZMH is the only military hospital in the United Arab Emirates. ZMH has 365 beds capacity and provide medical services to more than 100,000 people. ZMH is a tertiary type hospital and its departments are equipped with the the most modern equipment.

6

King Abdulaziz Medical City (KAMC), Saudi Arabia

Saudi Arabia health sector is highly developing sector with vast economic resources being devoted towards providing safe and better medical facilities for all citizens. Saudi Arabia health facilities have constantly been improving with the opening up of many new medical institutions with the latest state-of-the-art facilities provided by them. One of the earliest initiatives undertaken by the King was to establish free health care opportunities for both the native citizens as well as for pilgrims who came to visit the religious sites in the kingdom. Consequently, the medical facilities started improving in Saudi Arabia and major developments were made through the five-year plans. In the initial years, emphasis was laid towards the development of hospitals, clinics, research facilities, laboratories and clinical pharmacies. In 1990, the number of government operated hospitals stood at 258 with the total capacity of 36,099 beds. Out of these, 64 were privately owned and 163 were managed by the Ministry of Health. At present, the Saudi Arabian people can avail the best quality medical services and have an access to all modern health care facilities.

KAMC

Saudi Arabia has excelled in setting up big hospitals and medical cities in the kingdom, in the recent years. National Guard Health Affairs (NGHA) is a large health organization providing modern medical care to National Guard employees and their dependents, as well as to Saudi Nationals with tertiary health problems. Under the umbrella of NGHA, there are four hospitals and sixty primary and secondary health centres around the Kingdom. The four hospitals have expanded over the last few years to become major medical cities; namely, King Abdulaziz Medical City (KAMC) in Riyadh, King Abdulaziz Medical City (KAMC) in Jeddah, King

Abdulaziz Medical City (KAMC) in Dammam (known as the Imam Abdul Rahman Al-Faisal Hospital) and King Abdulaziz Medical City (KAMC) in Al Ahsa. The four medical cities provide an extremely high standard of medical services including international Pediatric Surgery, Open-Heart Surgery, Oncology Centre, Organ Transplantation, Laparoscopic Surgery, Trauma Surgery, and many high-calibre tertiary and quaternary medical specialties. A recent project completion sees a new, 3,200-square-metre E.R unit including a trauma section, an adult clinic, a pediatric clinic, and an Obs/Gynae clinic.

KAMC Riyadh

It commenced its operations in May 1983. Since then, it has continued expanding, while providing services for a rapidly growing patient population in all of its catchments areas. The King Fahad National Guard Hospital has evolved to be part of the King Abdulaziz Medical City with many other prominent medical centres. Since its inauguration in February 2001; and within a short period, KAMC has been recognized as a distinguished health care provider. At KAMC, the bed capacity increased to 690 beds in addition to 25 beds allocated for expected surgical operations, and 132 beds for admission of emergency cases. The Emergency Care Centre at KAMC continues to be the best Trauma Care Centre in the Kingdom of Saudi Arabia. It is ranked as the 4th Emergency Care Centre outside the United States of America, to provide (PHTLS) Pre-Hospital Trauma and Life Support program. Ambulatory Care Services and Primary Health Care Services provide Preventive Health Services including health education and behavioural modifications to adopt healthy lifestyles. Surgical and Critical Units include an outstanding Burn Unit, Surgical ICU, Endoscopy Unit, Operating Rooms, and Neuro-Surgical and Surgical Units. The Neurological Rehabilitation Unit for Handicapped was inaugurated in mid 2003. In addition to that in September 2004 there has been an expansion and renovation of the Rehabilitation Department with both occupational and physiotherapy units along with the IVF clinic and OB in 2003, and Medical Imaging, Laboratory, Pharmacy, and continuous renovation of patients' wards. King Abdulaziz Medical City in Riyadh continued its success by providing the lowest mortality and morbidity rates among the patient population despite the fact that the Emergency Care Centre is located close to the Riyadh-Dammam highway and receives plenty of cases with acute injuries.

JCI Accreditation

To improve health care quality it has passed the requirements for accreditation under the (JCI) Joint Commission International. This accreditation included all of its hospitals, namely, King Abdulaziz Medical City in Riyadh, King Abdulaziz Medical City in Jeddah, Imam Abdul Rahman bin Faisal Hospital in Dammam and King Abdulaziz Hospital in Al Hassa. In 2004 Saudi Government established the College of Medicine and the College of Nursing and Allied Medical Sciences. It added to its mission an academic dimension through the establishment of King Saud bin Abdulaziz University for Health Sciences, which will comprise all academic activities and will be the core of the medical scientific university for future generations.

KACC

The King Abdulaziz Cardiac Centre (KACC) is located within the King Abdulaziz medical City (KAMC) complex in Riyadh, Saudi Arabia. KACC has emerged as a rapidly expanding successful cardiac program committed to patient focused care, serving 4 million inhabitants as well as referral from other cities. KACC participates in training medical students in medical university campus (King Saud bin Adulaziz for Health Sciences). KACC started operations in 1999 and moved to its present dedicated centre in 2002. The centre provides a complete range of services including Adult Cardiology, Pediatric Cardiology, Cardiac Surgery and Cardiac Anesthesia.

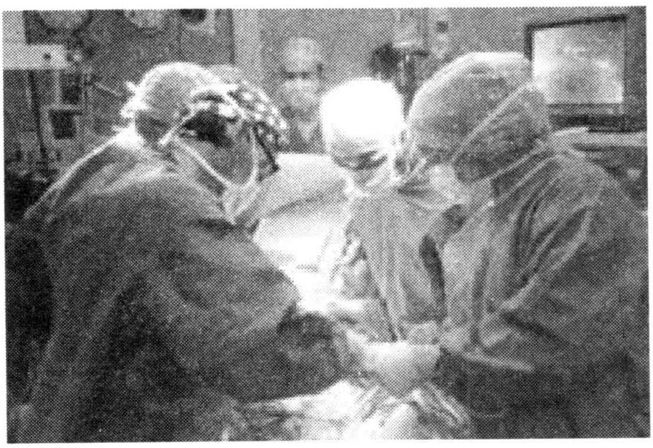

In 2002, the centre opened with 60 in-patient beds, 3 catheterization laboratories and 3 operating rooms. All beds are in private single rooms with windows open to natural sunlight. There are dedicated independent Intensive Care Units including adult cardiac surgical, pediatric cardiac surgical, medical cardiac and coronary care. As the centre built a local and international reputation the volume rapidly expanded resulting in full utilization of all available in and outpatient resources. With this success the need to expand the service became an urgent priority. A major expansion was approved in 2005 to double the beds and provide dedicated clinics. To immediately address the lack of beds an additional 15 telemetry beds were added in an adjacent building. This unit will be utilized for the care of congestive heart failure patients when the new centre opens. This unit will have a dedicated team of physicians and nurse specialists who will coordinate CHF clinic and in-patient care to insure optimal management of this, the most expensive of cardiac diseases. This unit will be a model for CHF disease management for the region. When the expansion fully opens, more than 150 beds will be available 60 of which will be critical care. The facility currently operates 4 Catheterization Laboratories, 4 Operating Rooms (OR's). A fifth OR in the existing theatres area will open in 2010. The new east wing has three 3,400 m^2 floors (10,000+ m^2) that will include 75 telemetry beds and an enhanced outpatient facility including a Lifestyle Modification Program.

Heart Transplantation

A Heart Transplantation Program is planned to be included as part of the enhanced CHF program. Currently, KACC has an advanced Nurse-Based Physician-supervised CHF and Atherosclerosis clinic. This comprehensive, multi-disciplinary program is unique to this region and has enrolled more than 1000 patients. A large research room, monitored recovery room, and a Lifestyle Modification Program are part of the enhancements for this program. Construction of a dedicated advanced cardiac imaging building will commence following opening of the expansion. This purpose designed building will accommodate high tech equipment including a Cardiac PET/CT Scanner, MRI, Nuclear Gamma Cameras, Image Fusion Technology, and a Robotic EP/Intervention Cath Lab System. This facility will be the most advanced, integrated cardiac imaging facility in the region. In 2006, the centre introduced pediatric and adult cardiac MRI and 64 slice CT scan examinations. Two Cardiac MRI/CT qualified consultant specialists supervise these procedures. One was trained at Toronto General Hospital and the other at Mayo Clinic. They have up-to-date echo machines including 10 3D Philips IE33 systems which are connected to an advanced cardiac imaging storage system (PACS) system (Xcelera).

Electronic medical records

The cardiac centre has implemented a comprehensive data driven reporting system that will soon automatically send information from cardiac systems to the Misys electronic medical record. In addition, this system will help with quality improvement and research. An ICU chartless system—Carevue is now implemented in CCU and Medical Cardiac ICU beds. This system is being expanded to other cardiac and hospital ICU areas. The main hospital (KAMC) introduced a full radiology PACS system which is also a great success. The cardiac service was originally a consultant based service in the 1990's with no junior staff. Due to the major increases in the workload and advances in the hospital, assistant consultant posts were generated. All assistant consultants are highly qualified and experienced. There is a handover meeting every morning where the cases of the previous evening are discussed by the cardiac team. Education and research is a priority with ongoing programs and new initiatives reflecting the interests of the growing staff. The centre produces many publications annually and there are ample opportunities for staff to participate in studies. A new separate major research building for Medical City has been approved this year and will house the cardiac research programs. KACC is supervised and run by Cardiac Executive Board. The board has representatives from all the cardiac sub-specialties. The Cardiac Centre was selected to organize the most recent Saudi Heart Conference. This event was a great success and included very successful live transmission of cardiac interventions from the National Guard Hospital and from France.

Department of Emergency Medicine

The Department of Emergency Medicine at KAMC is committed to the provision of quality emergency care, Resident and Fellowship training, and continuing Medical Education, Saudi-ization of the workforce and customer satisfaction in line with the mission statement of NGHA. Department of Emergency Medicine's mission is also to provide evidence-based, quality care to those who are in need of treatment, while ensuring efficiency and the proper utilization of resources. The state-of-the-art facility has more than 88 active beds, in 6 Clinical Divisions operating 24/7 all year round, divided into the following categories:

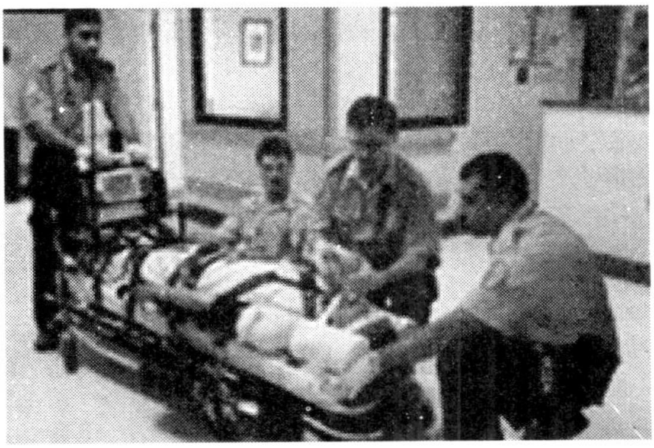

Front Desk Area

All patients received in this department are initially seen at the front desk. Patients that have acute critical conditions are placed into Critical/ Pediatric Care Areas expeditiously and patient registration is performed at the bedside. The more stable patients are initially triaged at the front desk and then proceed to Registration and formal physician triage.

Triage Area

The Triage Away of non-eligible patients, and those eligible ones with minor ailments, is done in the confined space (2 exam beds) of the Vital Signs Area of the ED, to the surrounding Primary Health Care Units is an important but stressful function. This function is performed by the ED staff physicians guided by the department's established Triage Away Policy and ongoing monitoring.

On average, > 40-50% of patients is actively, but appropriately, triaged away to respective NGHA, PHU or external centres where they are eligible.

Critical Care

This is a 16-bed unit with state-of-the-art equipment, which is needed to resuscitate the acutely ill and injured patients, excluding pediatric (PC Area) as well as gynecological emergencies (AC Area). A dedicated room in Critical Care is used for decontaminating patients with any chemical exposure before they access the clinical areas of the Emergency Department

Adult Care

This is a 25-bed unit where patients with intermediate medical and surgical conditions are treated. This area has two dedicated fast track beds to deliver expeditious care to those patients that are signed into the department, especially during peak hours. Obstetrical and Gynecological patients are initially assessed in this area. Includes a nebulization room and an acute psychiatric patient care room.

Pediatric Care

This is a 26-bed unit for the care of Pediatric patients with critical, intermediate, and low acuity as well as resuscitation cases. Includes a nebulization room, hydration area and an observation area.

Urgent Care Centre

This is an 8-bed unit for the care of eligible urgent cases with minor urgencies. It includes a suture room and nebulization rooms.

Observation Area

This is a 10-bed unit, dedicated for the care of patients that need an extended period of observation (< 24 hrs) in the emergency setting, to prevent premature disposition and discharge of patients or minimize unnecessary costly hospitalizations. This area operates utilizing strict clinical protocols, treatments (e.g. IV hydration, asthma, etc.) or reassessment (e.g. chest pain, abdominal pain, etc.) with predetermined clinical outcomes. The idea of EDOU is to decrease the number of unnecessary admissions thus decreasing the patient load of admissions to the hospital from the Emergency Department. Additionally, preventing pre-mature discharge and improving the quality of care provided

Emergency Medical Services Division (EMS)

EMS has several roles; one is an ambulance service provider for all NG locations and transport of discharged patients in need inside and outside of Riyadh city. The EMS personnel play an essential supporting in-hospital role in assessment of all incoming cases of accidents, trauma or non-ambulatory/stretcher cases whether brought in by ambulances or private vehicles; and initiating immobilization protocols if indicated. They also participate as a team member in responding to in-hospital code green cardiac arrest cases.

Disaster Management

The rapid changes in the physical layout of KAMC-Riyadh necessitated a revision of the organization's original Disaster Plan, available to staff via the intranet since April 2006. It was first activated during the May 2003 bombings and on several subsequent incidents since. A Disaster Coordinator position was created and a permanent Saudi candidate assigned.

Residency, Interns and Medical Student Training Programs

The rapidly evolving changes in the vision and direction of KAMC-Riyadh necessitated a corresponding response to meet the needs of a newly emerging academic training department. Since October 2001, the department has achieved and maintained unconditional approval designation for its residency training programs in both the Saudi Board in Emergency Medicine and the Arab Board in Emergency Medicine.

Pediatric Emergency Medicine Fellowship Training Program

Our program is under the umbrella of Saudi Council for Health Specialization. It is a joint venture between KFNGH, KFSH and KKUH; five fellows are currently in the training program (3 in the first year, 2 in the second year) with three graduated from program.

Adult Emergency Medicine Fellowship Training Program

We have accepted two new fellows into the Adult Emergency Medicine advanced training fellowship; which aims to train Board Certified physicians from general specialties such as Family Medicine and General Surgery, in Emergency Medicine. The target group is people already working in an emergency department who seek further training to optimize their practice.

Emergency Department Quality and Performance Improvement Programs

The rapidly evolving changes in the vision and direction of KAMC necessitated a corresponding response to meet the needs of a newly emerging quality improvement and management performance activities like morbidity and mortality case reviews; documentation, patient triage away/signed-in audits. The division has been working on these and other indicators since 2000. A full-time QM Specialist oversees these activities, assisted by three technicians PCT's.

Intensive Care and Burn Units

The new state of the art Intensive Care and Burn Units have been built and equipped through a generous philanthropic donation made by the Custodian of the Two Holy Mosques, King Abdullah bin Abdulaziz Al

Saud, in the name of his late mother, Fahda Bint Alasi bin Shraim. The new unit, which was opened in May 2000, has been dedicated and named in her memory. The Intensive Care Department is organized to provide a unified, multidisciplinary approach to critical care in a state-of-the-art, Intensive Care Unit (ICU) and Intermediate Care Unit (IMCU) and to support critically ill patients throughout the hospital via the Critical Care Response Team (CCRT).

Intensive and Critical Care

Critically ill medical and surgical patients are managed in a consultant based system 24 hours a day, 7 days a week by Critical Care Board certified Intensivists who are also qualified in the fields of Internal Medicine, Anesthesiology, Pulmonary Medicine, Infectious Diseases and Emergency Medicine. Working collaboratively with a multidisciplinary team of critical care fellows, critical care nurses, respiratory care practitioners, clinical pharmacists, nutritionists, physical therapists and others, the department strives to provide the best evidence-based care at the highest safety and quality standards. The consultant-based coverage has been a role model worldwide. In addition, the department has become a centre for promoting critical care education throughout the country and the region. The department has active clinical research program and has conducted and participated in multiple international Randomized-Controlled Trials.

The Mission of the Intensive Care Department is to provide exemplary care for critically ill patients at the optimal safety and quality standards, conduct cutting edge research related to critical care medicine, and educate tomorrow's leaders in the management of acute life-threatening illnesses and to promote critical care profession locally and worldwide. The Home Health Care Program is playing a major role in providing a high standard medical, psychological, and nursing care for already discharged long-term care patients.

Transitional Care Unit

The Transitional Care Unit in Ward 22 consists of 26 beds, usually provides medical chronic complex type of care (Chronic Ventilation, Hemodialysis, Tracheostomy, and Wound Care) to medically stable patients who step down from the acute bed setting and yet need some time in a sub-acute care setting in order to maximize their physical function and promote possible independence if any.

Rehabilitation Unit

The Rehabilitation Unit is consists of 18 beds and it provides care for neurosurgery and medical patients who require rehabilitation.

Long-term Care Unit

The Long-term Care Unit consists of 44 beds. It provides basic nursing and medical care for patients whose clinical condition is stable, chronic, terminal or non-curable. These patients have marked mental and physical impairment and lack adequate socioeconomic and family support that is needed for home discharge.

Department of Medicine

It is the primary goal of the Department of Medicine to ensure that every possible effort is directed to fulfil its role in meeting the mission of the National Guard Health Affairs in providing National Guard personnel and their eligible dependents as well as all other eligible patients with the highest quality of safe tertiary health care while ensuring efficacy and proper utilization of resources. Equally important to the mission are the components related to medical and health education and the scientific research.

The Department of Medicine's vision is to create a professional standard where the highest caliber medical staff are recruited and retained, and up-to-date medical equipment are purchased and maintained while the appropriate rules and ambitious plans are set to ensure that the Department of Medicine provides patients with nothing but the best available practice, residents with the best attainable training, and employees with the best possible working environment.

Divisions

The Department of Medicine is composed of eleven divisions which provide specialized high-standard medical care. These divisions are as follows:

- Division of Dermatology
- Division of Endocrinology
- Division of Gastro-enterology
- Division of Infectious Diseases
- Division of Internal Medicine
- Division of Mental Health
- Division of Nephrology and Renal Transplantation
- Division of Neurology
- Division of Physical and Geriatric Medicine
- Division of Pulmonology
- Division of Rheumatology

Department of Pediatrics

The Department of Pediatrics' mission is to strive for excellence in the management of childhood diseases and to develop a program of postgraduate training to meet the future needs of the medical services in the National Guard and to generate the future leaders in the field of Pediatrics and Child Health for the Kingdom of Saudi Arabia.

Main Objectives of Pediatrics Department

- *Patient Care*: By supporting and enhancing the pediatric component of patient care in the hospital.
- *Medical Education*: To create Postgraduate Residency and Fellowship Programs in Pediatrics which will be comprehensive, earning recognition for its excellence throughout the Kingdom.
- *Biomedical Research*: To encourage individual talent and develop biomedical research activities.
- Community Health Awareness.

The department of pediatrics continues to set the pace for phenomenal development and growth in this difficult economic environment as it raises the standards for excellence in each of the core mission areas—patient care, medical education, research, and community health awareness.

All Staff have participated equally in the provision of tertiary health care in their subspecialty as well as general pediatric care. The Department continues to serve as a major resource for children with complicated health problems that require high-quality skills of consultants with various subspecialties. There are 45 consultants, of whom 83% are Saudi. On average, there are 2-3 consultants in each pediatric subspecialty. These subspecialties include Allergy/Immunology, Endocrinology, Gastroenterology/Hepatology, Genetics/Metabolism, Infectious Diseases, Intensive Care, Nephrology, Neonatology, Neurology, Respirology, Rheumatology, Adolescent medicine in addition to Ambulatory Care and General Pediatrics. The department has seen incredible refinement in the quality of services delivered by pediatric subspecialty divisions. The department continues to excel in it steadfast commitment to provide high quality health care to our patients despite all the day-to-day challenges it faces. There has been a significant annual increase in the clinical quality and acuity.

The Primary care

King Abdulaziz Medical City, Riyadh provides primary, secondary and tertiary service with a capacity of 690 beds and has approximately 1.4 million outpatient visits a year. It has established itself as a centre of excellence as it has the largest Emergency Care Centre in the Middle East, a state of the art Hepatobiliary Sciences and Liver Transplant Centre, a state of the art Cardiac facility, Dental Care Services Department with various specialties, Long-term and Extended Care Services for patients requiring long-term nursing care, and the recently commissioned Oncology Unit. The Department of Pathology and Laboratory Medicine is a large and modern medical laboratory accredited by the Commission on Laboratory Accreditation of the College of American Pathologists (CAP) and the American Association of Blood Banks (AABB). The Department has maintained its CAP accreditation and JCIA. The Department of Pathology and Laboratory Medicine, in this tertiary referral centre, supports the King Abdulaziz Medical City, Riyadh and provides selected laboratory service to the other regional hospitals, including King Abdulaziz Medical City, Jeddah, King Abdulaziz Hospital, Al Hasa, Al Imam Abdul rah man Bin Faisal Hospital, Dammam, as well as many primary health care clinics and polyclinics located throughout the Kingdom.

Department of Oncology

The Department Of Oncology was established in 2005 to state of the art care for patients diagnosed with cancer. Currently the Department of Oncology has five divisions including: Adult Hematology, Adult Medical Oncology, Gynecology Oncology, Pediatric Hematology/Oncology, Palliative Care and Radiation Oncology.

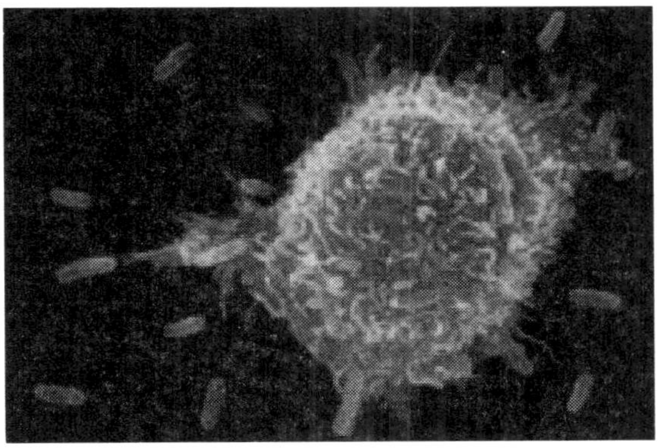

- A new Radiation Centre was developed to add this important modality to our Cancer Centre.
- All our consultants have trained in North America and are highly qualified in their field.
- Our goal is to provide multidisciplinary care following the most advanced approaches in cancer care.

KAMC Cancer Centre vision is to be the leading regional cancer centre and rank among the nation's premier comprehensive cancer centres by providing:

- World-class research in the prevention, detection and treatment of cancers and their related conditions.
- Comprehensive and compassionate care, in a multidisciplinary approach that is responsive to the needs of our patients and their families.
- Renowned teaching to ensure exceptional cancer care and research for future generations.

- Information and education to improve the health and welfare of our community.
- A dynamic and progressive atmosphere responsive to the needs of our patients and community.
- To provide a comprehensive clinical service through a multidisciplinary approach that focuses on physical, emotional, social and environmental aspects of care on each patient and their family during active treatment and end stage.
- To enhance the community education on the identification of the early signs and symptoms of cancer and increase awareness on cancer screening.
- Participate and collaborate with other agencies in the development of "Support Group".
- Provide educational opportunities to physicians and allied health professionals who wish to specialize in cancer field.
- Conducting research related to detection, diagnosis and treatment of cancer.
- Collaborate with National and International organizations to fight cancer.
- Sponsor high quality educational symposia and workshops.

Department of Anesthesia

The mission of the Department of Anesthesia is to provide patients requiring anesthesia care at the King Abdulaziz Medical City with the highest standard of comprehensive anesthesia care, utilizing the services of our highly trained staff and the use of the latest in anesthesia technology. We shall provide a comprehensive pre-anesthesia evaluation, intra-operative care and post-operative follow-up.

Department of Anesthesia being involved in a training and development program which trains staff in all aspects from administration to anesthesia technicians, the department also has a residency training program which is responsible for training excellent anesthetists within Riyadh and Saudi Arabia in addition to training fellows on sub-specialty in Pediatric and Cardiac Anesthesia.

These goals are achieved through the recruitment of the most qualified staff, the continuous education of all staff, medical research and audit of our practice, utilization of the most current of medical technology, and planning.

Divisions and Staff

- *Cardiac Anesthesia*: Provides anesthesia care for patients undergoing cardiac surgery, or cardiac catheterization for diagnostic and therapeutic interventions. The division provides 24 hours emergency call in-house.

- *Pediatric Anesthesia*: Provides anesthesia care for neonates, infants and children up to the age of 14 years, for surgical and non-surgical procedures. The division provides 24 hours emergency coverage only as back-up support to the on-call anesthesiologist in the main OR in cases of neonatal emergencies or very sick small children. The pediatric anesthesiologist does not reside in-house, and will come to the hospital only if called by the in-house consultant anesthesiologist. The pediatric anesthesiologist also provides other clinical services upon request from the Pediatric ICU or the Pediatric ER, mainly for insertion of central lines or to manage difficult intubation.
- *Hepatobiliary and Liver Transplant Anesthesia*: Provides anesthesia care for patients undergoing cadaveric or living-related liver transplant. It also covers major Hepatobiliary surgery. There are twc consultants (or one consultant and one associate consultant) on-call on 24/7 basis. In addition, another separate anesthesia team is on-call 24/7 for kidney transplant.
- *Pain Management*: Provides Acute Pain Service for all patients, mostly for post-operative pain relief on a 24/7 basis. The division also runs three Chronic Pain clinics per week and three half-day sessions per week for interventional chronic pain procedures.

Obstetric Anesthesia: Is not yet officially constructed, however, a group of anesthesiologists are assigned to obstetric anesthesia and one candidate is identified as "In-Charge" of the service. Hopefully when the manpower and space requirements become available, the division will officially be launched. At this point of time we provide anesthesia coverage by a consultant and a junior anesthetist (resident/staff physician/assistant consultant) during working hours. After working hours, one consultant covers both the Main OR and the obstetric ward. We aim at providing separate consultant coverage during the night for this important area. The division provides anesthesia care for c-sections and Statistical Data

During the year 2007, the department of Anesthesia had 16057 Anesthetics, 1787 pain management cases and 10211 patients at the Pre-Anesthesia Clinic.

Achievements

Our Division of Pediatric Anesthesia has performed the largest series of conjoined twins separation in the world with the best outcome. This clinical achievement has made our department famous around the world. The conjoined twins anesthesia team leader wrote a chapter in a famous Pediatric Anesthesia text book about anesthesia for conjoined twins.

Dental Services Department

The mission of the Dental Services Department at King Abdulaziz Dental Centre (KADC) is to provide the National Guard personnel and their dependents with the highest quality of primary, secondary and tertiary dental health services while ensuring efficiency and proper utilization of available resources. It also functions as a referral clinic as well as diagnoses and provides treatment to oral diseases and dental trauma cases. The King Abdulaziz Dental Centre (KADC) functions as a complete dental treatment facility and as referral clinics that diagnoses and treats cases of oral diseases or dental trauma cases that require the services for one or more dental specialties.

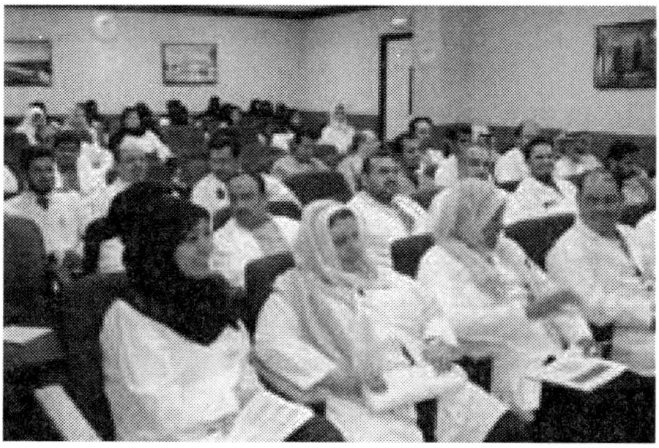

As a tertiary dental health care provider, the available dental specialties KADC include Pedodontics, Prosthodontics, Restorative Dentistry, Endontics, Periodontics, Orthodontics and Maxillofacial Surgery. KADC top priority is to provide primary dental care to National Guard personnel and their dependents through the various primary health care centres throughout the Central Region. KADC also provides emergency tertiary dental care for in-patients as well as patients in the main hospital's Emergency Room. Additionally, KADC is providing routine and tertiary dental public health care for the medically compromised patients (MCP). An active program in dental public health care has been put in motion by giving preventive dental health care among children and by raising the level of dental health awareness among the National Guard population. Four brand new and sophisticated dental mobile vans with two dental chairs per van are being utilized to compliment this program.

A state of the art Dental Laboratory is also housed at the King Abdulaziz Dental Centre (KADC). The laboratory deals with the design, fabrication and repair of artificial dental restorations. Dental devices prepared in the laboratory include crowns, prosthesis, maxillofacial prosthesis, dental bridges and other dental appliances according to dentist's specifications. Laboratory training programs are also provided to NGHA's Saudi Career Development Program (SCDP) participants, technology interns and summer training students.

Other dental supports which are essential and important contributors to the successful and comprehensive dental services are the Dental Hygienists and Dental Assistants. We are proud of our Saudization process as 96% of our dentists are Saudi while 23% of our support staff is Saudi.

In the academic front, they are providing advance training to young dentists through Advance Education in General Dentistry (AEGD) Program. We are also participating in the Saudi Council Programs such as Saudi Specialists Certificate in Advance Restorative Dentistry [SSDDent (ARD)], Saudi Specialists Certificate in Orthodontics [SSD-Dent (Ortho)] and Saudi Specialists Certificate in Prosthodontics [SSC-Dent (Pedo)]. Recently, we extended our participations by providing Saudi Specialists Certificate in Endodontics [SSC-Dent (Endo)].

KADC has set its sight also on Continuing Education by providing seminars, lectures and workshops presented by both local and international speakers. Under the auspices of NGHA, KADC successfully launched its first ever Dental International Symposium entitled New Dental Era on January 2006 at the Marriot Hotel in Riyadh. Schedules are now in place for other future Continuing Education events.

Liver Transplant Program

Since the inauguration of the Liver Transplant Program at KAMC in 1994 it is expanding constantly. Its active staff and cases being treated are in a constant increase. It has expanded to include the surgical operations and necessary interferes for liver, gallbladder, pancreatic diseases. Such increasing activities necessitated the establishment of a new Centre to satisfy the program's expansion and the pressure from all facilities Kingdom-wide. In 2001, Hepatobiliary Sciences and Liver Transplant was transferred to its new Centre.

Services provided by the centre

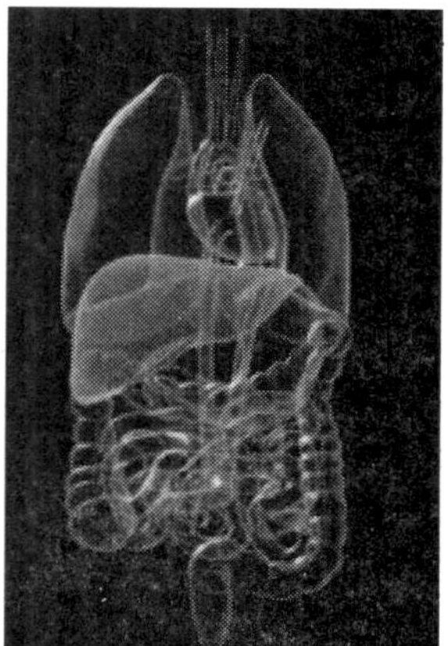

The Centre comprises an admission suite for investigation, treatment and surgical operations for liver cases, e.g. tumor excision and liver transplantation. It comprises out-patient clinics with its ancillary services in which the referred patients are screened and followed up. The Centre receives hundreds of medical reports for review and provides consultation either to the patients or the referring centres Kingdom-wide. Therefore, the Centre is serving the Kingdom as being a main centre for treating liver diseases, as it comprises qualified staff in the different fields related to adult and pediatric hepatology, including liver transplantation and Pancreatic and Hepatobiliary surgeries.

The Centre developed many important programs e.g. liver transplant program through brain-death donors, or partial-liver transplant from living-related donors, from patient's relatives.

Kidney Transplant Centre

- Achieved the highest number of kidney transplants ever done in this hospital and more than double what it was 5 years ago.
- Improved integration of the Hepatology service into the department.
- Significant improvement of the interpersonal harmony between the staff in the department and with all other departments in the hospital. This is evident by testimony of many departments and medical staff.
- The department was (and still is) a major contributor in the successful JCI accreditation process.

Medical Imaging Department

The Medical Imaging Department mission is to provide the finest diagnostic and intervention imaging service to the eligible National Guard Health Affair Patients and Physicians. The highest caliber imaging service will be provided, within budgetary restraints in a modern, patient-friendly atmosphere utilizing state of art equipment. The department will provide a work environment that is pleasant and safe, and affords dignity and respect for all. The department is totally committed to improvement of standards and to committing sufficient resources into continuing education, audit and research.

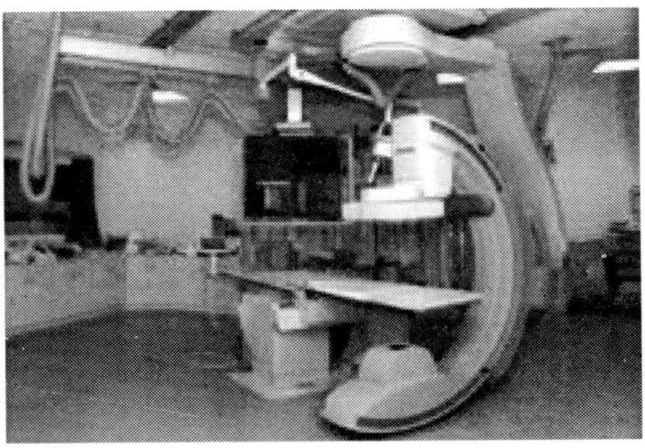

The department of imaging is the premier and largest imaging facility in the Middle East and is built upon a system of competence, teamwork, and innovation and provides the finest diagnostic and intervention imaging service to the eligible National Guard Health Affair patients, and physicians. The department is totally committed to improvement of standards and to committing resources into continuing education, audit and research. The radiology team is composed of board-certified radiologists from prestigious international institutions who represent every specialty and subspecialty of radiology from Neuro-radiology, Siamese twin separation radiology, cardiac radiology and interventional angiography to trauma and women's imaging. Over 100 technologists and allied science personal trained to international standards are employed.

Intervention

- Radiofrequency Ablation of Osteiod Osteoma
- Fallopian Tube re-canalization for infertility
- Coil embolization of cerebral artery aneurysms
- Coil embolization head and neck arterio-venous malformations
- Thrombolysis for strokes
- Vertebroplasty for osteoporotic and metastatic fractures
- Colonic Stenting
- Tracheal Stenting

Computed Tomography

- Virtual colonoscopy
- Carotid CT Angiography
- Cardiac CT
- CT Venography

MRI

- Perfusion brain imaging
- ADC mapping
- Spectroscopy

Nuclear Medicine

- FDG SPECT
- In 111-Octreotide for neuroendocrine tumours
- MIBG for neuroendocrine tumours

Musculoskeletal Radiology Intervention and Therapy

- Hip injections
- Subtalar Injection Block
- Knee injection
- Epidural Injection
- Sacro iliac joint injection
- Shoulder injection

- Greater trochanteric bursitis therapeutic injections
- Lesser trochanteric bursitis therapeutic injections
- Gangrene injection
- Bone biopsy and Spine biopsy under CT guidance
- Soft Tissue Biopsy

Department of Obstetrics and Gynecology

The Department of Obstetrics and Gynecology at KAMC—Riyadh is the busiest department in our medical city with more than 40% of admission and discharges, and 8,697 total deliveries for year 2008. The department consists of three sub-divisions with sub-specialist consultants.

Divisions

- *General Obstetrics and Gynecology*
  Provide care for general obstetrics and gynecological patients via outpatient in Clinic 101, inpatients services in Wards 1, 2, 3 and 4 and nursing and midwifery care is performed in our Labour and Delivery unit.

- *In-Vitro Fertilization and Reproductive Endocrinology*
  Provide In-Vitro Fertilization treatment to patients with the inability to become pregnant. With assisted reproduction, a man's sperm and woman's egg are combined until fertilization occurs and thereafter, the embryo is transferred back to the woman's uterus for development.

- *Perinatology: Feto Maternal Medicine*
  Perinatology is a subspecialty of obstetrics and perinatologist are physicians who have extensive training in the field of high risk obstetrics thus providing care for both mother and fetus with a higher than normal risk for complications. Under this division, many fetal abnormalities are detected at an early in pregnancy at high percentage accuracy rate.

Statistical Data

- Number of deliveries almost 9,000
- 50% of our patients are high risk patients
- Caesarean section rate + 20%
- IVF and Reproductive Endocrinology unit treats 900+ patients per year
- Almost 40,000 examinations performed last year (2008) in the ultrasound unit
  - o In the main unit, almost 8,000 ultrasounds performed with 133 invasive procedures.

Achievements

- Lowest perinatal mortality rate in the country, 5.7/1000
- Diagnosis of fetal abnormality is extremely high
- Our department has the highest passing rate of residents for the Saudi and Arab Board exams. Most of the gold medals were from our institution

Department of Surgery

The mission is to strive for excellence in the surgical management of all our patients ensuring patient safety, patient satisfaction and teaching residents to meet their future needs. To achieve our goals and objectives, we adapted the concept of shared decision-making to collect the responsibility of individuals, team accountability and professional collegiality. Furthermore, the Department of Surgery's eleven Divisions has been very pro-active and resourceful in which we are extremely proud of the Division's accomplishments for their continuing efforts and collaborative support.

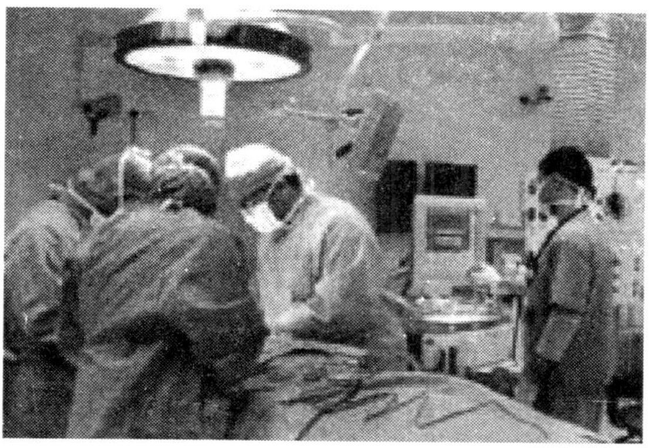

We believe that the Department of Surgery possesses an immense potential which allows us to survive some minor and major setbacks, but remain positive and strong, with a hope that we will continue to work hard to carry on with the ongoing process of striving for excellence!

Divisions

- Division ENT Surgery
- Division of General Surgery
- Division Neurosurgery
- Division of Ophthalmology
- Division of Oral and Maxillofacial Surgery
- Division of Orthopedic Surgery
- Division of Pediatric Surgery
- Division of Plastic Surgery

- Division of Thoracic Surgery
- Division of Urology Surgery
- Division of Vascular Surgery
- Podiatric Surgery Unit

Department of Infection Prevention and Control

The Department of Infection Prevention and Control is comprised of three main sections. Each section has its own objectives, goals, activities, and achievements, and each provides specific services to the hospital, affiliated clinics, and communities in the central region. It also oversees the activities and collaborates with the Infection Prevention and Control programs of the Western and Eastern provinces.

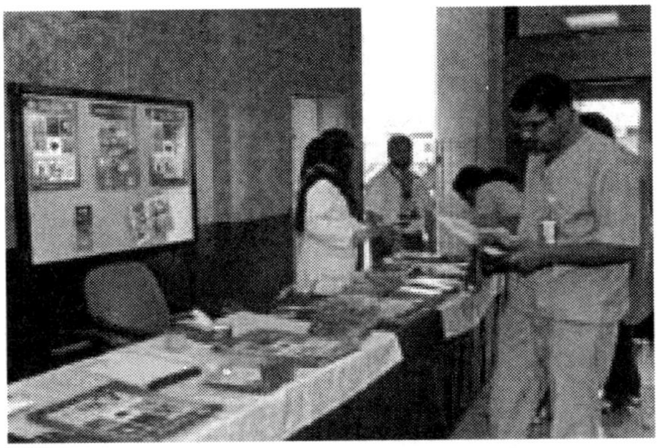

Divisions

The Department of Infection Prevention and Control has three directors one for each different division:

- *Hospital Infection Control Section*: To support the National Guard mission of promoting patient safety by reducing the risk of acquiring and transmitting infections; and to become a leader in our region in health care epidemiology and infection control.
- *Public Health and Field Epidemiology Section*: Public health section is focused on how to determine specifically the infectious diseases in National Guard community, promote health and prevent spread of infection.
- *Environmental and Occupational Health and Safety Section*: Our goal is to promote the health and productivity of employees of the NGHA KAMC by preventing and managing occupational and environmental injuries, illnesses and disabilities. We are committed to fostering a safe and healthful environment for patients, employees, visitors and communities.

NGHA Primary Health care Centres are working on providing the best precautionary and therapeutic services as well as contributing in serving patients and reducing pressure on the NGHA hospitals.

- Outside Riyadh:
  - Hail—Najran—Al-Qassim—Rafha—Arar
- Riyadh Region:
  - King Saud Residential City and Satellite Clinics (3 satellite clinics)
  - Crown Prince Palace, First Brigade Clinic
  - King Khalid Military Academy Clinic
  - Prince Bader Residential City Clinic
  - Second Brigade Clinic
  - Private Brigade Clinic
  - VIP Clinic, King Fahed Hospital
  - Employee Clinic, King Fahed Hospital
  - King Abdulaziz Residential City and Satellite Clinics (10 satellite clinics)
  - Family Practice Clinic, Al-Yarmok (King Abdulaziz Residential City)
  - Urgent Care Centre, Al-Yarmok (King Abdulaziz Residential City)
  - Health Care Specialty Clinic, Primary Health care Clinic
  - Health Care Specialty Clinic, Family Practice Clinic
  - Health Care Specialty Clinic, Urgent Care Centre
  - Health Care Specialty Clinic, Brigade and Battalion Clinics

King Abdullah Medical City in Makkah and Mina

Custodian of the Two Holy Mosques Saudi King Abdullah bin Abdulaziz inaugurated King Abdullah Medical City in Makkah and Mina Al-Wadi Hospitals. The two key health care facilities will serve the residents of the holy city of Makkah and Muslims performing Hajj (pilgrimage) and umrah (minor pilgrimage) all along the year. "The Kingdom of Saudi Arabia spares no efforts in providing the best possible medical service to the citizens, foreign residents and pilgrims," King Abdullah wrote in the official register of the medical city. "The Saudi authorities give top priority to the constant development and modernization of the health care sector within the framework of a visionary integrated approach," the monarch affirmed.

"Despite the challenges posed by the Influenza A (H1N1) pandemic, the health authorities, backed by King Abdullah, managed, thank God, to safeguard the safety of the pilgrims and control the outbreak of the fatal disease," the minister said in the inauguration ceremony. "This royal patronage embodies the keenness of the leadership on providing the best quality of health care for citizens, residents and pilgrims," he affirmed "King Abdullah's care for the health care sector is evident in three aspects, namely, the constant follow-up of the safety of citizens and residents, the endorsement of the medical cadre for all medical personnel at government hospitals and the support for the integrated health care strategy," Al-Rabee'a affirmed.

A row of medical cities

King Abdullah Medical City is the kingdom's third such key project after King Fahad Medical City in Riyadh and King Fahad Specialized Hospital in the north-eastern city of Ad-Dammam. With a total area of 800,000 square meters, the city is part of the national project for integrated and comprehensive health care. Its total bed capacity amounts to 1,500 beds, 500 of them for specialized hospital. The five-storey facility has all medical specializations including the rare ones such as radiology and digital radiography. It is equipped with the latest medical equipment in line with the world's most modern standards.

The maternity and pediatrics wards of the hospital have 500 beds. The hospital has rooms for additional bed capacity when other specializations are added in the future. With a total area of 3,400 sq meters, the three-storey Mina Al-Wadi Hospital has 200 beds for various specializations.

Saudi Arabia is leading the way with a total expenditure on health care construction projects of more than $6.6 billion, while the UAE and Qatar are closely matched at $2.9 billion and $2.8 billion respectively. Saudi Arabia has a total of 83 projects ranging from the $400 million King Saud University Medical City in Riyadh to the $5 million Qatif Central Hospital expansion in the Eastern Province. Qatar has two projects currently underway, but one alone is the region's biggest and most ambitious—the Sidra Medical and Research Centre which forms part of Doha's Education City development and budgeted at $2.3 billion. In the UAE, the biggest project is the $1.9 billion first phase of the Cleveland Clinic Al Suwwa Island development in Abu Dhabi and the second is the Mohammed bin Rashid al Maktoum Academic Medical Centre in Dubai Health Care City budgeted at $572 million. Kuwait has a one major hospital project under construction—the $1.2 billion Jaber Al Ahmed Al Sabah Hospital. Bahrain, meanwhile, is spending $130 million on the King Hamad General Hospital.

King Fahd Medical City (KFMC)

King Fahd Medical Centre was constructed from the year 1984 to 1995. The King Fahd Medical Centre is located in the Sulemanian area of Riyadh and covers an area of 50.50 hectares. The King Fahd Medical Centre is also known as King Fahd Medical City Complex and is easily accessible from all directions of the capital city. As stated in the beginning, King Fahd Medical Centre comprises of 4 hospitals with a total of 1095 beds and 33 Primary Clinics which also serve the purpose of an Outpatient Unit and provide the facilities of X-Rays, pharmacies, laboratories and screening patients. The four hospitals in the King Fahd Medical City Complex are—The Obstetrics and Gynecology Hospital, The Pediatric Hospital, The Specialist Hospital and The Rehabilitation Hospital.

- *The Pediatric Hospital*—It was officially inaugurated in the early summer of 2003 and has 246 beds. It has the latest state-of-the-art technologies and special care units for children.
- *The Obstetrics and Gynecology Hospital*—It was officially started on October 26th, 2003 and has 236 beds. There is also an Outpatient Department and special units for women's medical care.
- *The Rehabilitation Centre*—This centre has 154 beds and preparations are still under construction for the best quality of rehabilitation care.
- *The Specialist Hospital*—It has 459 beds and will have the latest medical technology for specialized medical care.
- *The King Fahd Medical Centre*—It will enhance the medical structure of Saudi Arabian country and will earn a high reputation for the countrv.

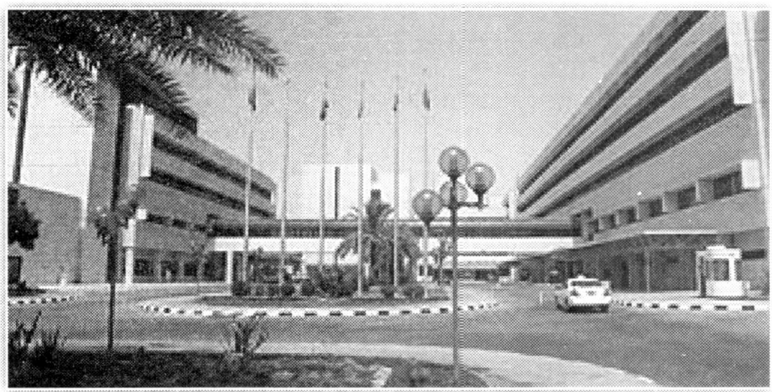

In addition to the hospitals there are a burns treatment unit, kidney centre, intensive care facilities and spinal cord treatment unit. The opening of KFMC coincided with the 23rd anniversary of Custodian of the Two Holy Mosques, King Fahd's accession to the throne. King Fahd donated SR53.98 million to purchase medical equipment. KFMC's yearly operating budget is estimated at SR300 million for medical and non-medical maintenance and catering contracts. It is expected to treat more than 50,000 in-house patients and more than 600,000 outpatients annually, the minister said.

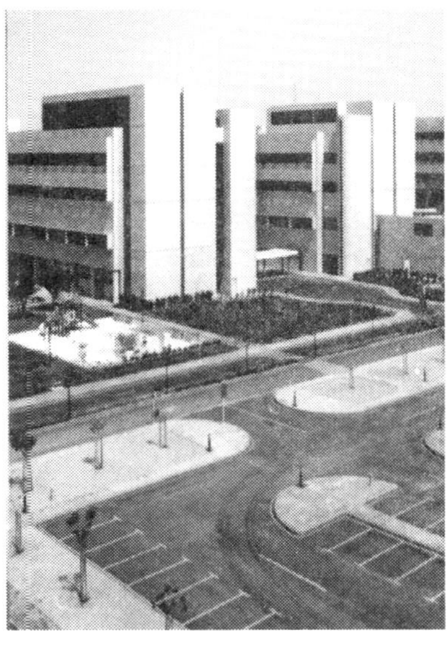

The Specialist Hospital (459 Beds) has the latest state of the art medical technology; will be the pioneer tertiary care centre providing third and fourth levels of specialized medical care. Commissioning will also include inauguration of specialized centres of excellence in every major medical specialty to serve as a hub for excellence in medical care.

- Main kitchen and staff dining (seats max. 436)
- Bulk Stores
- Pharmacies
- Central Sterile Supply Department
- Administration (Purchasing and Accounting Depts.)
- X-ray and M.R. Archives
- Mortuary and Autopsy Suite
- Imaging Dept.
- 50 Outpatient Clinics
- Accident and Emergency Facilities

The Obstetrics and Gynecology Hospital (236 Beds) Officially inaugurated and commissioned on October 26th, 2003, the Obstetrics and Gynecology Hospital with its latest state of the art medical technology is a pioneer tertiary care centre providing specialized medical care for women. There is also an Outpatient Department with the Obstetrics and Gynecology departments.

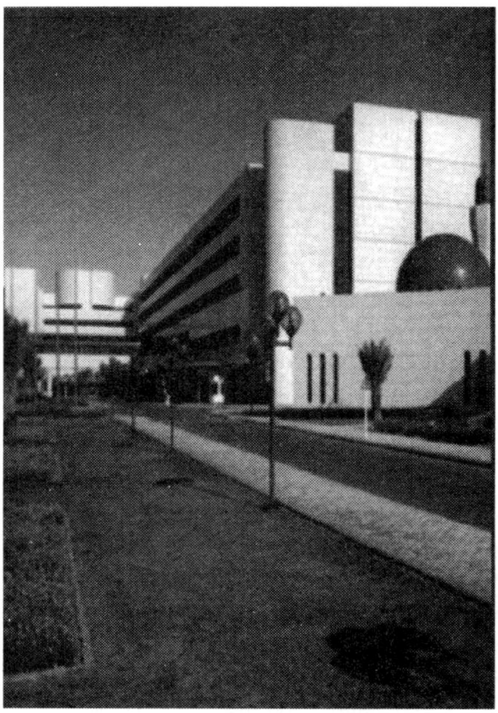

- Administration and Admissions
- Library and Medical Records
- Outpatient Dept. with Gynecology and Obstetrics Depts.
- Ultrasound Suite
- Dispensing Pharmacy
- Accident and Emergency Dept. plus Minor Operating Room

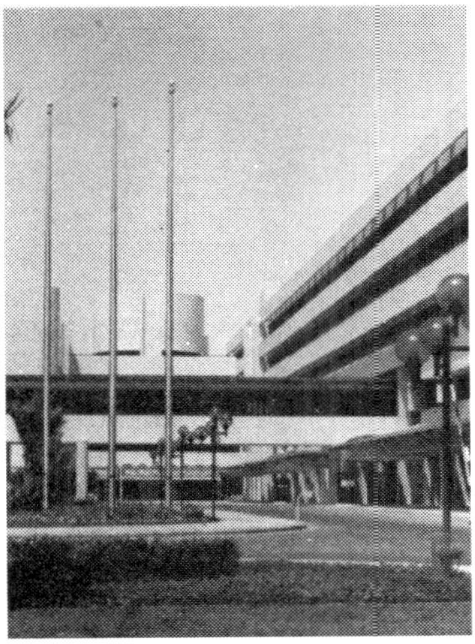

The Pediatric Hospital (246 Beds)

Officially inaugurated and commissioned in early summer of 2003, the Pediatric Hospital with its latest state of the art medical technology is a pioneer tertiary Pediatric care centre providing specialized medical care for children in every pediatric specialty and subspecialty. It has seven floors consisting of Sub-basement, Basement, and Ground and First through Fourth.

- Medical Library and Central Records
- In Service Training Facilities
- Administrative Offices
- Pharmacy
- Security Office
- Operating Theatres

Additional Laboratories (cont'd from General Labs).

The Rehabilitation Hospital (154 Beds)

With preparations underway for commissioning the latest state of the art medical rehabilitation technology; the Rehabilitation Hospital will provide high level tertiary rehabilitation care.

- Main Reception Concourse
- Physiotherapy Department with Hydrotherapy pool, Whirlpools and Activity Room
- 6 Outpatient Clinics

Incorporated in the Medical Complex on the site are Specialty and Facilities including:

- Burns Treatment Unit
- Kidney Centre
- Radiology
- Rehabilitation Facilities
- Intensive Care Facilities
- Spinal Cord Treatment Unit

Some other hospitals in Saudi Arabia in brief.

King Abdullah Medical City, Mecca, Saudi Arabia

King Abdullah Medical City is located in Mecca, Western Region of Saudi Arabia. KAMC consists of 3 hospitals and 10 Medical centres. KAMC is Ministry of Health Hospital and it has special budget from Government of Saudi Arabia

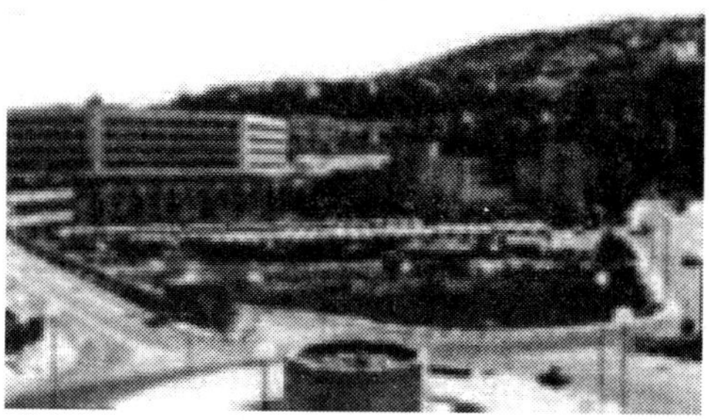

King Fahad Specialist Hospital—Dammam

King Fahad Specialist Hospital is located in Dammam, Eastern Provine of Saudi Arabia. It is a tertiary hospital and it is a Ministry of Health Hospital. The capacity of KFSH is 640 beds and it is equipped by the latest technology. KFSH in Dammam source for its staff from all around the World. All consultant physicians, Senior Nursing staff and Senior Paramedics must be qualified from North America and Western countries. KFSH in Dammam provide competitive salary and great benefits to its staff. In addition, employees are housed in hospital compound which it is well furnished, has swimming pools, gym, tennis, volleyball, basketball and other entertainment facility.

King Abdulaziz Medical City—Alahsa

Construction of King Abdulaziz Medical City, Alahsa was completed on June, 2002. It has 300 beds capacity and it provide primary, secondary and tertiary medical services to National Guard personnel and their dependents in the Eastern Province of Saudi Arabia.

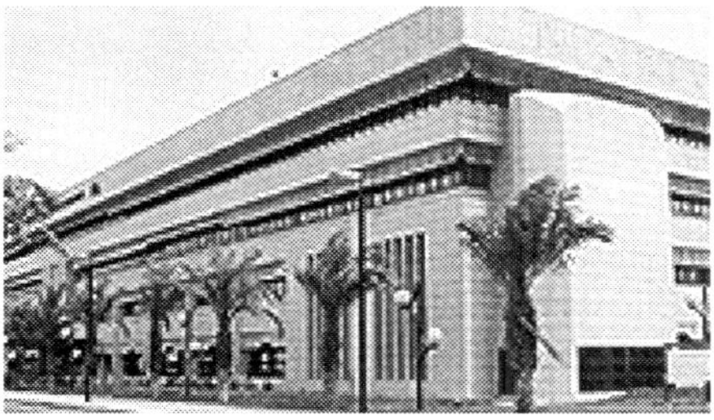

King Abdulaziz Medical City—Dammam

King Abdulaziz Medical City in Dammam construction was completed in June, 2002. The hospital has 100 beds capacity. It is equipped with the latest state of the art medical equipments and recruit its staff from all around the World.

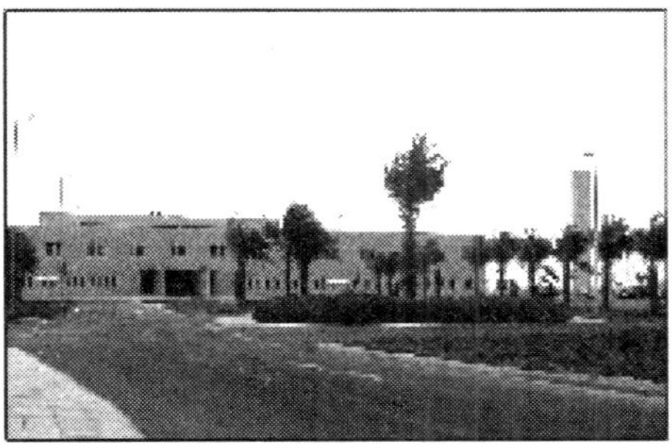

King Abdulaziz Medical City—Jeddah

King Khalid National Guard Hospital in Jeddah was founded in July, 1982. In year 2001, King Khalid National Guard Hospital became part of King Abdulaziz Medical Cities. King Abdulaziz Medical City, Jeddah is a tertiary type of hospital and its mission is to provide state of the art medical services to National Guard personnel and their dependents in the Western Region of Saudi Arabia. KAMC in Jeddah has around 350 beds.

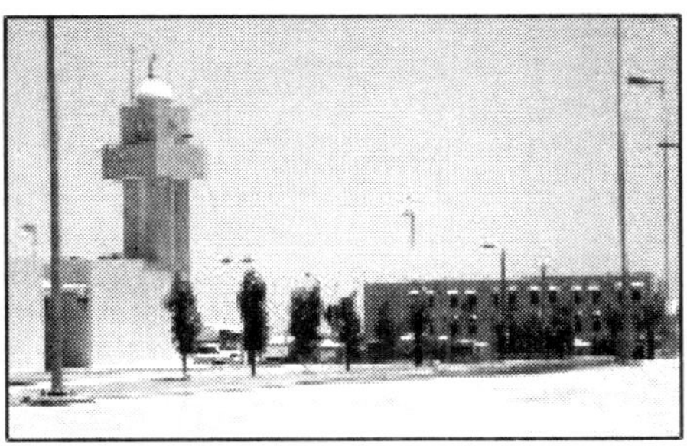

King Abdulaziz Medical City—Riyadh

. King Fahad National Guard Hospital in Riyadh commenced its operation in May, 1983. In year 2001, King Fahad National Guard Hospital became part of King Abdulaziz Medical Cities. King Abdulaziz Medical City in Riyadh beds capacity is 691. Since many years KAMC in Riyadh recruit its staff from many countries all around the World. Many physicians, nurses and paramedics are recruited from North America, Western Europe, Australia and South Africa. KAMC in Riyadh is a tertiary type hospital and conform to the highest International medical Standard.

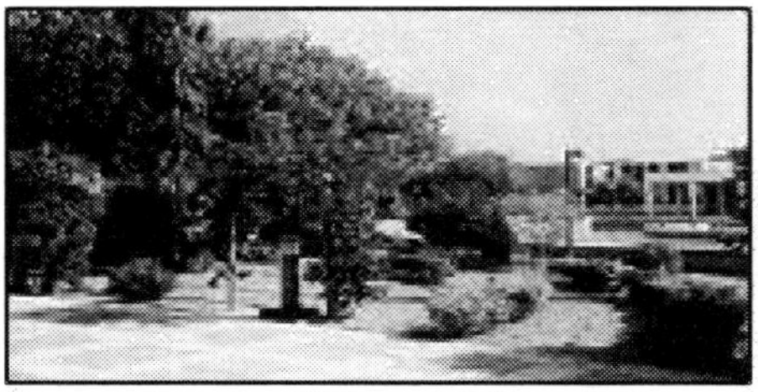

Sultan Bin Abdulaziz Humanitarian City

Sultan Bin Abdulaziz Humanitarian City (SBAHC) is a 400 bed rehabilitation hospital which was open on October, 2002, to provide inpatient and outpatient rehabilitation medicine. The city is located north of Riyadh in the Banhan area, Saudi Arabia. The patients are provided with the highest quality of medical services by well experienced medical staff, nurses, and rehabilitation specialist. SBAHC objective is to be a worldwide centre of excellence in rehabilitation, providing the highest standards of international health care in Kingdom of Saudi Arabia

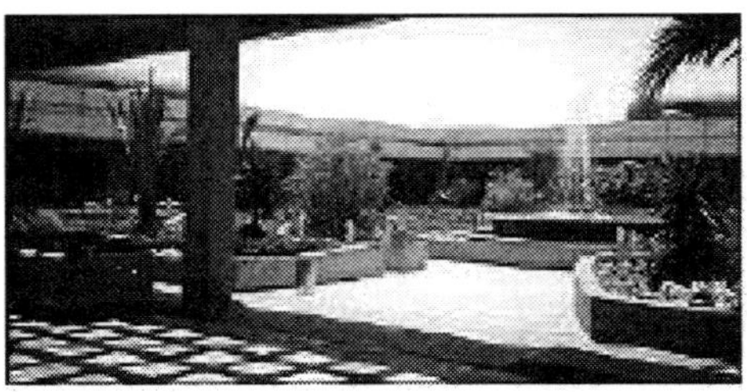

Saad Specialist Hospital (SSH)

Saad Specialist Hospital (SSH) was opened in year 2001. SSH main goal is to provide high quality of medical services to the local community. SSH provide modern tertiary medical services mainly to the Eastern Province population and to the Saudi population in general. SSH is located in Al Khobar in the Eastern Province of Kingdom of Saudi Arabia. It is located within few miles away from Demmam and Dhahran. SSH was built and constructed according to the highest international standards and it is accredited by Joint Commission International (JCI). Saad Specialist Hospital consists 600 beds hospital.

King Faisal Specialist Hospital and Research Centre in Jeddah (KFSHRC)

King Faisal Specialist Hospital and Research Centre in Jeddah (KFSHRC), commenced providing medical services to Jeddah city and to the Western Region of KSA in March 2000. It is 200 beds hospital equipped with the most modern medical equipment and medical technology available at present time. KFSHRC recruits many of his medical, nursing and paramedical staff from North America and Western European countries.

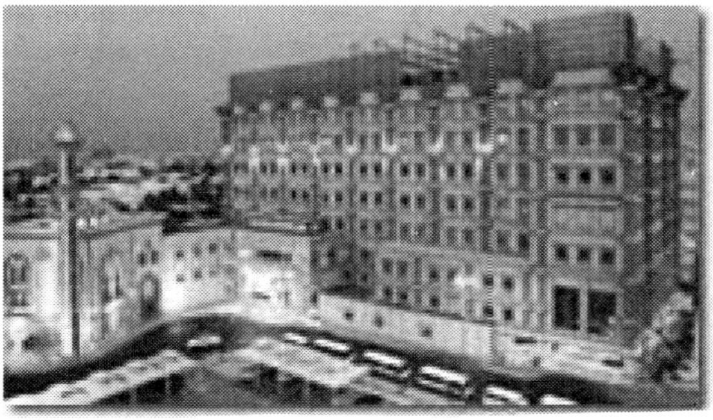

The hospital is accredited by Joint Commission International (JCI). KFSHRC is located on the coastal city of Jeddah on the Red Sea. City of Jeddah is a cosmopolitan city and it is the second largest city in KSA. It has 2 million population. In Jeddah, you will find modern shopping malls, variety international cuisine and many luxurious hotels spread all around the city.

King Fahed Military Medical Complex (KFMMC)

It is a little more than 300 beds, which provide primary, secondary and tertiary medical services. It is located in Dhahran. Its medical equipment contains the latest technology for expatriate staff, it is according to the Western standards and it contains recreational facilities. Furnished housing is provided for all staff.

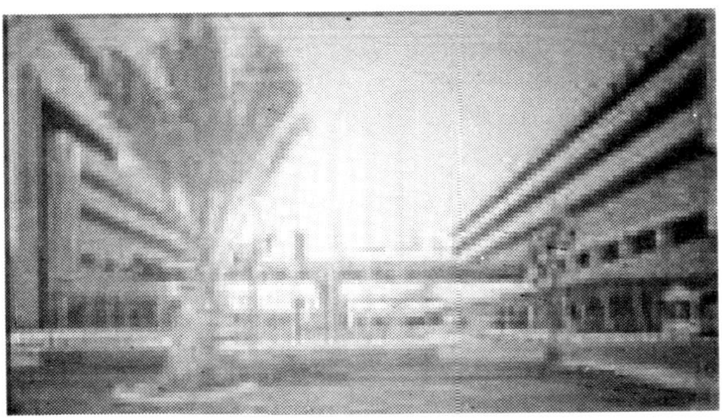

King Fahed Military Hospital, Jeddah

King Fahed Military Hospital in Jeddah is a 250 beds acute care centre providing medical care for Saudi Arabian Military personnel and their dependents. The hospital provides excellent housing facilities for its staff. It is located in Jeddah, a city of 2 million population.

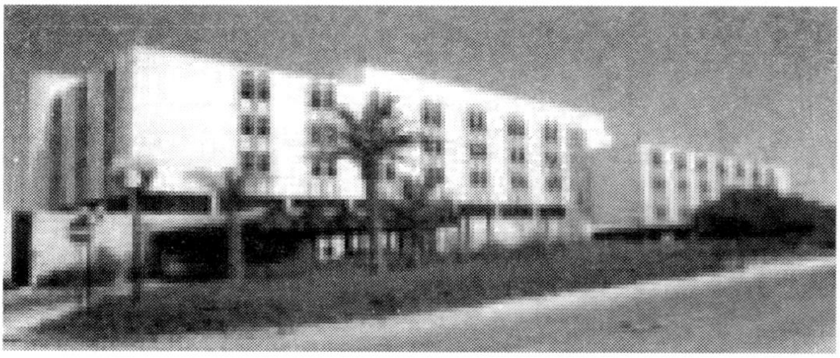

King Khalid Eye Specialist Hospital, Riyadh

The King Khalid Eye Specialist Hospital (KKHESH) is the largest eye hospital in the Middle East. Among the services offered by the hospital are Cataract Surgery, Corneal Grafting, Optometry, Clinical, Psychophysical and Electro Physical Laboratories, Ultrasonography and Pharmacies. There are 12 fully equipped operating theaters and 17 bed recovery rooms. The hospital provides excellent furnished housing for its staff. KKESH is located in Riyadh, the Capital of Saudi Arabia.

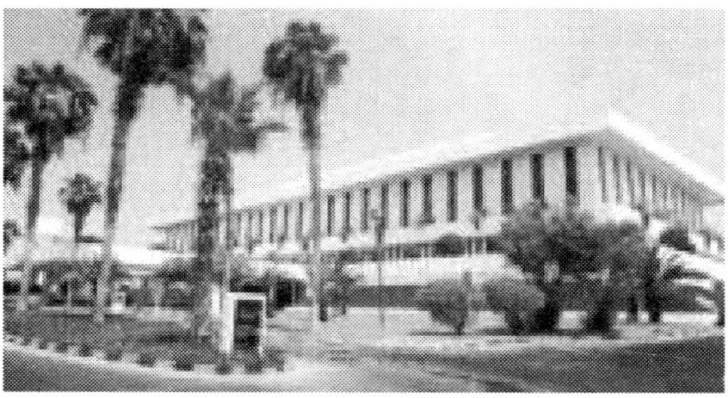

The Riyadh Armed Forces Hospital (RAFH)

It is located in Riyadh City, which is the capital of Saudi Arabia. The RAFH Hospital is approximately 770 beds. In addition to providing excellent care for patients, RAFH is heavily involved in training and educating Saudi Nationals. Furnished housing is provided for all staff.

Abdul Latif Jameel Rehabilitation Hospital and Specialty Clinics

Abdul Latif Jameel Hospital and Rehabilitation and Specialty Clinics is a non-profit hospital which provides excellent medical providing rehabilitation programs, neurological rehabilitation, musculoskeletal rehabilitation, artificial limbs, rheumatic rehabilitation, chronic diseases, sport injuries and various children programs. The Hospital is located in Jeddah, a city of 2 million populations. The hospital is a 10 minute drive from the Red Sea and 45 minute drive from Mecca (the Holy city for Muslims).

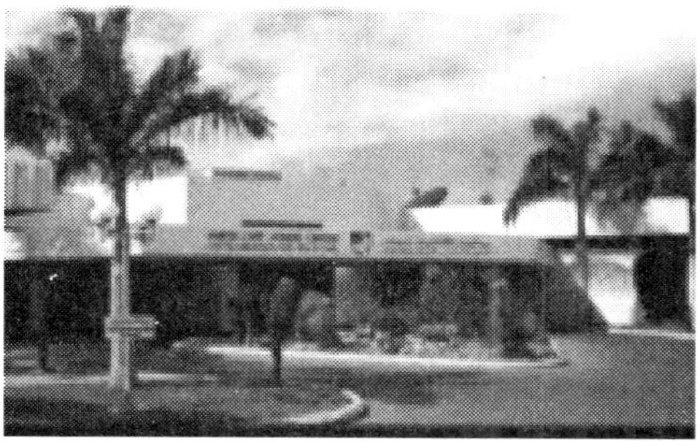

Armed Forces Hospital at Al-Hada, Saudi Arabia

The Armed Forces Hospital at Al-Hada is a 350 bed Hospital. This provides primary, secondary and tertiary medical services to the Saudi Arabian Military, personnel and their dependents. This facility is equipped with the latest technology in Western Countries. Housing for expatriate is located inside the Hospital's complex and it is within walking distance from the Hospital. The Hospital's complex contains excellent recreational facilities for its staff. The hospitals location is unique, it is a 45 minute drive from Mecca (the Holy city for Muslims), a 15 minute drive from Taif (population 300, 000), and 2 hour drive from Jeddah.

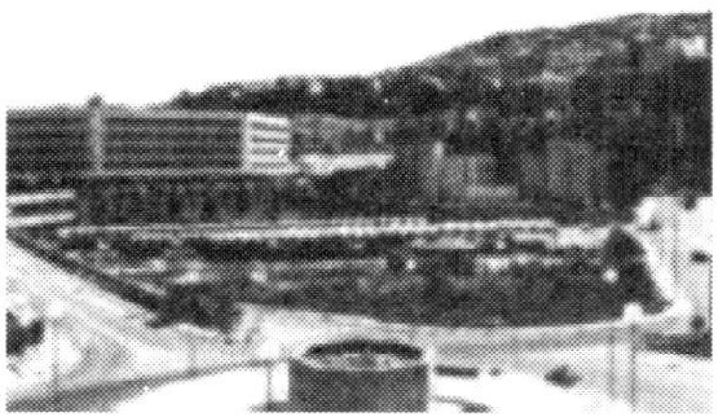

The Rehabilitation Centre in Taif, Saudi Arabia

The Rehabilitation Centre in Taif is a 100 bed Hospital facility which provides high quality medical rehabilitation programs to military personnel and their dependents. The Hospital is located in Taif, a 300,000 population.

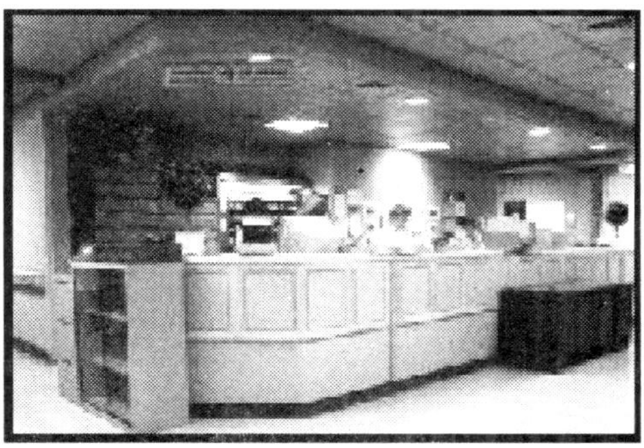

Mughrabi Hospital and Medical Clinic Centres in Saudi Arabia and Gulf States

There are more than 18 hospitals and centres for the diagnosis, treatment and surgeries of the eye diseases. It has more than 45 years experience and it is considered the pioneer in the provision of medical treatment for patients with eye disease in the Middle East and Africa. Mughrabi Hospital is the first institution to utilize modern technology from western countries. All medical consultants at Mughrabi hospitals and clinics hold the highest certification and degrees in the world. For instance; College of Bascom Balmer for Ophthalmology Wellmer College for Ophthalmology at John Hopkins University, Louisiana College.

Al-Mughrabi Hospital and Centres are located in all major cities in Saudi Arabia and Abu Dhabi. In Saudi Arabia Mughrabi Hospitals are located in the following cities:

1. Jeddah
2. Riyadh
3. Mecca
4. Demmam
5. Madinah
6. Taif
7. Khammis-Mushayf

Majority of Mughrabi Hospitals and Centres provides, Ophthalmology Ear, Nose, Throat and dental medical services. Mughrabi Hospitals and Centres provide the following procedures and services:

1. Glaucoma Unit
2. Cornea, External Eye Disease Unit
3. Vitro, Retina Unit
4. Cataract Unit
5. Retroactive Surgery Unit
6. Pediatric Ophthalmology Unit
7. YAG Laser
8. Argon Laser

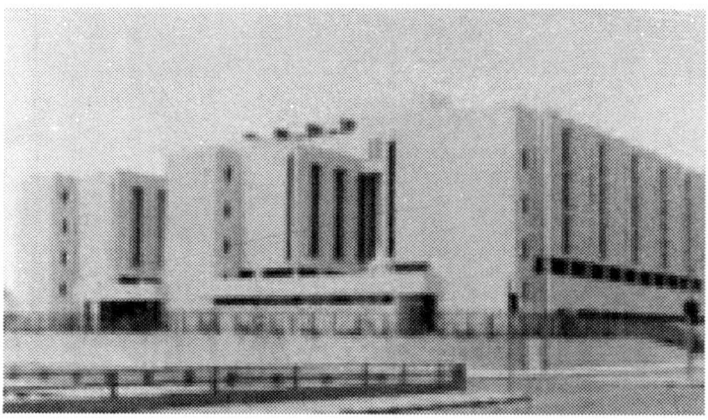

International Medical Centre (IMC), Jeddah, Saudi Arabia

The International Medical Centre (IMC) is a 300 bed private multidisciplinary hospital with several centre of excellence clinics in Jeddah, Saudi Arabia. (KSA) IMC is affiliated with the Cleveland Clinic Foundation in Ohio, USA. IMC will provide a "world class" holistic healing environment through the efficient well designed infrastructure, advanced technology equipment, sourcing and retaining competent physicians/surgeons, nurses, paramedics and support staff from across the globe; and through the continuous support of the management team, and the board of directors.

Key management staff at IMC is Harvard educated/trained and other American educated/trained professionals. IMC will offer competitive salary and benefits package to ensure the employment of highest quality staff. IMC will make a difference in health care paradigm in the Middle East. Jeddah has a population of 2 million with modern shopping malls, water sports, golf, equestrian clubs, museums, sea-side resorts, variety of international restaurants, international schools, active professional societies, and many world class 5 star hotels.

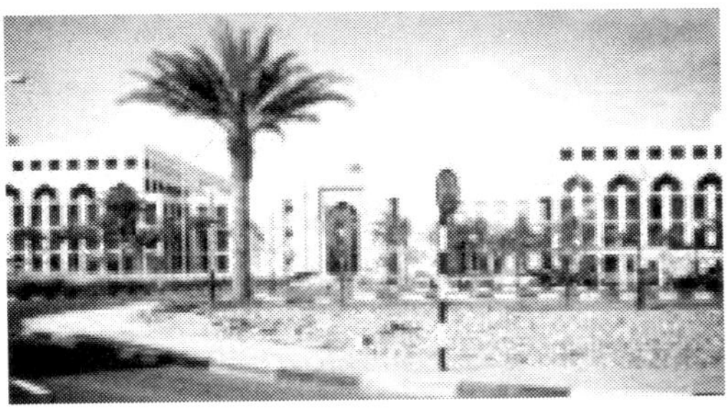

The North Western Armed Forces Hospitals Program, Tabuk

The North Western Armed Forces Hospitals are located in Tabuk city. It is considered as the northern western Saudi Arabia gate to Jordan and other neighbouring countries in the Middle-East. The city is famous with its agricultural production, mainly fruits and vegetables. Tabuk is located 2200 feet above sea level and has moderate climate in comparison with other Saudi cities climate. It has numerous supermarkets, restaurants and hotels with international standard. Tabuk city has an airport.

Al-Hada Armed Forces Hospital—Taif

Al-Hada Hospital, opened in 1980, is a modern, acute care facility with 368 beds located ten miles Northwest of Taif. Extensive medical and nursing services are offered including open-heart surgery and kidney transplant. The hospital provides the latest state of the art care in the renal medicine (dialysis), burn care, general intensive care and coronary care, obstetrics and gynaecology, neonatal intensive care, paediatrics; orthopaedics and various medical and surgical specialities.

The medical staff includes over 160 physicians, the majority of which are western educated and board certified with a resident staff of 25.

The nursing staff employs about 140 western nurses and an additional staff (about 250) of RNS, LPNs and aids under the direction of a strong nursing administrative staff. Ancillary services include comprehensive laboratory therapy, physical therapy and pharmacy.

Dallah Hospital and Western Region—Al-Kharafi

Dallah Hospital, a member of Dallah A1 Baraka Group, is the most specialised Medical Centre that Dallah Health Care provide. It has been established since 1987 with 220 beds in A1 Nakheel Quarter/North of Riyadh with an area over 40,660 m^2. The hospital is easily accessible by virtue of its closeness to the circular free way and the King Fahad high way. It is also very convenient for patients transferred from outside of the city or the Kingdom, as it is only 20 minutes drive from King Khalid International Airport. The hospital has been equipped in accordance with the highest international standards with regards to building specifications and safety procedures. Dallah hospital has acquired an excellent reputation as one of the best private hospitals in the Kingdom due to the high medical standards available in bath diagnosis and treatment fields in addition to the highly qualified and experienced staff. The hospital is also particularly proud of its competent group of consultants and specialists holding, American and European credentials, who have world wide experience through their work in different international medical centres. More than 75 physicians in various specialties provide optimum care to the patients.

Dallah Hospital has been keen on providing distinctive services in various medical fields by constantly updating its technical facility and selecting the most experienced medical staff. In its efforts to directly acquire the most updated medical practices, Dallah Hospital has conducted cooperative agreements with reputable Medical centres in the United States of America. The Dallah Diabetes Centre and most recently the Dallah Cardiac Centre were established in direct cooperation with Deaconess Hospital, one of the largest educational hospitals affiliated with Harvard Medical School, Other agreements were conducted also with California University Medical Centre, Los Angeles and LomaLinda University, California.

King Faisal Specialist Hospital and Research Centre in Jeddah (KFSHRC)

King Faisal Specialist Hospital and Research Centre in Jeddah (KFSHRC, commenced providing medical services to Jeddah city and to the Western Region of Kingdom in March 2000. It is a 200 bed hospital equipped with the most modern medical equipment and medical technology available at present time. KFSHRC recruits many of there medical, nursing and paramedical staff from North America and Western European countries. The hospital is accredited by (JCI) Joint Commission International. KFSHRC is located on the coastal city of Jeddah on the Red

Sea. City of Jeddah is a cosmopolitan city and it is the second largest city in Kingdom

Security Forces Hospital (SFH)

Security Forces Hospital (SFH) is one of the leading Health Care Providers in the Kingdom of Saudi Arabia. Founded back in 1984 with the primary focus to provide health care services to the employees of the Ministry of Interior. Its mission is to provide high quality health care service to all employees of the Ministry of Interior while promoting health care education, research, and the development of Saudi health care manpower, and optimizing the use of available resources. Security Forces Hospital with its advanced facilities, medical, clinical, and ancillary systems, including primary care clinics, specialty care clinics, and 500 beds inpatient facility combined with an integrated surgical facility and highly trained medical and other staff with various specialties are the key ingredient to the delivery of high quality patient care provided by the Security Forces Hospital Program.

Al Hammadi Hospital

Al Hammadi Hospital, in Riyadh is a Medical centre offering services in all medical specialization fields. Since its foundation and its opening in April 1985 the Hospital has been offering highly distinguished medical and therapeutic services, 24 hours a day And highly qualified Cadre covering all departments:—outstanding team of consultants and Specialists, Nurses and Technicians. Due to the fact that the Hospital covers all branches of medicine; medical and therapeutic Services in more than 24 medical specialization fields are offered in a unique way.

Patients are received around-the-clock in the following departments:

General Surgery—Vascular Surgery—Chest Surgery—Orthopedic and Traumatic Surgery—NeuroSurgery—UroSurgery—Obstetric Gynecological—Maxillofacial Surgery—Orthodontics—Dental Surgery—Plastic Surgery—E.N.T—Surgery—Also General Internal Medicine—Endocrinology—Cardiology-Psychiatry—Nephrology—Peadiatrics—Neonatology—Skin Care—Dermatology and Venerology.

Al Hammadi Hospital has also the most advanced therapeutic units equipped with the latest modern technology including: Lithotripsy (kidney stones—gallstones by shock waves—laser of ureter stones). Laser unit for ophthalmology—Laser unit for dermatology—Cardiac intensive care unit—Permanent and temporary pacemaker implantation—Surgical intensive care unit—Paediatric intensive care unit—Neonatel intensive care unit—Haemodialysis unit Electroencephalogram (EEG(unit—Portable Electrocardiogram unit—Coloured echo Doppler unit—Cardiac unit—Fluorescent Electrocardiogram unit and Exertion Electrocardiogram unit. Al Hammadi Hospital also has the latest technology fully equipped In-Vitro Fertilization (IVF) department, Intra Cyto-plasmic Sperm Injection (ICSI), plus facilities in micro-manipulation techniques.

7

Medical Cities in Jordan

Premier medical institutions like Al-Hussein Medical City, Jordan University Hospital and King Hussein Cancer Centre have achieved brilliant accomplishments. It excels in health care and health tourism in the Middle East. A country of almost six million inhabitants, Jordan is firmly rooted in the Islamic traditions. Courtesy and hospitality are among the most highly prized virtues, and the visitor is sure to be charmed by the genuine warmth and friendliness that awaits them. Jordan is a Kingdom steeped in history and culture and its rich heritage, all around are remnants of ancient civilizations long since past, yet they still remain, stamped into the very fabric of this amazing Kingdom and etched into the soul of the people who live here. The major cities of Jordan are Al'Aqabah, Ramm, Amman, Wadi Musa, and Irbid,

MEDICAL TOURISM IN JORDAN

Jordan is an emerging medical tourism destination housing an abundance of top-notch health care providers. The kingdom was rated as number one in the region and fifth in the world as a medical tourism hub in a study by the World Bank. Also, the government has implemented processes to make immigration for inbound medical tourists to be quick and easy.

Treatment costs in Jordan can be as low as 25% of costs in the US (and even 10% in several cases) while the quality of care is equal or superior compared to the United States. Get FREE price estimate for any medical procedures in Jordan.

Jordan medical tourism is popular in the areas of organ transplantation (kidney transplants), orthopedic surgeries, cardiac procedures, neurological surgeries as well as dental treatments.

Health-base, medical tourism facilitator in USA, is the trusted source for global medical and dental choices, connecting patients to leading health care facilities worldwide. They arrange a variety of medical tourism services from basic consultations to full service treatment abroad. Health-base caters to the needs of individual consumers, self-funded businesses, insurance carriers, benefit consultants, insurance agents, and third party administrators seeking affordable medical travel and dental travel options. Our state-of-the-art, easy to use, information rich web-based system makes it easy to coordinate international medical care including necessary travel and accommodation for patients and their companions, all at one place. Health-base arranges first class services for patients at major internationally accredited hospitals in Thailand, India, Singapore, Malaysia, Philippines, South Korea, Turkey, Belgium, Hungary, Costa Rica, Panama, Brazil, Mexico, USA and is expanding to Canada, UK, Jordan, Taiwan, Argentina, New Zealand, Australia, El Salvador and Guatemala.

They offer over two hundred medical, dental and cosmetic procedures in various categories: Orthopedic procedures such as hip replacement, Birmingham hip resurfacing, artificial knee replacement, rotator cuff repair, knee surgery; Cardiac and Vascular procedures like heart bypass (multiple coronary artery bypass graft or CABG), aortic aneurysm repair, heart valve repair, heat valve replacement, angioplasty, RF Ablation; Spinal procedures such as spine fusion, laminectomy, disc replacement; Weight-loss procedures like gastric bypass, lap band, gastric sleeve; Eye procedures like LASIK; Cosmetic and Plastic surgery procedures such as breast augmentation, face lift, rhinoplasty (nose surgery), liposuction; Dental procedures such as orthognathic surgery, dental bridges, dental implants, dental crowns; dental veneers; and hundreds of other procedures in the departments of Urology, General surgery, Wellness and many more. The savings are up to 80% of typical US hospital prices.

Medical Tourism, also termed as Medical Travel, Health Travel, Health Tourism, Global Health care, Medical Vacation, Medical Value Travel, Medical Treatment Abroad, International Medical, Surgical Tourism, Surgery Abroad, Surgical Trip, Health care Abroad, Medical Outsourcing, offshore Medical and Overseas Medical, is the act of traveling abroad to receive medical, dental and cosmetic care. Significantly lower cost for best practice care is usually the primary motivation behind medical tourism although some medical tourists go abroad for immediate availability of procedures and to seek treatments that are not available in their home country. Patients frequently also take advantage of the opportunity to vacation and tour inexpensively in the foreign country while they are visiting for health care.

Some important facts

Population—6 million, Area—34,578 sq mi (89,556 sq km), Currency—Jordanian Dinar (JOD, symbol: JD), each comprising 1000 fils or piastres, Flight times—From London to Amman is 5 hours, Cities—Amman (capital), Irbid, Az Zarqa, Aqaba, Time Zone—GMT+2, Weather—Dry and hot desert, with a rainy season in the west from November to April,

Languages—Arabic, English and French, Religion—Sunni Islam (over 90%), Christian 6% (majority Greek Orthodox), other 2% (several small Shi'a Muslim and Druze populations), Electricity—220 220V/50Hz (Continental round pin and UK plugs).

The capital city of Amman and some other cities

Amman, the capital of Jordan is a sprawling city spread over 19 hills. It is the modern, as well as the ancient capital of the Hashemite Kingdom of Jordan. The ancient city now boasts a population of around 1.5 million. Amman offers a variety of historical sites. The site which is known as the Citadel includes many structures such as the Temple of Hercules, the Omayyad Palace and the Byzantine Church. At the foot of the Citadel lies the 6000 seat Roman Theatre which is a deep-sided bowl carved into the hill and still used for cultural events. The three museums found in the area offer a glimpse of history and culture, they are the Jordan Archaeological Museum, The Folklore Museum and the Museum of Popular Tradition.

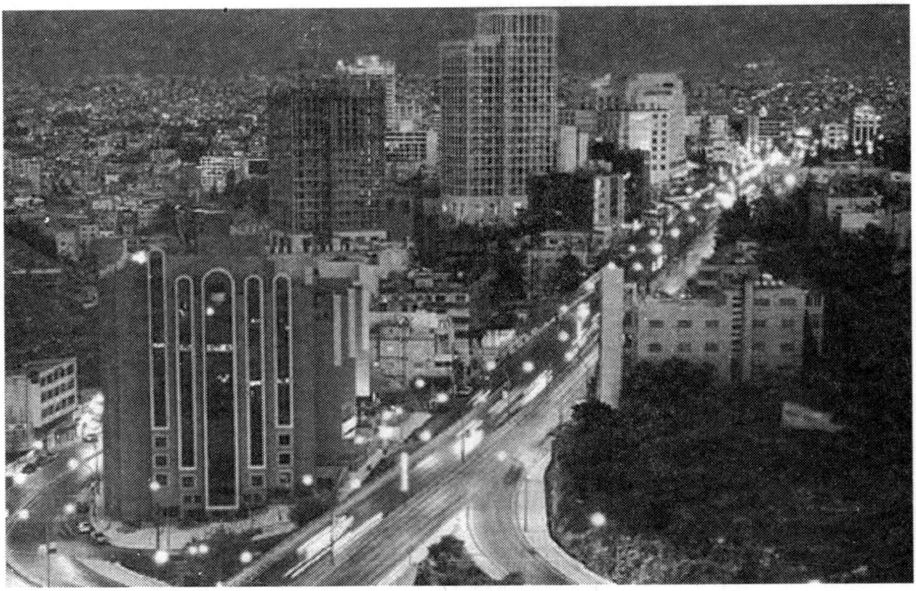

Madaba, "the City of Mosaics", is best known for its spectacular Byzantine and Umayyad mosaics, is home to the famous 6th century mosaic map of Jerusalem and the Holy Land. With two million pieces of coloured stone, the map depicts hills and valleys, villages and towns as far as the Nile Delta. Other mosaic masterpieces found in the Church of the Virgin and the Apostles and the Archaeological Museum, depict a rampant profusion of flowers and plants, birds and fish, animals and exotic beasts, as well as scenes from mythology and everyday pursuits of hunting, fishing and farming.

Petra, The ancient city of Petra is one of Jordan's national treasures and by far its best known tourist attraction. Located approximately three hours south of Amman, Petra is the legacy of the Nabataens, an industrious Arab people who settled in southern Jordan more than 2000 years ago. Admired then for its refined culture, massive architecture and ingenious complex of dams and water channels, Petra is now a UNESCO world heritage site that enchants visitors from all corners of the globe. Much of Petra's appeal comes from its spectacular setting deep inside a narrow desert gorge. The site is accessed by walking through a kilometre long chasm (or siq), the walls of which soar 200 metres upwards. Petra's most famous monument, the Treasury, appears dramatically at the end of the siq. Used in the final sequence of the film "Indiana Jones and the Last Crusade", the towering facade of the Treasury is only one of myriad archaeological wonders to be explored at Petra

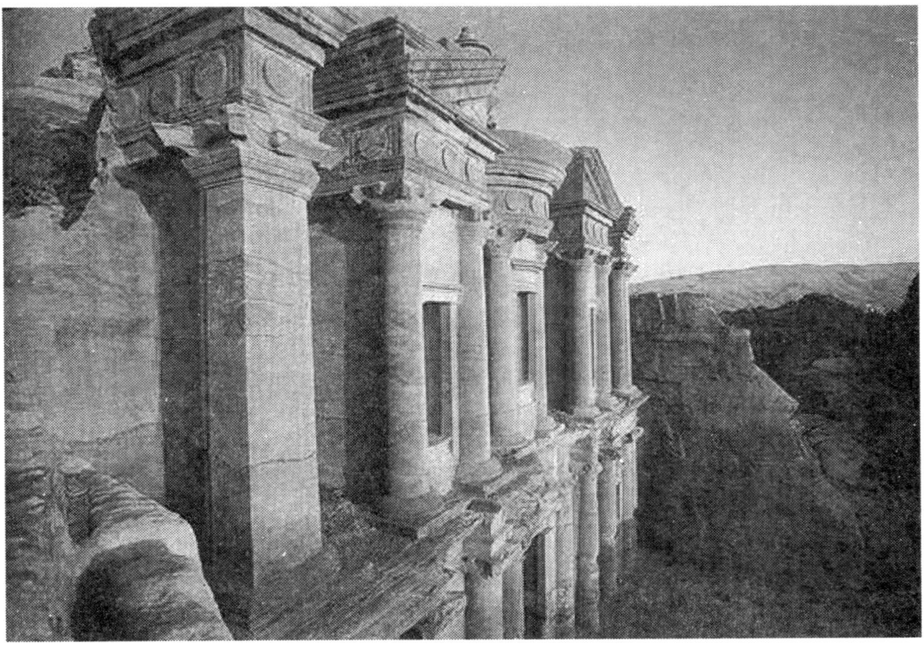

Jerash, the ancient city boasts an unbroken chain of human occupation dating back more than 6,500 years. The city's golden age came under Roman rule and the site is now generally acknowledged to be one of the best preserved Roman provincial towns in the world. Hidden for centuries in sand before being excavated and restored over the past 70 years, Jerash reveals a fine example of the grand, formal provincial Roman urbanism that is found throughout the Middle East, comprising paved and colonnaded streets, soaring hilltop temples, handsome theatres, spacious public squares and plazas, baths, fountains and city walls pierced by towers and gates.

Queen Alia International Airport (AMM) is located 32 km south of Amman. Metered taxis are inexpensive and readily available. There is also a public bus service.

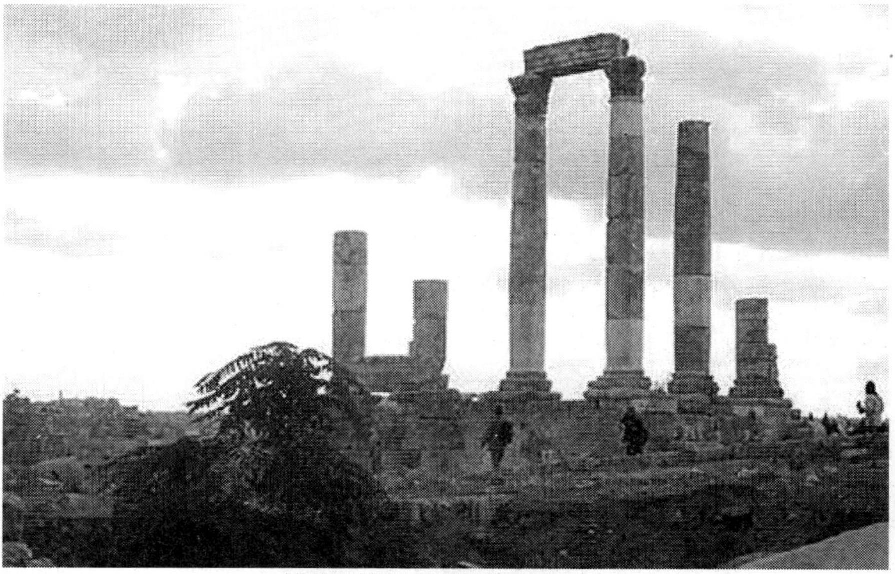

Ruins of The Citadel, Amma

Health tourism and economy

More 250,000 patients from other countries sought treatment in Jordan in the year 2007. This included an estimated 45,000 Iraqis and approximately 25,000 patients each from Palestine and Sudan. An estimated 1,800 US citizens, 1,200 UK citizens, and 400 Canadians also sought treatment in Jordan that year. It has been estimated to bring in revenues of approximately $1 billion USD annually and has been witnessing a yearly steady increase of around 10 percent of foreign patients. Treatment costs can be as low as 25 percent of costs in the US. The kingdom was rated as number one in the region and fifth in the world as a medical tourism hub in a study by the World Bank. Jordan also happens to be the only country that generates more money than it spends on Health care. There are close to 60 private hospitals in Jordan out of 100, an indicator of the sector's development. Jordan hosts outstanding resorts and spas, which include the five-star Angsana Resort and the five-star Jaz Tala Bay Resort that opened in November 2008. With spa and hotels populating areas such as the historic city of Petra and other significant religious sites in Jordan, it seems the future of health and wellness tourism looks very bright.

The kingdom has a relatively young population with a median age of 24.3 years old and has a 2.264 percent growth rate. The country ranks in the top six of 17 Middle Eastern countries for having a good business environment and relations between the West, particularly the U.S. The U.S. and Jordan have been close for six decades. The GDP per capita of Jordan is estimated to be around $3,369 USD in 2009. Total GDP, based on purchasing-power-parity or PPP valuation, is expected to grow from $25.79 billion, using current international dollar units, in 2006 to an estimated $40.96 billion by 2012. Of this GDP, the services sector, which includes tourism and health care, made up 86.3 percent (based on 2008 estimates of the total).

Pelloid, a mineral-rich alluvial sediment—saturated with sulphide components is one of the rare minerals found within the sea. With its multitude of therapies and healing qualities, the Dead Sea has a strategic advantage in the health and wellness area. Dead Sea's by-products are found in many spa and skin-treatments and there is some evidence in the literature that balneotherapy spa treatments have had some success with osteoarthritis, difficult pregnancies and stress.

History of Jordan's medical developments

People started learning about Jordan's medical developments since 1972, when, the first open-heart surgery was conducted at the Al-Hussein Medical City; in 1975 the first kidney transplant took place and in 1985 the first heart transplant was performed. This became more evident during the 1980s and 1990s as many private hospitals were built," Jordan is also self-efficient when it comes to competent doctors and nursing cadres—over 17,000 doctors—which is in turn a high turn up for a population of five and half million. "Easy procedures, including same language and similar traditions, are also among the reasons that encourage Arab patients, especially those from neighbouring countries, to seek medical help in

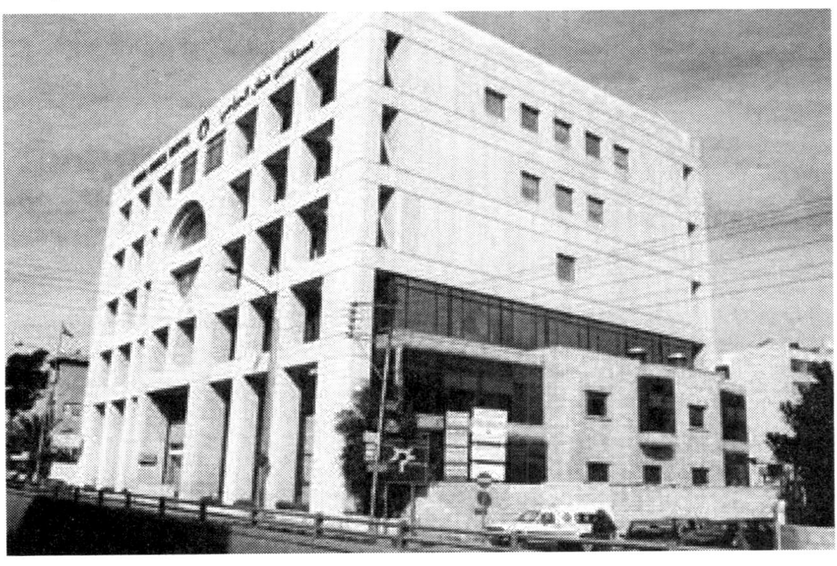

Jordan.' Over the years Jordan has become a medical hub for patients arriving from neighbouring countries. Patients from 46 countries come to Jordan. Foreign patients, who work in countries like Iraq and Palestine and come to Jordan for treatment."

King Hussein Medical Centre is the largest and most prestigious multidisciplinary medical institution in Jordan dedicated to providing the utmost in patient care and professional training. It is comprised of five centres: Although a military hospital it offers its services to military personnel and their families as well as civilian citizens from Jordan and beyond. It has an excellent emergency department with three nearby helipads and is at the forefront of all mass casualty situations in the country.

One of the top medical tourist destinations

Jordan is ranked by the World Bank as the number one medical tourism destination in the region, followed closely by Dubai and Abu Dhabi in the United Arab Emirates, and Israel. All major JCI accredited hospitals, namely, Jordan Hospital, King Hussein Cancer Centre, Al-Essra Hospital, and Specialty Hospital have the high quality standards with excellent western atmosphere luxury patient rooms. They have not only the latest technologies and medical devices but also have well trained, qualified English speaking staffs giving the best care of service. The quality of care provided truly exceeds the expectation of any accreditation standards and it's far better than hospitals, based elsewhere. This international exposure combined with their high quality treatments and low cost puts Jordan one of the top most medical tourist destinations in the world. There are six

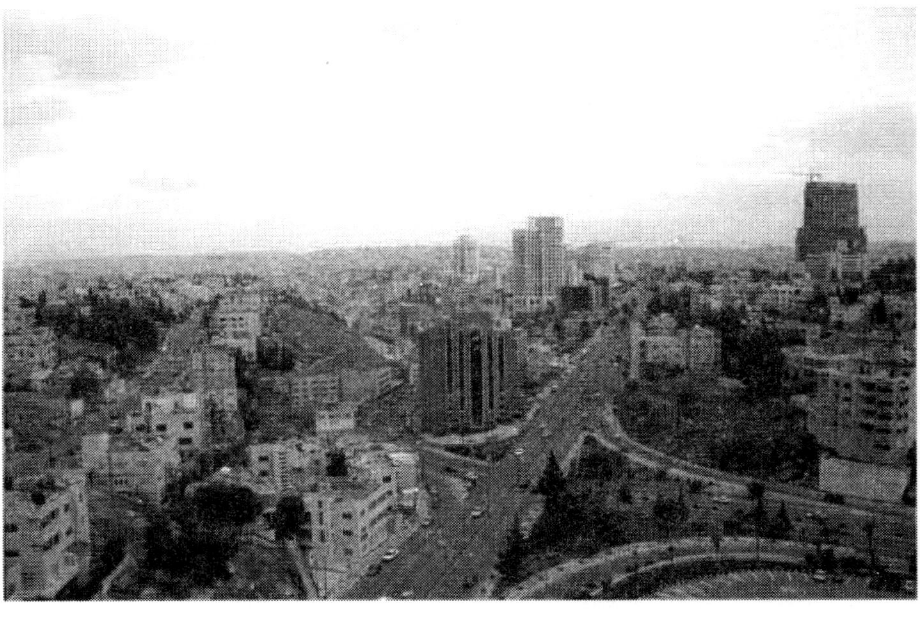

hospitals that are accredited by the Health Care Accreditation Council and four Joint Commission International (JCI) accredited hospitals in Jordan (all in the city of Amman) as of 2009. The JCI accredited facilities are:

- Al-Essra Hospital, first accredited back in May of 2008.
- Jordan Hospital and Medical Centre, first accredited back in June of 2007.
- King Hussein Cancer Centre, first accredited back in February 2006.
- The Specialty Hospital, first accredited back in April of 2008.

King Hussein Cancer Centre is a comprehensive cancer centre offering everything required for cancer diagnosis, treatment, management and social care. The hospital offers cancer surgery, radiotherapy, chemotherapy, pediatrics, psycho-oncology, palliative care, pain management, child play, back to school programs with in-house teachers and more. This hospital not only has JCI accreditation but it has the only oncology specific accreditation (first certified in December of 2007) outside the United States.

Another well-known facility is The Specialty Hospital which is a 250-bed multi-specialty hospital that is equipped with some of the latest medical technologies, such as an Open MRI, a 3T MRI, and 64-slice CT. In addition, the hospital has ten theaters with state of the art technology and telemedicine facilities and six specialties—general surgery, gynecology, pediatrics, general medicine, radiology and anesthesia.

Also, an upscale, prestigious multi-specialty hospital, which boasts up to 20 percent of its patents are foreigners (apparently coming mostly from Saudi Arabia, Sudan, and Palestine), is the Arab Medical Centre. The 142-bed hospital, which was established in 1994, has a consultant set-up where independent physicians, in private practice, use the hospital for surgery, radiology and other procedures.

Jordan's English-speaking doctors, who are trained with top U.S. institutions such as the Mayo Clinic, Cleveland Clinic and Johns-Hopkins are a big draw, especially at a time when health care costs are climbing and the global meltdown is forcing many to tighten their purse strings. A total of 56 hospitals in Jordan are involved in medical tourism. The majority of

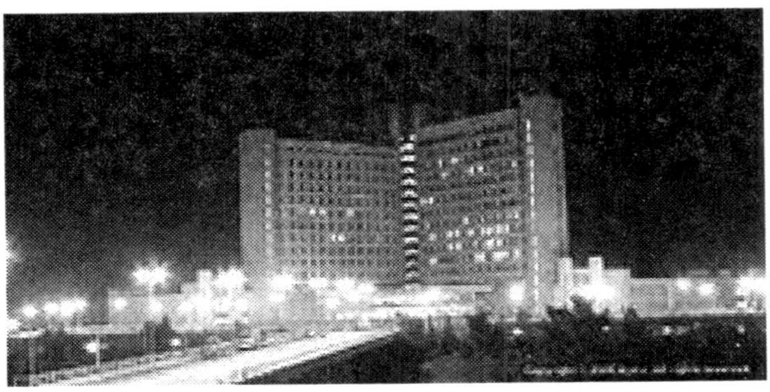

these are currently running at full capacity, and huge sums of money from private investors and government sectors are being invested into the expansion and further development of these existing facilities as well as in providing world-class training for Jordanian doctors. (See Appendix II, p. 270 at the end of the book, 'Common Surgical Interventions Sought by Foreign Medical Tourists'.

Location Map

The Abu Dhabi Fund for Development (ADFD) is financing the expansion and improvement of Al Basheer Hospital in Jordan. The development loan given by ADFD to the Jordanian Government has a total value of Dh89.7 million. Al Basheer is one of the largest hospitals in Jordan and has a 800-bed capacity. The hospital, located east of Amman, caters to mainly people with limited income.

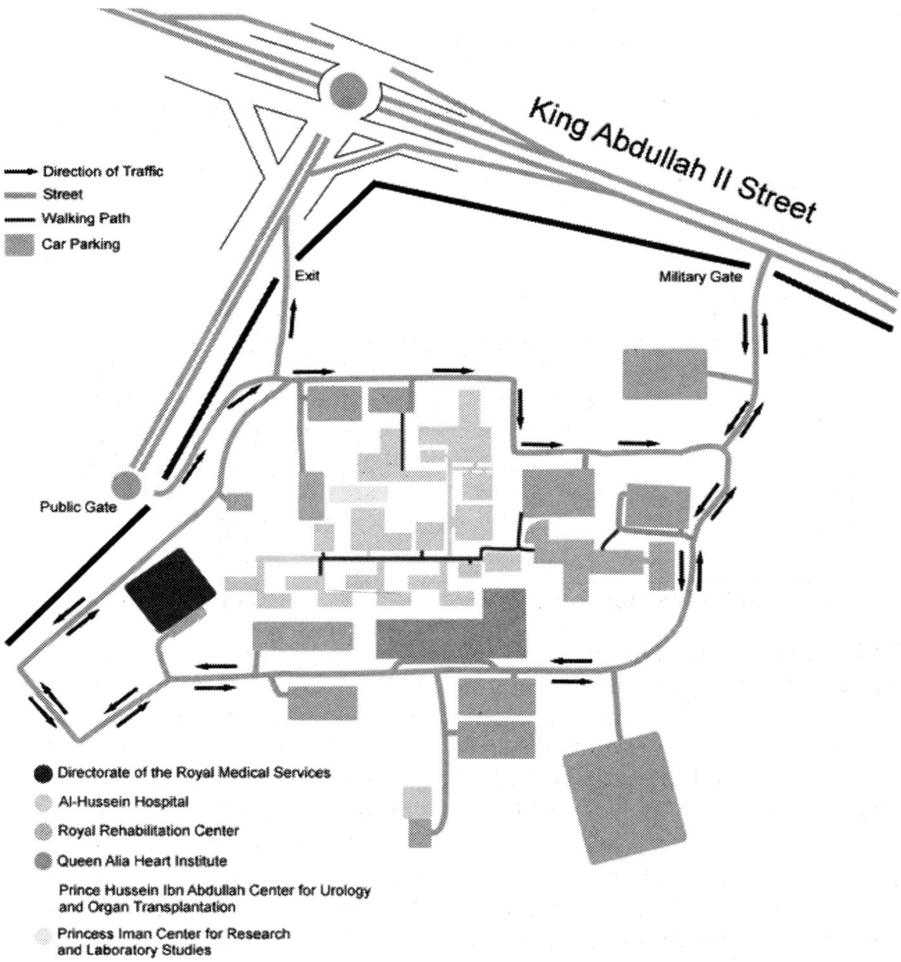

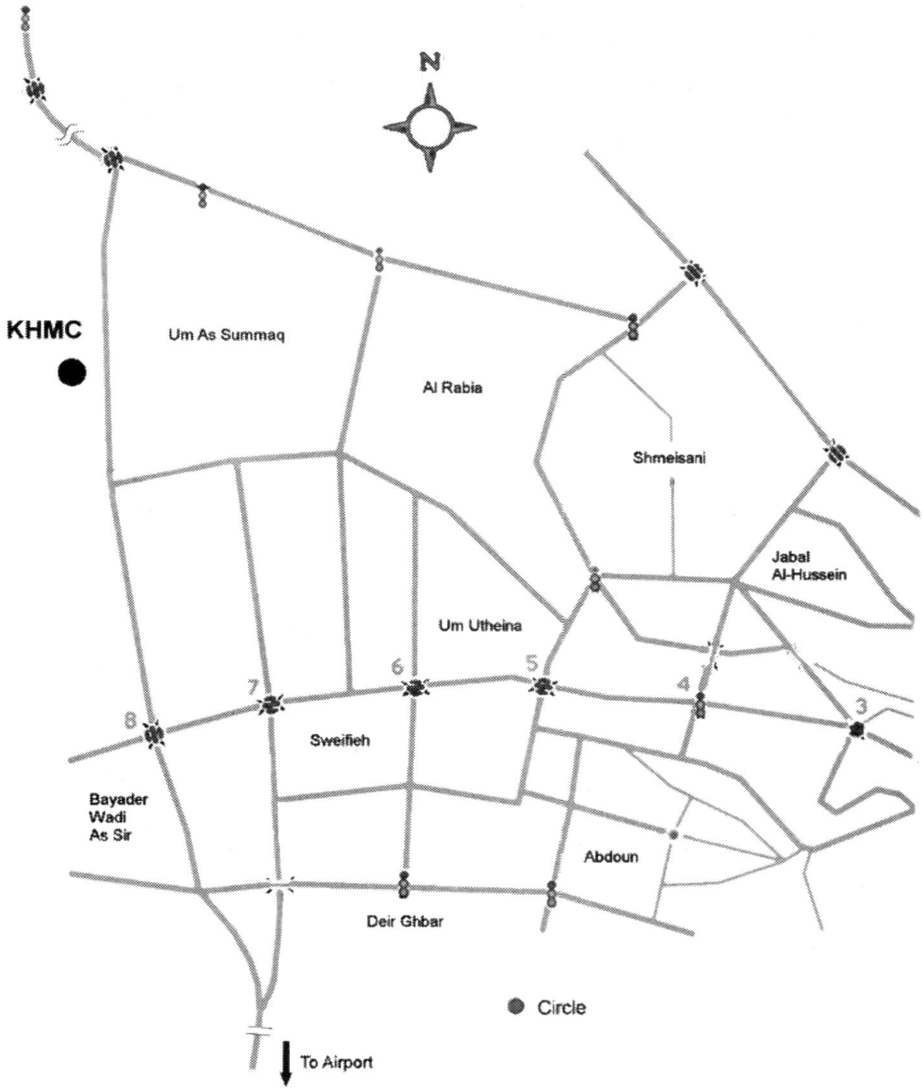

Kuwaiti investor's interest

Kuwaiti investors submitted an application for the Jordanian government to obtain approval for setting up a medical city near the capital, Amman at a total cost of between $3 billion and $5 billion, the *Jordan Times* reported. The project, which is expected to start operations in 2012, will include hospitals with the latest medical technology, hotels, entertainment centres, swimming pools and gardens. According to Jordanian medical officials, the project will offer a wide range of high-quality services to patients from Jordan and the Middle East region. The Kuwaiti investors have also offered a partnership deal for the project with Jordan's Social Security Cooperation, one of the largest financial institutions in the Kingdom. Knowledgeable medical officials described the project as "a new type of service to the region including organ transplant, stem cell research and new methods in treating complicated diseases. Investors from the Gulf, mainly Kuwait, Saudi Arabia and the United Arab Emirates have been flocking to Jordan over the past three years to invest oil revenues in development projects mainly in real estate and education.

Therapeutic Tourism

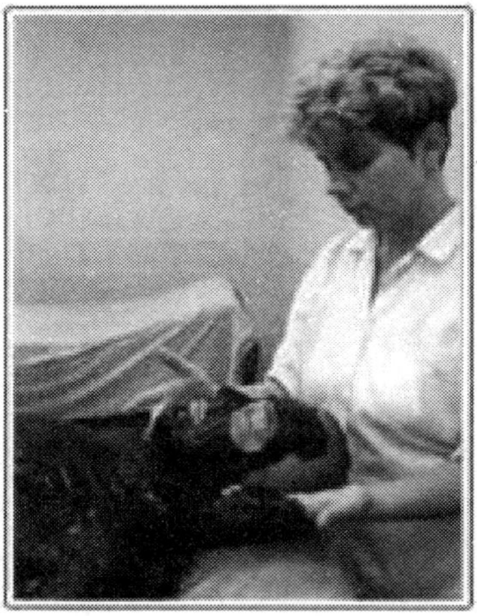

So few are the places where man can find both physical and emotional healing together. Perhaps Jordan is one of these few places where physical ailments vanish along with emotional. Due to the gracious nature that has been bestowed upon Jordan with all it's healing resources from hot water, rich with minerals to volcanic mud to moderate weather and breathtaking natural scenery. Jordan is considered one of the leading countries in therapeutic healing. For in addition to its natural healing resources from mineral-saturated waters and hot waterfalls and volcanic mud, it is also gifted with a lot of groundbreaking hospitals, prolific doctors that have established a well known status all over the world.

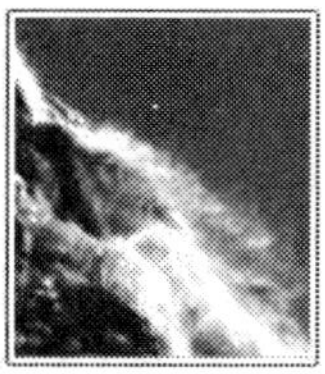

Natural Healing Areas

A lot of tourist sites are rich with mineral-saturated water and volcanic mud, which makes them healing spas that many ailing people come to visit. Here are some of the most important healing spots

The Dead Sea

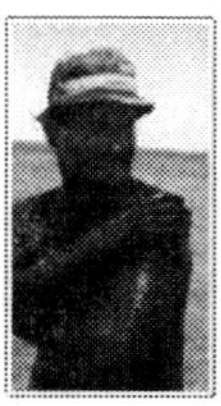

This area is warm and sunny all year through, where the average temperature is 30.4 degrees Celsius. The rays of the wonderful sun in the Dead Sea are not harmful to humans in this area. As for the air, it is dry and saturated with oxygen. The Dead Sea is famous for its black mud that is highly rich with salts and minerals.

The waters in the Dead Sea have high levels of natural minerals, especially Calcium, Magnesium and Bromine. The unique blend of salts and minerals in these waters is one of the most important resources for natural healing that is supervised by specialized people at the available spas

Ma'een Falls

Fifty-eight kilometres south of Amman lies Ma'een, 120 meters below sea level. Well known for it's spas and it's natural clinics that provide treatment for people with skin diseases, blood circulatory problems and bone, joints, back and muscular pains. For the clinics in the area also provide physical training activities.

Jordanian Hummah

Al-Hummah lies 100 kilometres north Amman, it is one of the most vital therapeutic and tourist places in the area. A spa and some clinics have been established there to offer many services to the visitors of this area. A centre for respiratory problems and diseases is also available in addition to centres that provide treatments for skin diseases and diseases related to the nervous system and joints. On the other hand, the Hemmah Hotel can provide lodging for those who wish to stay longer than a day.

Afra Falls

In the south of Jordan, 26 kilometres away from Al-Tafilah, the hot waters erupt from over 15 sources to fill the aura of the place with healing minerals. Experts say that this water in specific has tremendous power to heal infertility, varicose, anaemia and rheumatism. A centre for general services has been built next to the restaurant and natural clinic.

Hospitals

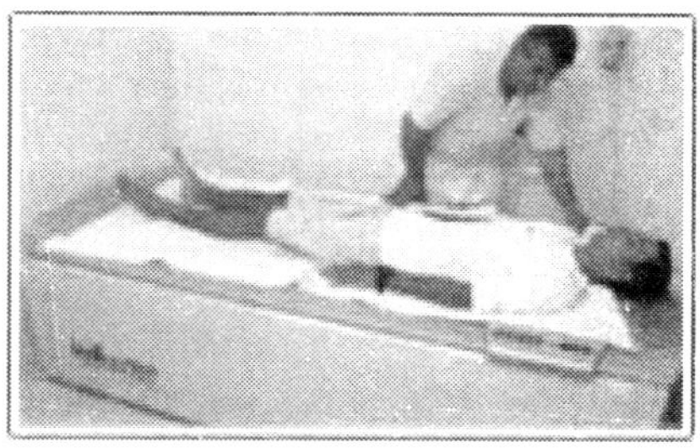

Jordan has a exclusive medical network in both the public and private Sector. Medical services in Jordan are well known for their novelty and the presence of some of the most important names in different medical fields. In Amman, the Jordanian capital, there is a large number of specialized hospitals that treat cancer, heart problems, optical diseases, infertility and family medicine in addition to other areas of specialization. Al-Hassan Medical City is one of the most respected medical centres in the region and world. For it holds a large number of the most important doctors and surgeons all over the world.

- King Hussein Cancer Centre—The First Hospital in Jordan achieved (JCI) accreditation. The First Hospital outside the United States of America achieved Health care (JCI) Disease—Specific Certification in the area of Cancer Treatment (DSCC) Queen Rania Street—Amman-Jordan
- Al-Mahaba Hospital—Al-Mahaba Circle, Petra Street-Madaba
- Al-Mowasah Hospital—North Marka, Amman

- Jordan Hospital—JCI accredited hospital, Queen Noor Str. between Abdali and 4th Circle—Amman
- Specialty Hospital—University Street near the Royal Cultural Centre—Amman
- Ebn Haitham Hospital—Amman
- Al-Khalidi Medical Centre—between 3rd and 4th Circles—Jabal Amman-Amman
- Arab Medical Centre—5th Circle—Amman
- Jordan University Hospital—University Street—Amman
- Istaklal Hospital-Dakhlia Circle—Jabal Hussein—Amman
- Istishari Hospital—King Abdullah Gardens Street intersection—Shmeisani—Amman
- Jerusalem Hospital—Amman
- Al-Israa Hospital—Sweileh—Amman
- Italian Hospital—Amman
- King Hussein Military Hospital—Medical City—Amman
- Farah Maternity Hospital—3rd Circle—Jabal Amman—Amman
- Al-Amal Maternity Hospital—Dakhlia Circle—Jabal Hussein—Amman
- Palestine Hospital—University Street near Dakhlia Circle—Amman
- Bashir Government Hospital—Amman
- Brazil Hospital—Amman
- Islamic Hospital—Abdali—Amman
- Shmaisani Hospital—Shmaisani—Amman
- Princess Basma Hospital—Irbid
- Princess Rahma Hospital—Irbid
- Princess Badee'ah Hospital—Irbid
- Jordanian Red Crescent Hospital—Amman
- King Abdullah University Hospital (KAUH)—Irbid

The King Hussein Cancer Centre (KHCC)

It is one of the most prominent comprehensive cancer centres in the Middle East that treats both adult and pediatric patients. KHCC treats over 3500 new cancer patients each year from Jordan and the region. It is equipped with state-of-the-art medical equipment and services. Hundreds of highly-qualified oncologists and health care professionals work tirelessly to ensure that patients receive the latest in comprehensive cancer care. KHCC has established programs that focus on all stages of comprehensive cancer care: from prevention and early detection, through diagnosis and treatment, to palliative care.

The King Hussein Cancer Foundation (KHCF), founded in 1997, undertakes various fundraising activities to support and maintain the mission of KHCC as a comprehensive cancer centre of excellence. KHCF is a free-standing, independent, non-governmental, not-for-profit organization established by a Royal Decree to combat cancer in Jordan and the Middle

East region. The Foundation and Centre is run by a Board of Trustees consisting of a dedicated group of prominent volunteers and chaired by HRH Princess Ghida Talal. The Director General of KHCF is HRH Princess Dina Mired and Dr. Mahmoud Sarhan is the Director General of KHCC.

Prior to the mid-1980s, there was no infrastructure for treating cancer patients in Jordan. For quality care, wealthy patients sought treatment abroad, while those without means were treated locally, with limited resources and poor results. In 1997, the Al-Amal Centre, meaning "The Centre of Hope", opened its doors. This much-need cancer-specific hospital was established to provide the many patients in Jordan with quality care comparable to that offered in the West. To honour the late King Hussein, who lost his sadly lost his courageous battle with cancer, the Centre was renamed the King Hussein Cancer Centre in 2002. From 2002-06, the hospital intensely focused on areas of quality control, and the recruitment of highly-qualified staff. Patients, patient services, programs and staff exponentially increased at a rapid pace. The focus, from its inception, was to deliver the highest level of care in a safe environment. These efforts were recognized in 2006 when the Centre earned its first international accreditation from the Joint Commission on Accreditation of Health care Organizations (JCAHO). The Centre was the first hospital in Jordan to achieve such recognition.

In 2006, Dr. Mahmoud Sarhan became the Director General and CEO of the King Hussein Cancer Centre. Dr. Sarhan, a former Professor of Pediatrics in the Bone Marrow and Stem Cell Transplantation Program at Duke University, was an instrumental figure in the Centre's establishment. He founded KHCC's BMT program in 2003, a program which has become one of the largest and most successful BMT programs in the Middle East. It is one of the largest (performing approximately 100 bone marrow transplants each year) and most successful programs in the Middle East, achieving cure rates compatible with international standards. The program oversees both matched allogeneic and autologous transplants and performs transplants utilizing cord blood, making it the only program in Jordan and the second in the region that offers such a highly specialized procedure. Other non-cancer cases are also treated through the KHCC BMT program including thalassemia, aplastic anemia and other metabolic diseases. After just one year under Dr. Sarhan's leadership, KHCC received additional valuable international accreditation, again from JCAHO, as a cancer-specific centre based on a review of compliance with international standards, clinical guidelines and outcomes of care. KHCC became the first centre outside the US to earn this prestigious distinction.

Additionally, the Department of Pathology and Laboratory Medicine was awarded an international accreditation from the College of American Pathologists (CAP), recognizing the exceptional high quality of KHCC's pathology and laboratory services. This honour bestowed upon the Centre was also the first in Jordan and only the fifth in the Arab world to achieve such accreditation, confirming that KHCC laboratories meet and exceed regulatory requirements, yielding the highest accuracy levels of laboratory results. KHCC continues to achieve accreditation from both international and national organizations for its ongoing pursuit of excellence—a world-class comprehensive Centre with services comparable to those in the West. In 2007, KHCF and KHCC were entrusted to lead the first national breast cancer program, Jordan Breast Cancer Program (JBCP), in partnership with the Ministry of Health and other stakeholders. The main objectives of the program are to reduce morbidity and mortality from breast cancer through awareness campaigns, early detection and access to screening for all women in Jordan in order to shift the current state of diagnosis to the early stages of the disease, when it is most curable with high survival rates. The mission of the King Hussein Cancer Centre is to: o provide state-of-the-art comprehensive cancer care to the people of Jordan and the Middle East region o offer access to education, training and public awareness aimed at the early detection and prevention of cancer o supply access to research in order to decrease mortality and alleviate suffering from cancer with the highest ethical standards and quality of care

Centre of Excellence

To transform the King Hussein Cancer Centre into a leading institution in oncology care, training and research that will be a pillar in elevating health care in the region and beyond. In accordance with its stated mission, the King Hussein Cancer Centre, in its ongoing efforts to remain a Centre of excellence, tirelessly works to assure: Excellence in Clinical Care The primary goal at KHCC is to ensure excellence in clinical care by its comprehensive approach to treating patients, focusing on patients' individual physical, emotional, social and environmental needs. A multi-disciplinary approach for delivering cancer care is what distinguishes KHCC from other cancer care centres. Excellence in cancer education, training and public awareness KHCC has advanced programs and initiatives to promote education and public awareness. These include, but are not limited to, the establishment of: Oncology Fellowships and Residency Programs, the KHCC USAID Medical Library which offers the largest on-line resources in the Region, multiple community outreach programs from its Office of Cancer Communication and Public Awareness, a hospital-based Cancer Registry, a toll-free Cancer Information Helpline and clinics which promote healthy lifestyle changes, such as the Nutrition Clinic and Smoking Cessation Clinic.

King Abdullah University Hospital (KAUH)

It is the largest hospital in northern Jordan, serving the approximately one million inhabitants of the Irbid, Ajloun, Jerash, and Mafraq governorates. It is also the teaching hospital affiliated with Jordan University of Science and Technology (JUST)[1], located within the campus adjacent to the university's Medical Faculties Complex.[2] The hospital is staffed with full time physicians and surgeons who are faculty members of the Faculty of Medicine, in addition to many others from the Ministry of Health, and the Royal Medical Services (RMS). The overall area of various hospital buildings is 95583 m^2, in addition to a double story car park of 9000 m^2 area. The hospital has a bed capacity of 683 which can be increased to 800 beds in an emergent situation. Structurally, the hospital is composed of a 15 story high-rise building, in which all hospital beds are located, and a 3 story low-rise buildings in which patient clinics, diagnostic and other services are located. The hospital is connected to various health science faculties via the ground floor of the low-rise building.

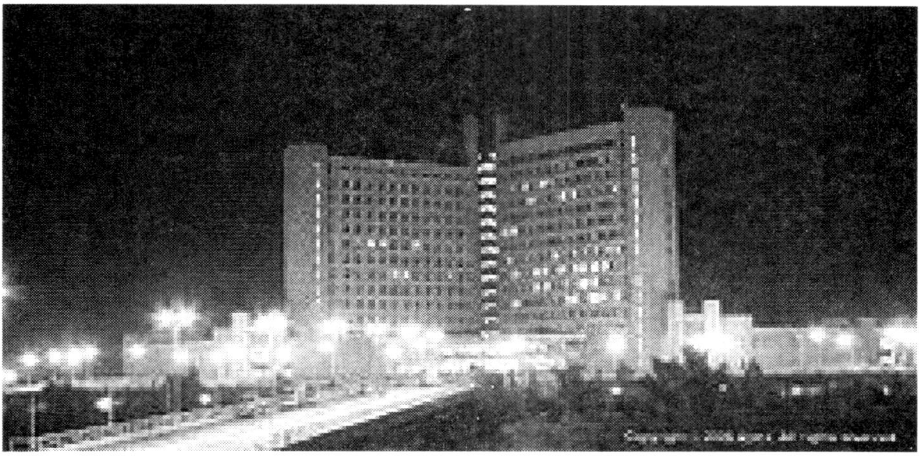

Built by Acciona at a cost of approximately $120 million, the King Abdullah University Hospital was the culmination of efforts inaugurated by the late King Hussein bin Talal to address the critical lack of central, advanced medical facilities serving the population of Northern Jordan. Though King Hussein laid the cornerstone in a 1994 ceremony, he himself did not live to see the completion of the massive hospital, named after his grandfather, the founder of Transjordan, King Abdullah I. KAUH which was inaugurated by his Majesty King Abdullah II on 28th November 2002, has become, within short period of time, one of the most prominent and reputable non-profit hospitals in Jordan and the region. It opened with founding departments in obstetrics—gynecology, pediatrics, internal medicine, and general and special surgery, in addition to emergency facilities including a medevac heliport. JUST medical, dentistry, and nursing students complete laboratories, practicals, internship, and residency at or in close conjunction with KAUH and its extensive facilities.

KAUH is located near the Northern Jordanian town of Ramtha; the hospital and the larger JUST Campus[1] are located 20 km east of Irbid and 80 km north of Amman. The hospital's main building, a modern 15-storey structure with a capacity of 683 beds, is a distinctive landmark in the region, impossible to miss from the main highway linking Irbid to Syria to the North, and even visible from the city of Irbid.

The hospital includes the following departments:

- General Surgery
- Special Surgery
- Emergency Department
- Pediatrics
- Obstetrics and Gynecology
- Internal Medicine and Dermatology
- Cardiac Centre
- Diagnostic X-Ray
- Pathology and Laboratory
- Endoscopy Unit
- Physical Therapy and Rehabilitation
- Physiology Function Test
- Neuroscience
- Nursing
- Information System Department

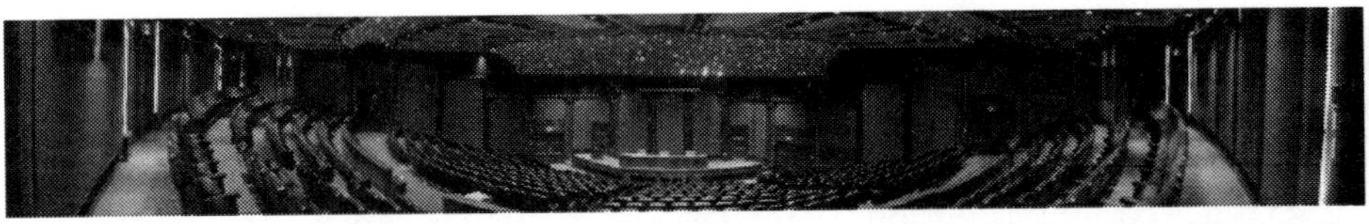

The Red Hall (conference room) in King Abdullah University Hospital

Private Hospitals' Association (PHA)

It is a private, voluntary, non-profit organization that was established in 1984, representing the private hospitals in Jordan. Its membership is open to all private hospitals in Jordan.[1] PHA applies quality standards and general guidelines on its members in order to maintain and perhaps raise the Jordanian health care reputation. Recently, the association applied the national accreditation program to all medical sectors that belong to the association. And now, Jordan's high tech hospitals, such as the Specialty Hospital, the Arab Medical Centre, Al Khalidi Medical Centre and many others, with their high class health care at costs significantly less than those of Europe and the US, gained the PHA a high reputation for its work and progress for reaching its aim. PHA main aim is for the hospitals that are members of its association become globally competitive with the medical service that they offer. With that aim in mind, PHA attempt to make the Jordanian hospitals to become amongst the medical service leaders on a global level.

USAID-funded SABEQ Program

USAID-funded Sustainable Achievement of Business Expansion and Quality program (SABEQ) is a five year broad economic development initiative implemented by Bearing Point Inc. and a team of international and Jordanian partner firms. By both supporting improvements in the business environment and offering assistance to increase productivity in Jordanian medical services' businesses, it supports the primary objective of building up the private medical sector as a high profile powerful engine of economic growth.

USAID/SABEQ program signed Memoranda of Understanding with the PHA in October 2007. Ever since the program started, the PHA have received support in various forms, most of the support was directed towards technical assistance.[3] The association started participating in international medical travel conferences more extensively, and that is to pursue the goals of the program. The goal of the funding is to enhance the quality of services provided, increase their market access internationally, increase the number of incoming patients, help develop medical professionals, and train PHA members and staff to the standards compliant with international certifications, such as JCI's standards.

eHOpe

A Leading Hospital in Jordan Implements eHOpe to accommodate its big expansion and success. The story of this hospital began in 1978 with a small clinic specialized in obstetrics and gynecology serving around 25-30 patients daily. This small modest clinic was founded and run by a Jordanian doctor who established the hospital later on. In 1985, and just a few years after the birth of the world's first In-Vitro Fertilization (IVF) baby in Great Britain, the doctor decided to venture into a journey that proved to be indeed difficult and challenging at the beginning, yet sweet and rewarding at the end. This was the journey of introducing IVF to Jordan and the region. The first IVF baby was born in Jordan May 1st, 1987. This day indeed changed the lives of thousands of couples in the country and the region and continues to do so. This is when the hospital started searching for an integrated and comprehensive information solution that can provide efficient and up-to-date information that enhances the ability of health care professionals and improves patient care, as well as organize financial transactions.

In 2002, eHOpe (electronic Hospital Operations Management Information System) was implemented to accommodate the big consecutive expansions the hospital has been going under through; back in 1987, a small clinic was established and today, the hospital consists of 100 rooms of which many of them are royal suits. eHope includes over 40 modules serving administrative, medical, financial and MIS departments of the hospital, and was implemented to promote the use of technology in order to provide better health care, increase hospital output and reduce operational costs. One of the biggest challenges faced during the implementation of eHOpe, was the need to develop an IVF module that could enable the hospital to handle IVF cases from the first visit of the couples all the way through till the baby is born. This included different IVF cases such as sperm preparation, pick-up, denudation, ICSI, fertilization, development, embryo transfer, embryo freezing, PGD (Pre-Implantation Generic Diagnoses) and destruction. eHOpe was designed to accommodate all stages of IVF, thus keeping track of all charges resulting from these services, while being fully integrated with all other financial, medical and administrative modules.

Jordan Hospital

It is a 300-bed comprehensive state of the art multi-specialty medical centre providing advanced medical services comparable to those provided by the best-reputed health centres worldwide.

Jordan Hospital's Commitment to Excellence

- JH is a JCI accredited hospital.
- JH was found to be compliant with the international society for quality in health care ISQua accredited Jordanian Hospital accreditation standards.
- JH is ISO 9002-2000 Certified.
- Jordan Hospital has Partnership as Agreement with George Washington University Medical Centre.

Jordan Hospital Is a Main Referral Medical Centre of the Middle East and North Africa (MENA)

- It has the most highly qualified consultant physicians in all medical specialties.
- Most have received training in the USA, UK, Europe and Canada.
- It has very highly-skilled staff.
- Utilizes up-to-date medical technology and techniques. .
- Has a high ratio of doctors (and other medical professionals) to its population size.
- Is considered very cost competitive as it is :
- One-tenth of US cost
- One-third of European cost
- The speed with which medical procedures are preformed.

Jordan Hospital: a Comprehensive Medical Centre Providing...

Surgery

- General Surgery
- Cardiac Surgery
- Neurosurgery
- Pediatric and Neonatal Surgery
- Orthopedics
- Urology
- Plastic Surgery

Internal Medicine

- Endocrinology
- Nephrology
- Rheumatology
- Pulmonary
- Hematology/Oncology

Pediatrics and Neonatology

Anesthesia Department:

- Obstetrics, Gynecology and Infertility
- Radiology Imaging Department
- Ophthalmology
- E.N.T.

Special Centres

Specialized Therapeutic Units:

- Emergency Department
- Radiology : Imaging and Interventional
- Laboratories and Pathology
- Nuclear Medicine
- Renal Dialysis Unit
- Lithotripsy Unit
- Physiotherapy
- Respiratory Therapy
- Gastrointestinal and Respiratory Endoscopy
- Cardiac Catheterization
- Intensive Care Unit

Medical Centres:

- Diabetes and Endocrinology
- Osteoporosis
- In-Vitro Fertilization
- Men's Diseases
- Obesity Centre

Quality management meeting the requirements of ISO 9002 .

- Provision of general and specialized medical services including all diagnostic and therapeutic support, medical education and training.
- Sincere commitment to quality and quality system.
- A written policy statement specific to the organization's goals, expectations and needs of our customers.

- Understood and implemented policy at every level.
- Organizational responsibilities and authorities defined.
- Adequate verification resources.
- Quality system periodically reviewed.
- Management Representative and an executive management headed by the Director General deals with all quality matters.
- Quality System fully documented and implemented.
- Quality manual well maintained.
- Procedures documented and implemented.
- Full considerations are given in preparing the quality plans.
- We have adopted (ISO 9002) 1994 since 1998 and will upgrade to (ISO 9000) in September 2001.

Executive Department:

- Quality Management
- Nursing Department
- Pharmacy and Medical Supplies
- Medical Department
- Administration
- Finance Department

Nursing Department:

- Provides a high level of competent nursing care for patients.
- Implements and develops the nursing manual procedures and quality assurance.
- Constantly guides, instructs and trains the nursing staff during the regular rounds made to the sections and units.
- Documents the forms and nursing reports.
- Strengthens cooperation with the universities and colleges in activating the training process of the student nurse.
- Cooperates with other departments to obtain, provide and deliver patients' needs.
- To maintain the safety of the nursing staff and patients.
- To maintain the proper professional conduct of the nursing staff.

Pharmacy and Medical Supplies
Special Services:

- Responsible for procurement as well as dispensing all medications and medical disposables.
- Supply the patient with the medication according to the price list of the Ministry of Health.
- All systems within this department are fully authorized and computerized according to international standards.

- This department includes 2 pharmacies: An in-patient pharmacy responsible for dispensing medications for all in-patients and an out-patient pharmacy that mainly sells medicines to our patients and customers. All prices are according to Jordanian Ministry of Health regulations.
- Jordan Hospital is mainly concerned with quality service. All items such as medicines and disposables are of top quality and only high standard items are procured

Medical Department:

- Supervision of all medical departments.
- Recognized for postgraduate training by:
    - The Jordanian Medical Council in the fields of surgery, medicine, Obstetrics and Gynecology.
    - Arab Board for medical specialties—pediatrics.
    - Training programs for consultants from Arab countries.
    - Training and education of students from Jordanian and Arab Universities and colleges.
    - Medical Library and Internet services.

Administration:

- Quality management and job description for all departments by-laws.
- Internal regulation approved by the ministry of labour.
- Education training and specialized courses to raise the standard of hospital employees.
- Hotel services complying with various economic needs of customers (suites, one-bed rooms, two-bed rooms and 3-bed rooms).
- Hotel services maintain a high quality standard of:
    - Cleanliness and sterilization.
    - Diet under the supervision of consultants and patient choice.
    - Patient satisfaction questionnaire to ensure patients' satisfaction.

Finance Department:

- Official charges approved by the ministry of health and medical association.
- Computerization of all procedures.

APPENDIX I

ASIAN HOSPITALS TAKE A LEAP FORWARD IN HEALTH TOURISM

The birth of new technologies, has transformed the globe's vast population into a boundary-less "Global Village Community." From a 'consumer' point of view, it is now possible to take advantage of both cheap airfares and often higher standards or more affordable medical treatment in foreign countries, than those available in their own countries. From a patient perspective, the benefits of global health care are numerous. Though cost is the over-riding factor, the wait for surgeries in some developed nations can also be annoying. USA, Canada and Great Britain have reported a surge in the number of people traveling outside the country to avoid long queues in the National Health Service, which can often be for a year or more for some surgical procedures. The South East Asian countries such as Thailand, Malaysia, Singapore, Korea and Philippines are the popular destinations for medical treatment. India is positioning itself as the primary destination for advanced medical procedures in the world. Some of Indian hospitals are also competing with their Asian peers to get a slice of the cake in the booming health tourism market for international patients.

Asia leading

Health tourism is a promising new industry in Asia, offering prospects for private hospitals facing saturation in patient growth. It is with a clearer view of the addressable market potential, internal strengths and limitations, as well as the level of external competition, that health care providers may best move forward to realize this potential. Health care providers may now consider the medical quality of their services, how non-medical services are key to encouraging patient access, and the various marketing options available to them. Thailand's Bumrungrad Hospital was among the first in the region to focus on attracting foreign patients. Thailand's Bangkok Medical centre is also excelling in health tourism. The Malaysian Government has successfully exerted its leadership to facilitate and encourage hospital industry development, with the formation of National Committee for the Promotion of Health Tourism. The Hong Kong Government is starting to consider to possibility of marketing its Traditional Chinese Medicine (TCM) capabilities to the region, while concerted efforts have similarly been launched by government agencies in Singapore to market its world-class medical capabilities. In countries such as Thailand, the onus remains on the private sector to analyze available opportunities, spearhead sectoral development, and formulate strategies to improve their competitiveness.

With the tightening of immigration rules and security checks, the US has seen a decline in the number of foreign patient visits. More patients, especially those in the Middle-East, are moving towards alternatives like Thailand. Over 100,000 foreign medical tourists visit Malaysia annually, while Singapore and India are also starting to experience positive growth in patient visits as a result of their aggressive marketing initiatives to source countries like Indonesia. However, Thailand leads the Asia-Pacific region. Thailand is able to attract a large volume of patients as it has a variety of existing tourist attractions for recuperating patients, a relatively low cost of living, expat-friendly locals, and a respectable quality of health care, in cosmetic surgery.

Industry's best practices for International patients

Medical tourists expect the highest possible quality of care, having traveled great distances to seek world-class doctors and hospitals. Many leading hospitals have expounded on this by branching their medical expertise into super-specialization. For instance, some Australian hospitals focus not only on cancer, but perhaps on specific variations of skin cancer. This also builds credibility and buy-in, when the referring doctors are trained in the post-procedural stage to provide a continuum of patient care. Even nursing teams are trained to specialize as oncology nurses, while the cross-fertilization of medical teams such as with dermatologists, radiologists and oncologists ensures that all complications are completely accounted for. Medical quality is also supported by hardware and software investments. Hardware investments include the purchase of cutting-edge technology such as MRI or Gamma Knife machines. Software refers to the intellectual output of the hospitals as demonstrated by the latest medical research.

Non-medical services

Many hospitals offer airport pick-up services for patient convenience. Hospital reception areas are fitted as luxuriously as five-star hotels; Bumrungrad Hospital in Thailand for instance even features a Starbucks café and McDonald's outlet. Bangkok's Piyavate Hospital may even feature spa facilities that offer a holistic wellness experience. Western-style hospitals such as in the US, UK or Australia feature their own on-site accommodation, both for patients in the aftercare stage, as well as for their relatives. Similarly, many Asian hospitals that do not manage their own accommodations also offer link-ups with different hotels, hostels, etc. Apart from bedside manners, hospital staff members are also being recruited to accommodate to their religious, dietary and cultural needs.

Hospitals that are successfully attracting foreign patients enlarge their geographical footprints with representative offices or agencies in other countries. For example, Cromwell Hospital in the UK has representatives in India and Pakistan, while hospitals in Singapore are also setting up offices such as in Indonesia or the Middle-East. These agents help establish and maintain relationships such as with local hospitals, doctors, embassies, sponsor corporations, or insurers. Participating in different events also facilitates such relationships. For instance, trade shows, exhibitions or training seminars allow health care providers to share their medical expertise.

With budget air travel and the Internet providing access to information about cheap or specialist treatment overseas, medical centres across Asia are vying with each other to become regional or even global hubs for health care. Singapore is aiming to attract one million foreign patients per year by 2010 while India is gunning to be a top medical tourist destination, benefiting from its huge base of medical professionals and low costs. Pioneering stem or embryonic cell work is attracting patients to South Korea and China to undergo treatment that is not available, or legally permissible, in many other countries. The work may be controversial but it is providing new hope to paralyzed patients.

Medical tourism as an engine of economic growth

In the past 30 years or so, the costs of health care have soared in developed countries, especially the United States. Americans and, to some extent, the British, Canadians, Australians began to look for ways to reduce these expenses. Certain services and procedures in American hospitals are now being contracted out to Third World countries, from transcriptions of medical records to the reading of X-rays. Medical tourism presents an opportunity for hospitals to fuel economic growth by tapping the potential of the international patient market. To attract foreign patients, health care providers may consider leveraging on both business and clinical considerations. The advancement in medical technologies, increased patient mobility and demand for immediate quality health care is arousing interest among health care providers globally. To set-up world class medical tourism centres, massive investment in health sector is called for. This will not only improve health care for the countrymen, but also attract patients from all over the world on the strength of quality, promptness and economy.

However needs can vary widely between the 'essential' health care seekers—traveling by necessity, because treatment is not available or unaffordable locally—and the 'premium' medical tourists, who are typically looking for wellness or cosmetic procedures and may want first-class flights and exclusive add-ons. Pacific Health care Holdings Patient Relations Manager Alison Lim says, our International Patient Liaison Centre has seen an increase in these "premium" medical tourists seeking high end elective treatments like titanium dental implants, complex cosmetic procedures as well as deluxe health screening. An emerging trend is the bundling of five-star health care services with unconventional post-operation treatment. India is providing traditional recuperation forms such as yoga and naturopathy, while Thailand is promoting its ancient Thai herbal remedies to the West, Middle East and Far East. To create awareness and market their medical services, Singapore's Raffles Hospital works with 50 agents in 12 countries. Parkway Group Health care has marketing offices in 15 countries including China, India, Bangladesh, Sri Lanka, Vietnam, Brunei, UAE, Brittan, Russia, Canada, Indonesia and Malaysia, which last year helped attract over 17,000 indoor patients and 140,000 outpatients.

Top 10 in medical tourism:

- Bumrungrad International Hospital in Bangkok
- Buchinger Clinic in Germany
- All India Institute of Medical Sciences in Delhi
- The Fyodorov Clinics in Russia
- A Technology Prescription: Denver Health
- Brigham and Women's Hospital
- Sourasky Medical Centre in Tel Aviv
- Hôpital Edouard Herriot in Lyons
- Hospital for Tropical Diseases in London
- Mount Sinai Medical Centre

The medical tourism policy can draw strength from recommendations that the corporate sector has been making in India, and specifically from the "Policy Framework for Reforms in Health Care", drafted by the Indian prime minister's Advisory Council on Trade and Industry, headed by Mukesh Ambani and Kumaramangalam Birla. Certain other Asian countries have taken Giant strides in promoting medical tourism in their respective countries. However, the current market for medical tourism in India is mainly limited to patients from the Middle East and South Asian economies, besides the NRIs from all over the globe. Analysts say that as many as 150,000 medical tourists came to India in the year 2005 and over 200,000 in the year 2006. Afro-Asian people spend as much as $20 billion a year on health care outside their countries—Nigerians alone spend an estimated $1 billion a year. Most of this money is spent in Europe and America, but it is hoped that this would now be increasingly directed to developing countries like India.

The foreign patients come from SAARC region, Afghanistan, Ethiopia, Nigeria, Tanzania, other parts of Africa, CIS countries and the Middle East, especially Oman and Yemen As per New trends from 2003, patients from the US, UK and Canada, escaping high costs and waiting lists are coming to India. Also from Europe, Australia and New Zealand for procedures not covered by insurance such as cosmetic surgery, obesity treatment, and new techniques like hip resurfacing. Around 30 private tertiary hospitals, mainly in Delhi, Mumbai and Bangalore; but also Chennai, Calcutta Thiruvananthapuram, Coimbatore and Hyderabad. It Includes hospital groups like Apollo, Wockhardt, Fortis, Max, Escorts. At an Indian medical tourism expo in the UK last year, 25 per cent of visitors were seeking medical treatment in India India's Apollo is setting up hospitals in joint ventures in Dhaka and Colombo; and clinics in Yemen and Saudi Arabia

Parkway Holdings of Singapore in tie-up with Apollo in Calcutta; with Asian Heart Institute and Research Centre in Mumbai; International chain Columbia Asia has a 75-bed multi-speciality hospital in Bangalore.

Indian corporate hospitals have a large pool of doctors, nurses, and paramedics ensuring individual, personalized care for all. The highly skilled personnel, with wide experience and international exposure excel in cardiology and cardio thoracic surgery, joint replacement, orthopedic surgery, gastroenterology, ophthalmology, transplants and urology to name a few. The various specialties covered are Neurology, Neurosurgery, Oncology, Ophthalmology, Rheumatology, Endocrinology, ENT, Pediatrics, Pediatric Surgery, Pediatric Neurology, Urology, Nephrology, Dermatology, Dentistry, Plastic Surgery, Gynecology, Pulmonology, Psychiatry, General Medicine and General Surgery.

Bangkok; the hub of medical tourism

Catch some sun, take in a few golden temples, and get a new hip- a new slogan coined by the Thailand Tourism, to promote medical tourism. It's an increasingly popular itinerary for foreign visitors who are flying into Thailand in ever greater numbers to get quality hospital care at bargain prices, part of a 'medical tourism' boom that is turning into a multi-billion dollar industry in Asia. The kingdom is one of several countries in the region cashing in on its ability to use cheap but highly skilled labour, affordable hospital accommodation and offer specialist treatments. Of a total of one million patients each year at Bumrungrad, nearly 50 percent are foreigners with Americans making up the biggest group, followed by patients from the United Arab Emirates, Bangladesh, Oman, Britain, Japan, Australia, Cambodia and Myanmar. Among Americans, back surgery and hip and knee replacements are the most popular procedures at Bumrungrad, while many Australians seek plastic surgery. Bumrungrad International Hospital offers a full spectrum of services from executive health tests to cardiac packages, cancer therapy, eye surgery, liposuction and other cosmetic options. Bumrungrad has more than 700 internationally-trained and board-certified doctors, and a complete range of health care services and facilities.

Which Thai Hospital is Best: Bumrungrad *vs.* Bangkok Hospital

Charles Runckel writes about two leading hospitals in Bangkok, Thailand. Thailand is the world leader for medical tourism, but which hospital within Thailand is best for you? This article, part three of a series on Medical Tourism, explores the top two choices. While there are many hospitals in Thailand that cater to medical tourists, these are two full-service facilities that have strong reputations for quality and experience with foreigners. The aspiring medical tourist should consider these two before any other Thai hospitals, even ones with a slightly lower cost, as they are the gold standard for medical tourism not only in Thailand but worldwide.

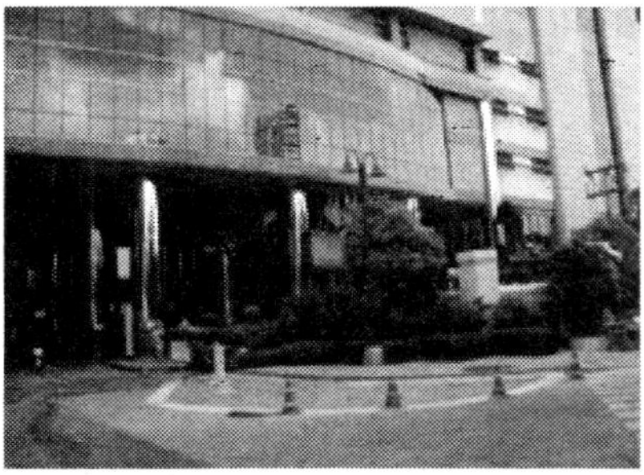

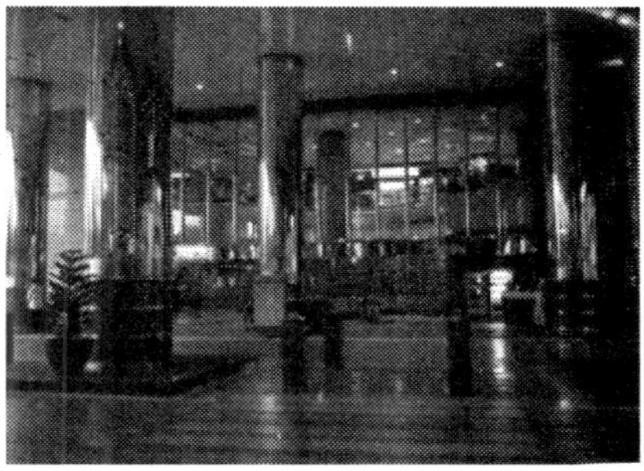

Pictures (top) Bumrungrad Hospital's main building and entrance

Pictures (below) Bangkok Hospital's Buildings and one of their entrance

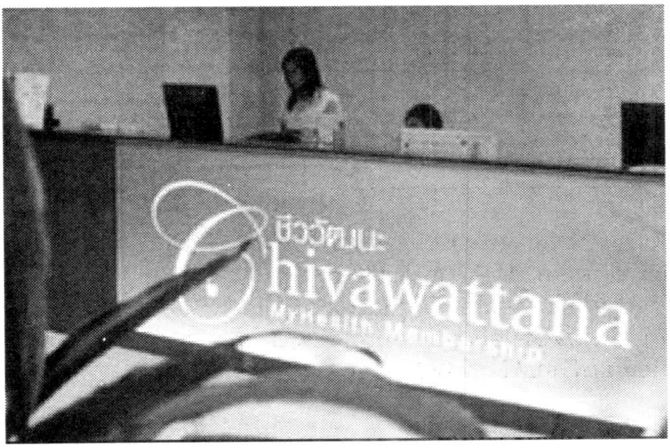

Background and Location

Bumrungrad Hospital treats over 400,000 foreign patients every year and has made medical tourism its major focus. The monolithic hospital consists of a large tower and several associated buildings adjoining, all conveniently located in downtown Bangkok. The hospital is within walking distance of Bangkok's Skytrain (light rail system) but only barely, and given the heat usual in Thailand most patients are strongly advised to take a taxi. International patients are so much a part of Bumrungrad's focus that they recently broke from their single tower architecture and built a separate International Tower that caters specially to foreigners with a brand new Physical Exam wing and upgraded VIP rooms.

Bangkok Hospital Group is a network of Thai hospitals focused on Bangkok and sprawling into the provinces and even Cambodia, though the portion of this that is most important to foreigners is their Bangkok Hospital Medical Centre (BMC) complex. This campus consists of their International Hospital as well as their main General Hospital and a collection of specialty hospitals, including their Heart Hospital, Rehabilitation Centre and Dental Clinic. The BMC is a series of adjacent buildings connected by skywalks and, apart from the main General Hospital building, are new having been built in the past five years. The BMC is located near, but not walking distance from, several Sky-train and subways stations, so a taxi is in order in this case as well. While BMC and Bumrungrad treat about the same number of total patients each, a lower proportion of BMC's patients are from overseas and total only 150,000 annually, though these are often for more serious treatments.

Layout and Impressions

Bumrungrad Hospital is, as previously mentioned, monolithic. Visitors enter into the lobby of the main tower at the ground floor, but this and the next floor contain mostly restaurants, coffee shops and the cafeteria. The Hospital portion does not begin until the third floor, where the patient is greeted with a larger lobby and registration area. Elegantly uniformed staff register new patients with digital cameras—both Bumrungrad and BMC are very tech savvy hospitals with test results updated and delivered electronically and pictures of each patient checked at every stage to avoid foul-ups. This registration area is both the point of entry and exit, and next to registration are desks for checkout and a pharmacy.

On every floor of Bumrungrad runs a long, wide hallway with specialty clinics and divisions branching off, generally four to six per floor. Each has its own lobby, which looks out onto the hall. The older main tower and new international tower are quite different, with the older tower very much feeling like a mature hospital, with traditional waiting areas and layout, while the new wing is decidedly more modern and up-to-date, from the lobbies and hallways to furnishings in patient rooms.

Upon walking into BMC's main building, one is immediately greeted with the registration staff. They are far more eager to register you than those at Bumrungrad, though this has a strong basis in necessity. Upon registration, a patient's schedule will likely initially take them to another building, or several buildings if they have multiple appointments. The BMC staff then ensure that you are taken to the right building or floor of the main structure. There are enclosed walkways between the buildings, however most patients are initially led to the shuttles, which are over-sized gold carts or minivans that scoot patients around the campus.

Each division, clinic or specialty hospital at BMC has its own modular area with it's own independent registration and cashier services (so you don't have to go through the main lobby at all, if you know where you're going). These lobbies, especially in the newer buildings, are considerably more aesthetically appealing and pleasant to wait in than many of Bumrungrad's specialty clinic lobbies, mostly due to their smaller size, more updated furnishings and clever architectural design. Like Bumrungrad, there is a clear difference in ambiance between their older General Hospital building and the new, adjoining specialty centres.

The famed, or infamous, Bangkok Hospital Phuket is renowned as a world leader in sex-change operations, but is also a state-of-the-art hospital for more mundane purposes and nothing beats Phuket's beaches for physical therapy and recuperation after a surgery in Bangkok, which the Phuket Hospital supervises and coordinates.

One of many MRI scanners at the Bangkok Hospital

Unlike many other aspects of a hospital experience, the sheer technical capabilities of a hospital are somewhat easily quantified, and it is in this aspect that Bangkok Hospital most outshines its competitor. BMC has focused a tremendous amount of resources to being on the cutting edge of medical technology, and while Bumrungrad is certainly not unsophisticated, there is general agreement that Bumrungrad is a solid step behind BMC technologically. BMC's hi-tech drive falls into two general areas: advanced imaging and non-invasive surgery. Their advanced imaging options include at least seven MRI scanners in their main campus alone. Each department receives its own specialized diagnostic equipment, unlike many hospitals which must pool resources, including Digital Mammography and a brand new 128-slice CT scanner currently being installed. It is peerless in South-East Asia, and BMC boasts one of Thailand's only two clinical PET-CT scanners. The non-invasive offerings include state-of-the-art radiation systems such as the Novalis device for brain tumors and robotic laparoscopic surgery for both heart and joint operations (with different robots, of course). Bumrungrad simply does not compete in this field, which gives BMC a decisive advantage in the specific operations these advanced machines enable; reducing risk, discomfort and hospital stay time.

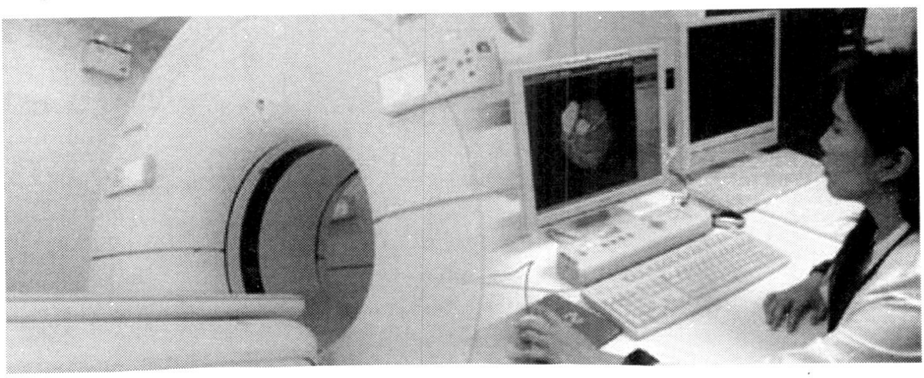

Reputation and Marketing

Bumrungrad is probably the best-marketed hospital in the world. Their fame is well deserved, but their marketing staff and management have put a tremendous effort in being "The" medical tourist hospital that potential patients in the Western world have heard of, specifically through news reports on ABC and CBS as well as multiple appearances in

Newsweek. BMC, in contrast, is more famous within Thailand and elsewhere in Asia and the Middle East. Both hospitals treat approximately the same total number of patients—about 1 million a year—however, Bumrungrad began courting foreign patients much earlier than BMC and now draws 400,000 foreign patients a year to BMC's 150,000-250,000. It is worth noting that different hospitals use different metrics to calculate these numbers (visits vs. patients) so these comparisons must be taken with a grain of salt, however, it is commonly accepted that Bumrungrad's proportion is higher than BMC's, though not by as much as the disclosed numbers suggest. While BMC's focus for the future includes increasing the proportion of foreign patients, the target countries of both hospitals will likely remain the same with Bumrungrad focusing on the US and BMC focusing on the Middle-East and Asia, affecting the level of marketing in each area.

Part of Bumrungrad's early marketing included aggressive pursuit of international certification, and as a result Bumrungrad correctly claims a number of regional "Firsts" with various international credentialing organizations. In many ways, Bumrungrad was a trendsetter and these certifications were necessary when no one had even heard the term "medical tourism" and there were serious doubts about the quality of a Thai hospital. Today, the first and second tier of Thai hospitals are firmly within international standards and rising acceptance of medical tourism make this less necessary. BMC has, itself, a slew of acronyms attesting to its quality, many of which overlap Bumrungrad's, and comparing certifications should be less important to the potential medical tourist than other aspects of reputation, but for a nervous first time medical tourist Bumrungrad's list of "firsts" can be welcome reassurance.

The savings on one 'major tooth repair' can pay for an economy level 2 week vacation including air:

- Root canal and cap front tooth 14,000 thb US $354. AUD $481. EU284.
- Significant dental work (2 teeth) would result saved money in your bank account + the vacation!
- Very simple but necessary dental procedures from cleaning to cosmetic .. available at significant savings..
  - Diagnostics, imaging, lab analysis, physical rehabilitation, cosmetic surgery, dental .. all 80% off US pricing.

    Anonymous violent crime/robbery, common in the West, is all but unknown in Thailand.
  - Most "Thailand Citizen US Educated Doctors" return to Thailand after graduation from their US Medical School.
  - Plus, access to top Thai specialists within 24 hours is pretty reassuring
- .. no waiting, ever, for anything! + a free tasty lunch!

- The Dell computer system at Bumrungrad is equal to any in the world.
- Orthopedic images, blood work, diagnostics, specialist notes .. all are available across the network.
- No carrying film/records to a specialist .. it's in the system and instantly available.
- Doc suggests additional imaging: .. OK, he orders it, the test is completed and you are back in his office getting his interpretation within 24-48 hours.
- Doc orders a CAT scan and it's completed the next morning and immediately it's in the computer system! .. !!
- Appointments are coordinated system wide .. smooth patient flow .. no bottle necks .. no waits, respect .. professional! + smiling happy Health care team and bilingual clerical staffing.

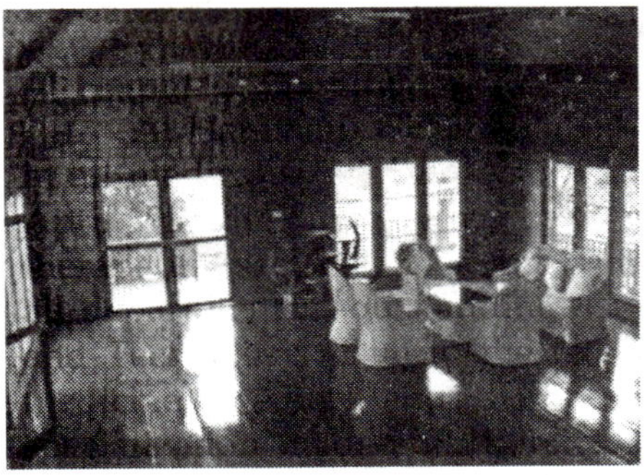

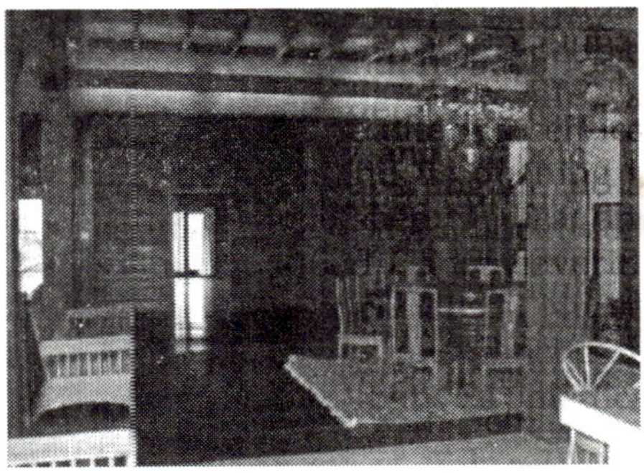

In the Chiang Mai/Chiang Rai area some incredible Lanni Thai style house are available for short-term rental .. quite marvelous houses built from 100% teak. The house above rents for 17,000 Thb (US $400, Euro 325 per month) .

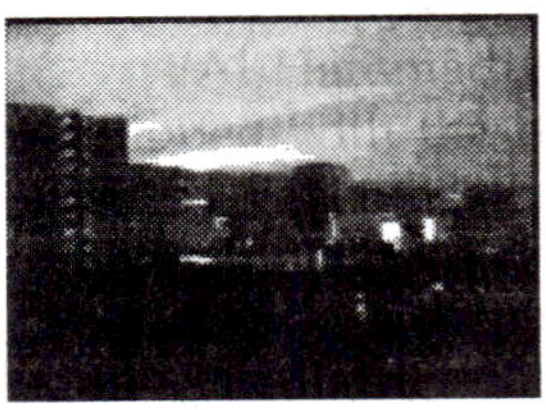

Golden Triangle

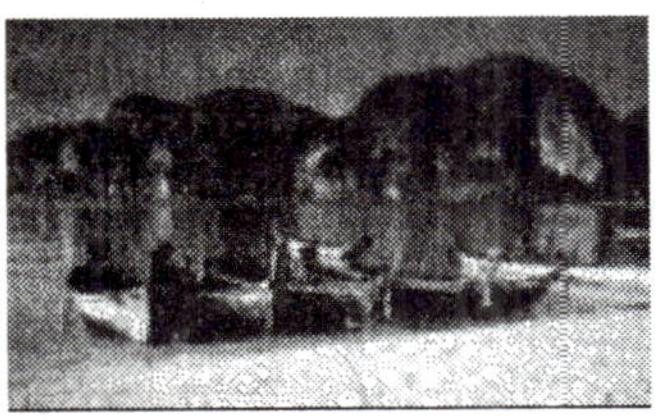

Beaches

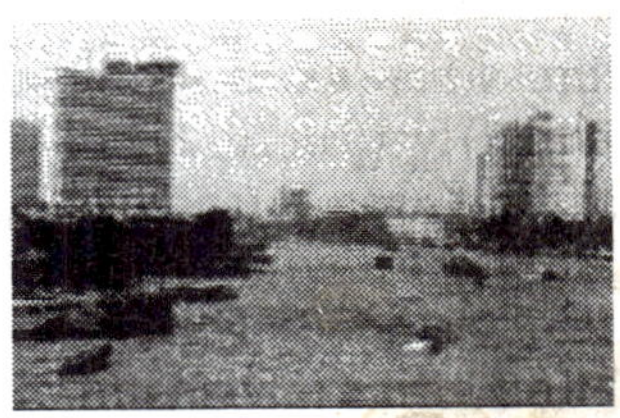

Bangkok

Bangkok is a wonderful mix of Ancient Far East and Ultra Modern West.

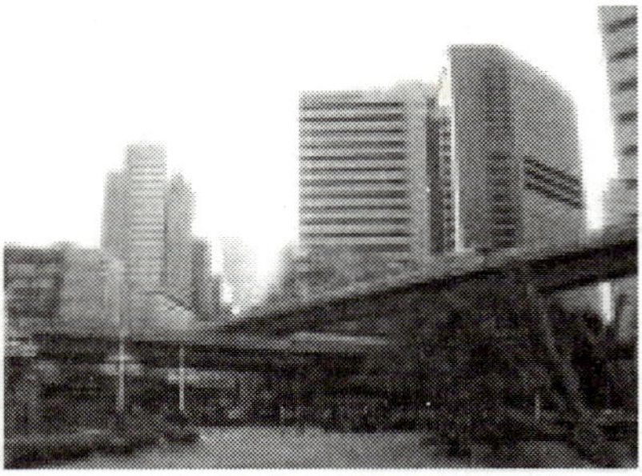
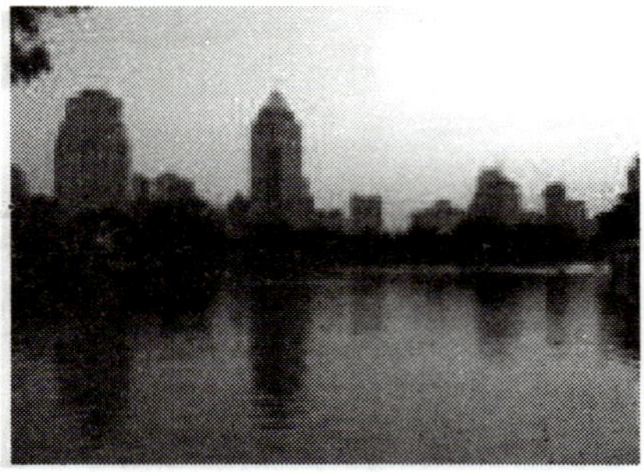
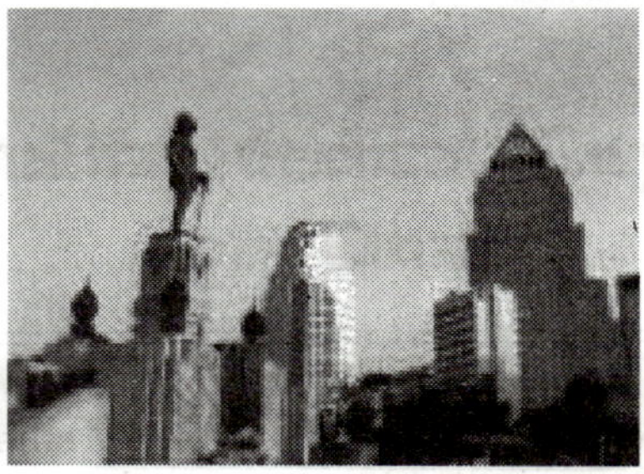

Thailand can provide an "extremely cost effective" Health Vacation.

- Grand Imperial Travel of Bangkok offers Executive Medical Tourism Packages!
  - o They assist with appointments and suggest hotels/ apartments near your medical provider.
  - o They pick you up at the airport, provide a cell phone for your stay, provide a personal guide for both tourist outings and medical appointments .. all for a flat fee.
- Bumrungrad and Bangkok Hospital compare well to US Med Centre Hospitals .. and far better than rural US hospitals.

Bumrungrad Hospital, is very foreigner-friendly. Said to be #1 in Asia! Bangkok Hospital, off New Petchaburi Road, is foreigner-friendly and comparable to most western hospitals. Private hospital room is $60. per day. A few extra days in the hospital, no problem. Many Japanese companies send their employees to Thailand for annual physicals as well as long-term medial care modalities. The savings on medical fees and the high quality medical care makes the air fare inconsequential. See attached appendix to this chapter for more details on Bumrungrad.

Dental experiences vary greatly. These clinics offer modern equipment and a full range of 'pain reduction techniques'.

- Asavanant Clinic.
- Bangkok Dental Hospital
- Siam Family Dental

- The Dental Hospitals on Suk Soi 55, Suk Soi 49 and Suk Soi 39 as well as the Dental clinics at Chula Hospital and Bumagard Hospital are professionally staffed and equipped well.
- Bumagard Hospital has serviced apartments adjacent to the hospital.. hospital staffed rehabilitation apartment suites for less than $100 per day.
- Affordable 24/7 out patient nursing. $100. per day can provide luxury hotel accommodations, gourmet meals and 24 hour 'private duty assisting provider' .

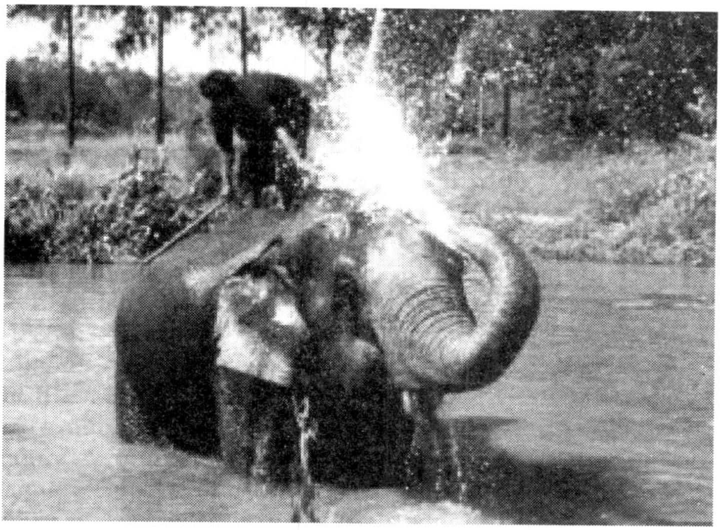

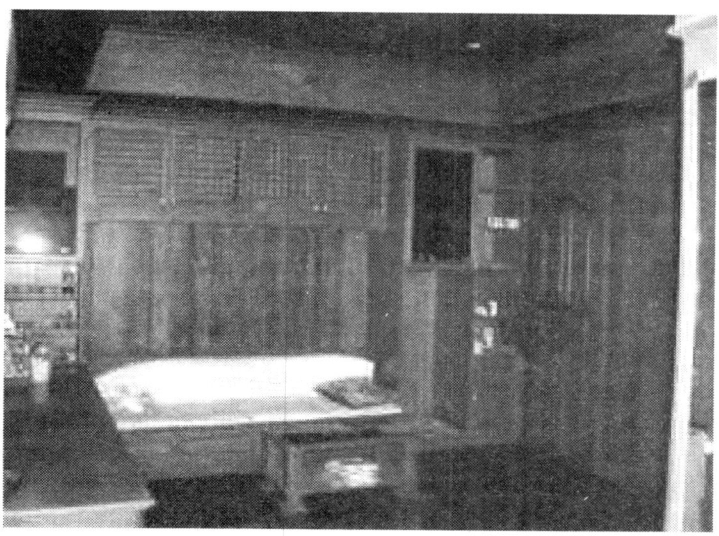

More than 150,000 North Americans and Europeans currently seek medical treatment overseas each year, estimates Josef Woodman, author of the forthcoming "Patients without Borders." For invasive surgeries, preferred destinations include India, Thailand, Singapore and Malaysia. Large hospitals, such as Bumrungrad and the Apollo chain in India, actively court American, European and Middle Eastern patients. Bumrungrad arranges limousines to pick up patients at the airport, and sheiks and princes congregate in the Platinum Lounge of Apollo's Delhi hospital. Abacas International, a leading travel facilitator, reports that medical tourism to Asia could generate billions of dollars.

Businesses are taking notice. At least 40 corporations have signed on to the overseas plan that United Group Programs, a health insurer in Boca Raton, Florida, began offering six months ago. Sending an employee abroad can save 80 percent of the costs of a procedure; a $50,000 angioplasty in the United States costs less than $6,000 in Mohali, Chandigarh, India, according to Global Choice Health care, a firm that arranges foreign medical procedures. Walk-in patients see a specialist in 17 minutes on average. Since 75 percent of hospital revenues are paid by patients directly, health and insurance companies have no say in treatment. Low labour costs allow Thai hospitals to employ more staff.

In Australia, Europe and North America, "complementary and alternative medicine" (CAM) is increasingly being used in parallel to modern medicine, particularly for treating and managing chronic disease. Concern about the adverse effects of chemical medicines, a desire for more personalized health care and greater public access to health information, fuel this increased use. For the past six years, persons from over two hundred countries with difficult and chronic conditions, i.e., diverticulitis, cancer, and incurable autoimmune diseases such as Systemic Lupus Erythematosis (SLE), Multiple Sclerosis (MS), Lou Gherigi's Disease (ALS), have been motivated to explore the options Traditional Chinese Medicine (TCM) offers them at Huai Hua Red Cross Hospital. Since these conditions are chronic and often times incurable, they have led many patients and/or their family members to seek and decipher complex, baffling, and, obscure medical information and to explore options encountered beyond the diagnostic and treatment scope generally available to them. Despite their diverse cultural backgrounds, many persons reach this intersecting destination at the time-honoured tradition of TCM and the Huai Hua Red Cross Hospital for Difficult and Chronic conditions.

Five million tourists for health treatment

According to the Tourism Authority of Thailand (TAT), at least five million tourists come to the country annually for medical treatment. Various plastic surgery clinics could attest that the number of both Thais and foreigners undergoing dental and plastic surgeries, lasik, and other physical enhancement procedures is increasing. Aside from these, Thailand has earned its reputation as an excellent location for spa services. "The growth of spa business is a good sign that tells us that we can respond to customers' needs," Mr. Apichai added pointing to Proud Asia 2008 as an excellent venue where the international community can actually see the advancements that Thailand has taken the field of medical tourism.

"Beauty business will continuously grow as both men and women care about their looks," President of Thai Society of Cosmetic Dermatology and Surgery, Dr. Thada Piamphongsan, said, adding that Thailand has more advantages than other countries in Asia when it comes to offering the best quality medical and beauty services but at cheaper rates.

"Proud Asia 2008 is definitely not just the usual exhibition event on beauty and health care products and services we see here and in other countries. What makes this event extraordinary is the fact that we are going to have a grand showcase of the latest innovations of products and services in the field of medical tourism, spa and wellness. Everybody will be here- the expert in medical tourism, the best spa and wellness providers, and the most highly interested buyers. "The event promises to be a big one for both suppliers and buyers and the most important thing is that it will be held right here in Bangkok. This means that the Kingdom will again have the chance to prove to the international community that Thailand has sufficient MICE infrastructure to be the best venue for this kind of trade exhibition and conference. Proud Asia 2007 is a huge event that will help the country achieve its goal of becoming a regional hub for exhibitions and conventions business and Mice market," said Mr. Vithaya.

Health tourism boom takes Singapore by storm

Singapore on the other hand makes world headlines for performing complex neurosurgical procedures and delivering cutting-edge medical treatment by the region's leading health specialists. The Republic's reputation for high quality medical facilities and well-trained doctors pulled in more than 370,000 visitors in 2004. The cost of treatments in Singapore, such as a hip replacement, can be less than a third of the price in the United States. In some cases, the cost is less than a tenth of what people would pay in America or Europe.

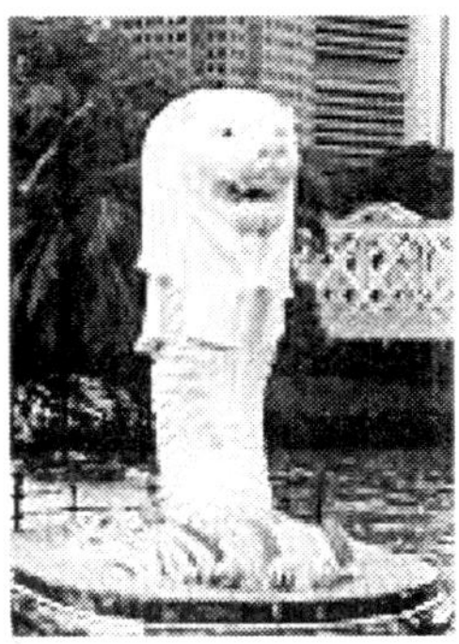

Raffles Hospital, has gained fame in recent years for highly publicized operations to separate conjoined twins, exemplifying the highly skilled expertise available.

The tiny island of Singapore, having a populace of 4.4 million, is fast positioning itself as a medical tourism hub. The authorities are ambitious of serving one million foreign patients annually by 2012 and generate USD 3 billion in revenue.

Parkway hospitals group is Singapore's largest private health care group in Asia, owning three tertiary care private hospitals: East Shore, Gleneagles and Mount Elizabeth. The magnificent façade of these hospitals are complemented by equally competent doctors and excellent services with world class equipment. Incidentally, quite a few patients come from India for liver transplant. Nitin Saxena, who brought his father all the way from Delhi to Gleneagles for a liver transplant, opines unlike Indian hospitals, the services and facilities value for money.

Stem cell transplant is yet another field developing rapidly on the health map of Singapore. The haematology and stem cell transplant centre of Mount Elizabeth Hospital has pioneered stem cell treatment for patients with advanced cancer tumours. Headed by director Dr, Patrick Tan, a world renowned specialist in the field of oncology, cost of treatment here ranges from USD 72,000 to USD 90,000 per person, compared to USD 235,000 for similar treatment in the US. Recently, a 12-year-old girl from Delhi underwent cord blood transplant at the centre. As a mark of hospitality, hospital staff goes to receive patients and their relatives from the airport, make arrangements for their stay and even provide with language whenever required.

The medical tourism boom is just not restricted to Singapore alone. Current trend of economic developments in the Asian region, higher life expectancies, an aging population and an ever-increasing awareness of the benefits of the quality health care have given a shot in the arm to the Asian health care industry, taking it to witness an unprecedented growth. Presently, there are only 140,000 hospitals serving an Asian population of 3.5 billion. With Asian population expected to grow to 5.6 billion by 2050, the consumer expenditure on health care services and goods will increase from US $90 billion in 1999 to US $188 billion in 2013. Malaysia is targeting the Middle East and China to generate whopping revenue of 2.2 billion by 2010. These emerging markets prove that there's immense potential in the Asian health care business, remarked Ms Tan-Hoong Chu Eng, MD, Parkway Promotions Pte Ltd., a subsidiary company of Parkway-Holdings Ltd. the largest private health care group in Asia.

Demand for health care is rising in the Middle East with millions of dollars spent in establishing specialised hospitals and clinics, expanding existing facilities and adopting world class technology in Bahrain, Kuwait, Yemen, Oman and Qatar. In the UAE, for instance, the government plans to double the bed capacity of public hospitals to achieve a target of one for every 300 people by the end of the decade.

The Philippines Faith healers

The Philippines beats other countries to this idea of medical tourism faith healing' for the last many years. I recall how in the 1970s, faith healers like Tony Agpaoa were already offering tour packages for people coming in from Europe and Japan who wanted the faith healers' services. Agpaoa even had his own little hotel in Baguio City so patients didn't have to look for their own accommodations. The faith healing packages eventually went into decline, and last I heard, it was our faith healers who were going to Eastern European countries to do their road-show healing.

Earlier this year, then-secretary of tourism Roberto Pagdanganan announced that the Department of Tourism was teaming up with the Department of Health, specifically the Philippine Institute of Traditional and Alternative Health Care, to promote medical tourism. At that time, he said only the St. Luke's hospital had been accredited for their program but Asian Hospital, Capitol Medical Centre, and Medical City had also applied. Our medical and nursing curricula are certainly tougher than many of our neighbours in Southeast Asia. Who knows, maybe medical tourism can convince a few more Filipino health professionals to stay rather than migrate.

Malaysia

Malaysia raked in RM 203.6 million in hospital receipts last year from nearly 300,000 foreign medical patients. Health Ministry parliamentary secretary Datuk Lee Kah Choon said Penang's portion of the takings amounted to RM129.9 million or 63.83 per cent of the total. The other cities involved were Kuala Lumpur, Malacca and Johor Baru. "We are expecting double-digit growth for hospital receipt figures this year," he said after witnessing the signing of a clinical research collaboration between YSP Industries Sdn Bhd and Penang-based Infor Kinetics Sdn Bhd here. Among the types of treatment sought are for heart ailments, cosmetic surgery, and wellness treatment at spas. "Patients include those from Indonesia and Singapore. The government is studying ways to make medical tourism more attractive to invest in." Health care tourism in Malaysia took-off in an aggressive manner in 2002 when Tourism Malaysia began promoting it overseas. "This includes tax-relief on the purchase of medical equipment or capital allowance on costs for new buildings," he said, adding that the proposed breaks were to reduce the "burden" on these institutions to enable them to continuously invest in upgrading their services. The Health Ministry is pursuing international accreditation for two Kuala Lumpur hospitals to boost medical tourism.

Several other countries in Asia and other continents are also working for medical tourism.

Appendix II

COMMON SURGICAL INTERVENTIONS SOUGHT BY FOREIGN MEDICAL TOURISTS

Globalisation has promoted a consumerist culture, thereby promoting goods and services that can feed the aspirations arising from this culture. This has had its effect in the health sector too, with the emergence of a private sector that thrives by servicing a small percentage of the population that has the ability to "buy" medical care at the rates at which the "high end" of the private medical sector provides such care. However, for patients and profits to increase, India must remedy negative first impressions and persuade doubters that millions of the country's poor and ailing won't be left behind.

The following services are visibly noticed.

Bone Marrow Transplant

Major hospitals in India have oncology units comprising surgical oncology, medical and radiation therapy as well as the crucial Bone Marrow Transplantation (BMT). The BMT unit with high-pressure Hipa filters has helped achieve a very high success rate in the various types of transplantation. Cord Blood Transplant and Mismatched Allogeneic Stem Cell Transplant have been performed successfully, a feat that is remarkable and significant, considering the fact that the treatment costs one-tenth of what it does in the west. Special surgeons are available for individual organs. Plastic surgeons of repute provide treatment for head and neck cancer, breast cancer and other malignancies. Facilities offered include tele-therapy, which includes simulation work stations to ensure high precision and safety during treatment at the 18 MV linear accelerator or telecobalt machines, brachy therapy and 3-D planning systems. In orthopedics, the Ilizarov technique is practiced for the treatment of limb deformities, limb shortening and disfiguration.

Cardiac Care

Cardiac care has become a specialty in India with institutions like the Escorts Heart Institute and Research Centre, All India Institute of Medical Sciences and Apollo Hospital becoming names to reckon with. These centres have the distinction of providing comprehensive cardiac care spanning from basic facilities in preventive cardiology to the most sophisticated curative technology. The technology is contemporary and world class and the volumes handled match global benchmarks. They also specialise in offering surgery to high-risk patients with the introduction of innovative techniques like minimally invasive and robotic surgery.

Having accomplished what he set out to do with Escorts, Trehan is planning a multispecialty hospital in Gurgaon, on the outskirts of New Delhi, that's patterned on the Cleveland Clinic in Ohio and the Mayo Clinic in Rochester, Minnesota.

Interventional Cardiology

Interventional Cardiology is a specialty which uses imaging techniques and strategies for the diagnosis of the diseases of the heart and blood vessel. These novel, minimally invasive, non-surgical procedures make use of mechanical treatments for the diseases of the heart and blood vessels. These procedures are mostly performed under local anesthesia, have a considerably short hospitalization and recovery period with minimal post-operative pain and discomfort. Interventional Cardiology includes a number of procedures that can be performed to the heart by means of inserting a 'catheter' either in your heart or in one of your blood vessels of the groin, neck or forearm. Established in 2000, the Krishna Heart Institute and Specialty Clinic is known for its innovative diagnostics and treatment procedures, and its extensive work in areas such as cardiology and joint replacement. Located in Ahmedabad, Gujarat, this institute is one of Gujarat's leading medical facilities. Initially specializing in cardiac care, the institute has grown into specialized areas such as hip and knee replacement surgeries, plastic and reconstructive surgeries, Onco-surgery, and other invasive and minimally invasive procedures. The institute has an excellent record for providing quality medical care for its international visitors at affordable prices. An air conditioned lounge is on each floor and there is a cafeteria with an expert chef serving a selection of cuisines. The institute provides continuous central monitoring and International standard water filtration and distribution systems for pure water, hot and cold. This institute is only one of the several cenres of excellence in the field of interventional cardiology.

Peripheral Angioplasty or Percutaneous Transluminal Angioplasty (PTA)

Peripheral Angioplasty is a minimally invasive procedure which is used to open narrowed arteries of the legs (most commonly iliac arteries causing cramps when walking, known as claudication), those to the brain known as the carotid arteries (causing stroke) and the arteries to the kidneys (causing high blood pressure). These conditions belong to the group of Peripheral Vascular Disease. Another condition may be ballooning of the artery called aneurysm. Aneurysms commonly occur in abdominal aorta where it manifests itself with abdominal pain or tenderness and a throbbing mass in the abdomen. Peripheral Vascular Disease is diagnosed by a procedure called angiogram which is similar to Coronary Angiogram. Peripheral Angioplasty is very similar to Coronary Angioplasty where arteries of the heart are narrowed due to atherosclerosis (Coronary Artery Disease). The blockage in the arteries is caused by deposition of fat in the form of plaques which accumulate along the arterial wall. Cost of procedure performed in the US: $18,171.

What does the procedure for Peripheral Angioplasty involve?

The procedure for Peripheral Angioplasty usually comprises of three steps: Step one of Peripheral Angioplasty, also known as artherectomy involves removal of blockage (plaque) from your peripheral artery either by laser or with specialized instruments to cut the plaque away and clear the arterial channel. The second step of Peripheral Angioplasty makes use of a balloon. An un-inflated balloon is inserted with the help of a guide wire to the site of blockage. The balloon is then inflated, which as a result enlarges the blood channel and increases blood flow through the artery. It is interesting to note that Peripheral Angioplasty can reduce a 70-90% blockage to about 20-30%. Step three of Peripheral Angioplasty consists of implanting a mesh stent which is tightly mounted on the Peripheral Angioplasty balloon into the walls of blocked artery.

If you have been diagnosed with intermittent claudication, i.e. aches, pain, cramps, or tightness in the calves, thighs, hips or buttocks when walking, which is relieved with a few moments rest, if you have leg ulcers or gangrene, if you have an aneurysm (abdominal aorta or cerebral artery), if you are a smoker who experiences numbness, tingling or coldness of legs and feet, if you suffer from high blood pressure, diabetes, high cholesterol, a family history of heart or vascular disease, and are overweight with symptoms of peripheral vascular disease, then you are an ideal candidate for Peripheral Angioplasty.

Peripheral Angioplasty has a success rate of almost 95% with the chances of re-stenosis occurring in 5% of the patients. This procedure is less painful and allows you to go back to your daily activities quickly. This means that you will not have the symptoms of Peripheral Vascular Disease any more. Insertion of Drug Eluting Stents have potentially improved the clinical outcome of the procedure of Peripheral Angioplasty. Peripheral Angioplasty has revolutionized the treatment of Peripheral Vascular Disease. Implantation of stents during angioplasty procedure reduces the chances of re-stenosis of the artery tremendously. The procedure of Peripheral Angioplasty is certainly not a treatment for Peripheral Vascular Disease however, accompanying lifestyle changes can definitely reduce your chances of further problems and complications. Cost of procedure performed in the US: $18,171.

What is Coronary Angiography?

Coronary Angiography is a procedure in which a non-ionic contrast dye is injected into the coronary arteries. This allows your cardiologist to visualize the coronary arteries on an x-ray and view the flow of blood through them. Cost of procedure performed in the US: $3,000 to $6,000. During the procedure of Coronary Angiography, you might experience some flushing and/or palpitation which will subside quickly. If you have chest pain which may or may not be increasing in intensity and duration, if you have unexplained pain in your jaw, neck or arm, if you have congenital heart disease or congestive heart failure, if you are planning to have heart valve surgery, if you have problems with your blood vessels like aortic aneurysm, if you have suffered a traumatic injury to your chest, then you are an ideal candidate for Coronary Angiography. Coronary Angiography is a relatively harmless procedure that can unfold tremendous amount of information and detail about the structure and function of your coronary arteries. Coronary Angiography is a diagnostic procedure that is used to confirm the diagnosis of the diseases affecting your heart and blood vessels. This procedure is also used to determine the extent and severity of your disease, and to help plan your treatment.

Risks of Coronary Angiography

- Allergic reaction to the contrast dye
- Irregular heart beat (arrhythmias)
- Heart attack and death during the Coronary Angiography procedure
- Stroke
- Injury to the internal wall of the artery where the catheter was threaded in
- Perforation of coronary artery.
- Kidney damage
- Excessive bleeding (hemorrhage)
- Infection
- Blood clots

Alternatives to Coronary Angiography

- *Magnetic Resonance Angiography (MRA)*—In this procedure detailed images of your heart are captured using radio waves in a strong magnetic field without the use of catheters or X-rays.
- *CT Angiography*—This method does not require catheterization within the heart reducing some of the risks associated with Coronary Angiography.
- *Digital Subtraction Angiography (DSA)*—This method combines the X-ray techniques of Coronary Angiography with a high-speed computer to improve the resolution of images obtained.
- *Cardiac Catheterization*—This procedure is very similar to Coronary Angiography and consists of passage of a catheter in the coronary artery

What is Coronary Angioplasty?

Coronary Angioplasty or Balloon Angioplasty is a minimally invasive procedure in which the blocked or narrowed coronary arteries are opened (widened) to facilitate perfusion of the heart muscle. Coronary Angioplasty reduces the need for medication and to some extent eliminates chest pain due to Ischemic Heart Disease. Cost of procedure performed in the US:

$35,000. The procedure for Coronary Angioplasty usually comprises of three steps: Step one of Coronary Angioplasty, also known as artherectomy involves removal of blockage (plaque) from your coronary artery either by laser or with specialized instruments to cut the plaque away and clear the arterial channel. The second step of Coronary Angioplasty makes use of a balloon (thus the alternative term Balloon Angioplasty). In this step, an uninflated balloon is inserted with the help of a guide wire to the site of blockage. The balloon is then inflated, which enlarges the blood channel and increases blood flow through the artery. It is interesting to note that Coronary Angioplasty can reduce a 70-90% blockage to about 20-30%. Step three of Coronary Angioplasty consists of implanting a mesh stent which is tightly mounted on the Coronary Angioplasty balloon into the walls of blocked artery. The balloon is then deflated and removed leaving the stent in place permanently to hold the artery open. In this procedure of Coronary Angioplasty, the coronary arteries are accessed through a puncture made in the groin (femoral artery) or arm (brachial artery). Usually the femoral artery is used. Depending upon the extent of coronary artery narrowing, all three steps may or may not be carried out. The procedure of Coronary Angioplasty can take 30 minutes to several hours depending on the number of blockages being treated.

Benefits of Coronary Angioplasty

- Quicker and less painful recovery
- Short hospital stay, does not require general anesthesia
- Small incision
- Coronary Angioplasty can be done under local anesthesia
- The chest cage does not need to be opened
- Chances of major post-operative complications like stroke are minimized as heart-lung machine is not used during the procedure of Coronary Angioplasty

Risks of Coronary Angioplasty

- Allergic reaction to the dye
- Ruptured coronary artery
- Bleeding and infection at the site of insertion
- Arrhythmia
- Stroke
- Heart attack
- Kidney failure
- Rupture or dissection of the coronary artery
- Re-stenosis of the coronary artery requiring Heart Bypass Surgery

Why is Coronary Stenting performed?

Coronary Stenting is performed to hold your coronary artery open to facilitate flow of blood to the heart muscle and reduce your chest pain due to angina. The coronary stents physically hold your artery open and create a channel for your blood to flow through it easily. Coronary Stenting is usually performed as part of the Coronary Angioplasty procedure. So if you are an ideal candidate for Coronary Angioplasty, i.e. if one or more of your coronary arteries are blocked, if your chest pain due to angina is not well controlled with medications or if it is severe enough to disrupt your daily activities and also occurs at rest, then you are an ideal candidate for Coronary Stenting. Coronary Stenting has a success rate of almost 95% with the chances of re-stenosis occurring in 5% of the patients. This procedure is less painful and allows you to go back to your daily activities quickly. This means that you will not have chest pain any more and that your tolerance to exercise will increase. Drug Eluting Coronary Stents have potentially improved the clinical outcome of Coronary Stenting.

Benefits of Coronary Stenting

- Quicker and less painful recovery
- Short hospital stay, does not require general anesthesia
- Small incision
- Coronary Stenting can be done under local anesthesia
- The chest cage does not need to be opened
- Chances of major post-operative complications like stroke are minimized as heart-lung machine is not used during Coronary Stenting procedure
- Implantation of drug eluting coronary stents dramatically decreases the chances of re-stenosis and the need for a repeat procedure.

In the procedure for Drug Eluting Coronary Stenting, the implanted stent is coated with a medication that prevents re-stenosis. This type of stent consistently releases a chemical substance that prevents clot formation and narrowing of coronary artery. Drug Eluting Coronary Stenting has been 20-30% more successful than bare metal stenting. Cost of procedure performed in the US: $37,000.

Benefits of Drug Eluting Coronary Stenting

- Quicker and less painful recovery
- Short hospital stay, does not require general anesthesia
- Small incision (Minimally Invasive procedure)
- Drug Eluting Coronary Stenting can be done under local anesthesia
- The chest cage does not need to be opened

- Chances of major post-operative complications like stroke are minimized as heart-lung machine is not used during the procedure of Drug Eluting Coronary Stenting.
- Implantation of Drug Eluting Coronary Stenting has dramatically decreased the chances of re-stenosis and the need for a repeat procedure.

Dialysis and Kidney Transplant

Common diseases like diabetes, hypertension and chronic glomerulonephritis can lead to permanent loss of renal functions—with dialysis and renal transplantation being the frequent outcome. The emergence of new therapeutic interventions has created opportunities in India to manage the progression of renal diseases. Major hospitals in India like Holy Family Hospital, Jaslok Hospital, Apollo Hospital, Sir Ganga Ram Hospital, Batra Hospital, Bombay Hospital and Hinduja Hospital have departments of Nephrology and Organ Transplant equipped with the latest computerised dialysis machines, reverse osmosis water plant to provide pure and trace element-free water supply, as well as state-of-the-art facilities in the operating rooms and Transplant Intensive Care Units.

For those who need renal replacement therapy, the following services are also available.

Patients can also avail of the bicarbonate dialysis facility at these centres. Round the clock service is available at these hospitals for the critically ill patients in the intensive care units who may need fluid, electrolyte management and renal supportive therapy.

The cost of getting a dialysis is around Rs. 1700 to Rs. 1800 per dialysis whereas the same costs about $300 in the U.S.A. Similarly a kidney transplant package in India is available for around Rs. 3 Lakhs, which is comparatively much cheaper than what it would cost abroad. Hemodialysis Chronic Ambulatory Peritoneal Dialysis (CAPD) Transplantation. In addition to the basic haemodialysis facilities, the patients' requirements for other modalities of treatment such as—Continuous Arterio-Venous Haemofilteration (CAVH) Continuous Veno-Venous Haemofilteration (CVVH) Continuous Cycler-Assisted Peritioneal Dialysis (CCPD).

Gynecology and Obstetrics

Leading Indian hospitals with gynecology departments and women's hospitals have facilities for the prevention and early detection of gynecological disorders. Many hospitals have women check-up programmes designed to detect the earliest signs of disorders of the breast and the organs of reproduction as well as catering to the contraceptive needs of women. A mammogram, an ultrasound of the pelvis and a pap smear of the cervix are an integral part of any good medical check-up for women. Specialist medical as well as surgical care is available for all types of gynecological problems like menstrual abnormalities, prolapse, fibroids and other tumors of the uterus and ovaries, tubal re-canalization by microsurgery and care of the infertile couple. State-of-the-art gynecological surgery is available with world-class equipment and expertise using minimally invasive techniques.

Ectopic pregnancies, ovarian cysts and tumors, fibroids endometriosis, tubal blocks and even hysterectomies can be performed laparoscopically. Hospitals like Apollo have state-of-the-art IVF labs backed by highly experienced doctors who have been involved in the field of infertility and assisted Reproductive Technologies (ART).

Joint Replacement Surgery

Shoulder/hip replacement and bilateral knee replacement surgery using the most advanced keyhole or endoscopic surgery and arthroscopy is done at several hospitals in India including the Apollo Hospital, Sir Ganga Ram Hospital and Holy Family Hospital in Delhi, Bombay Hospital, Leelavati and Hinduja Hospital in Mumbai and the Madras Institute of Orthopaedics and Trauma Sciences. Some hospitals like Apollo in Delhi have Operation Theatres with Laminar Air Flow System, which compares with the best in the USA and the UK. A knee joint replacement costs only a quarter of what it costs in the UK. In the last 5 years arthroplasty has got established and has changed the face of osteoarthritis patients. More than 10 million people are supposed to suffer from this ailment in India alone. Dr. Dholakia was the first to introduce the technique in 1986. Ranawat performed surgery on the knees of the then prime minister of India in 2000. Now further advancement has occurred and new techniques have come in giving better results.

Neurosurgery and Trauma Surgery

Other routine procedures performed with excellent results are replacement arthroplasty, diagnostic and operative arthroscopy, spinal surgeries including. Harrington Rod Instrumentation for scoliosis, corrective and reconstructive procedure for poliomyelitis and cerebral palsy, micro cascular surgical procedures and automated percutaneous lumbar distectomy. In addition, the advanced Luque technique is employed for the correction of complex scoliosis, and decompression and stabilisation of fractures of dorsal and lumbar spine with paraplegia, by neurosurgeons with excellent training and background. Many super-speciality hospitals in India like AIIMS, Ram Manohar Lohia Hospital, Vidya Sagar Institute of Mental Health and Neuro Sciences, Bombay Hospital, Jaslok Hospital, Nizam Institute of Mental Health and Neuro Sciences and Apollo Hospitals have advanced facilities devoted to the treatment of the entire range of brain and spinal disorders with highly experienced neurosurgeons, neurologists, Neuro-anaesthetists and Neuro-radiologists. Treatment of intra- and juxta-cranial, spinal tumours and vascular malformations, aneurysms and thrombolysis for brain attacks are done at these centres. Hospitals like Apollo employ state-of-the-art LINAC-based stereotactic radio surgery system outside the USA. The Clinic 6000SR Linear Accelerator with

XKNIFE system is a highly sophisticated computer-driven technology used for removal of appropriately selected brain tumours, arteriovenous malformations and other abnormalities.

Osteoporosis

Several drug therapies now easily available in the market have been shown to be clinically effective in slowing down or reversing the bone-loss process. Leading hospitals in India are well equipped to detect and treat bone loss in its earliest states, so as to prevent the disease or lessen its impact. Doctors in leading hospitals have the expertise for the diagnosis and treatment of osteoporosis that involves an objective, quantifiable measurement of the patient's bone mass or bone density. Advanced technology called the DXA for bone densitometry is available. During a comprehensive bone valuation with DXA, the patient lies comfortably still on a padded table while the DXA unit scans one or more areas, usually the fractured spine or the hip. The entire process takes only minutes to scan depending on the number of sites scanned. It involved no injections or invasive procedures and the patient remains fully clothed.

Refractive Surgery

Refractive surgery is gaining popularity in India both among the public as well as among ophthalmologists. Till a few years ago only a few centres performed high volume radial keratotomy. Today, the highest international quality of eye care for cornea, cataract, squint and glaucoma is available in over 40 centres all over India. When it comes to reliability, India has the best ophthalmic surgeons with clinico-academic expertise honed to perfection in the best possible institutions. Apollo Hospital, Gurunanak Eye Centre, Dr. Rajindra Prasad Centre For Ophthalmic Sciences and Mohan Eye Centre in Delhi, Shankar Naytralaya in Chennai, L. V. Prasad hospital in Hyderabad are just some of the more popular eye care hospitals. The No Stitch Cataract Surgery with the most modern way of removing cataract through the use of Phacoemulsification procedure can be performed in India for as little as Rs. 20,000, for both the eyes, whereas the same surgery costs $45,000 in the USA. Facilities for PRK, myopia and astigmatism are now available in almost all parts of the country. Hyperopic and LASIK are available and even supra hard cataracts are treated using just 1 mm incision instead of the 3 mm incision size. Photo-refractive keratectomy or PRK treats the surface of the cornea with the Excimer laser while LASIK treats the inner tissue of the cornea. For this reason, with LASIK there is less area to heal, less risk of scarring, less risk of corneal haze, less post-operative pain and vision often returns very rapidly.

Urology

Several super specialty hospitals in India offer comprehensive Urologic services to diagnose and treat stone disease, Urologic cancer, incontinence, infertility, impotency and other urinary difficulties. Advanced methods such as lithotripsy for treating kidney and ureteric stones without surgery are available with complementary methods of treating stones endoscopically. Advanced machines like the Lithostar obvert the need for anaesthesia in the treatment of kidney and ureteric stones. High tech facilities for the treatment of prostate, bladder cancers, urethral strictures are also available. Investigation and treatment facilities for impotence and male/female infertility exist with specialized facilities for pharmacotherapy, cavernosometry and cavernosography, in addition to doppler studies for the assessment of blood flow.

Other surgeries

Removal of the gall bladder, the spleen, the bowel and other organs like the adrenals, an operation for prolapse rectum and hiatus hernia repair have become fairly commonplace in almost all the major speciality hospitals in India. Experts are easily available and accessible and the workload at most of these hospitals ensures that the doctors have enormous experience. High intensive care treatment at much cheaper rates than in the west is available at most of these centres.

Preventive Health Care

Preventive health care has been introduced for the first time in the country by Apollo Hospitals with hospitals in the metros of Hyderabad, Chennai and Delhi, within easy international air access. The professional chain also pioneered the concept of lifestyle clinics, established the first organ registry in the country and introduced non-invasive technique for treatment of lesions and tumours of the brain—Stereotactic Radio Surgery and Radiotherapy in the country. It recently installed a state of the art Cobalt Unit. Apollo Heart Hospital provides a complete network for cardiac patients. It has a total bed capacity of 500 beds distributed between Apollo Chennai, Hyderabad and Delhi. Apollo is linked to the Mayo Clinic and the Minneapolis Heart Institute, a premier heart institute led by the team of doctors who pioneered the Jarvik artificial heart.

Imaging with MRI, a hypertension research centre and facilities for hemodialysis and kidney transplantation are available at Akila Hospitals at Trichy. The hospital boasts a transplant team with 8 specialists, bone marrow transplant team along with five specialists on call to Sri Lanka, Sharjah, Kuwait and major Indian cities.

In Chennai, the Vijaya Heart Foundation's 79 beds have a state of the art cardiology and cardio-thoracic surgical unit manned by competent and experienced staff. The Vijaya Health Centre with 270 beds offers diagnostic facilities in laboratory, X-ray, ultrasound, treadmill, Endoscopy,. C.T. Scan, M.R.I. and nuclear medicine.

Fasting

Naturopath doctors at such centres mean a minimalist diet of 300 calories per day—veggie broths and juices-for two weeks to several months, accompanied by blood tests, purges and other treatments. They say many hard-to-treat conditions, from arthritis to allergies and various skin disorders, benefit from the metabolic switch that takes place when the body starts living off its own reserves. Of the thousands guests who come to fast each year (half from southern Europe, America and the Middle East), about one third arrive with serious ailments—the rest come to lose weight or cut stress. Fasting has lately gotten a boost from medical research. Clinical studies in Scandinavia have shown that fasting is an effective treatment for rheumatism—especially if followed by a vegetarian diet. In one study, pain and swelling came down by a third in a week and stayed that way for a year. Other studies have shown success in lowering blood pressure and treating chronic pain like migraine or arthritis. They have shown that when patients fast, stress hormones levels go down and serotonin levels rise (which may explain the "fasting high" many patients report). "The more we look into it, fasting seems to work like a reset button for the body's own self-regulating mechanisms," say Naturopaths.

$800 vs. $18

In the U.S., organizations such as the Joint Commission International (JCI) on Accreditation of Health care Organizations, based in Oakbrook Terrace, Illinois, assess infection rates, the width of hospital corridors and the capacity of elevators. Dr. Trehan, Escorts' founder, says the hospital had a mortality rate of 0.8 percent and an infection rate of 0.3 percent in 2003. That compares with an observed mortality rate, or the rate of actual deaths, of 4.77 percent for heart valve surgery or coronary artery bypass surgery that included heart valves at New York—Presbyterian Hospital. Charging foreigners more than Indians is one way hospitals can make money to treat the poor, says Gautam Kumra, a McKinsey & Co. partner in New Delhi. An echocardiogram machine, used to picture the heart, costs about $200,000 anywhere in the world. Doctors can charge $800 per scan in the U.S.; in India, they charge 800 rupees, or $18, Trehan says. Fortis Health care plans is setting up two hospitals on the outskirts of New Delhi. One will cater to overseas patients and charge them higher prices, says Harpal Singh, who adds the hospitals haven't set fees yet. Fortis is owned by brothers Malvinder and Shivinder Singh, who control India's largest drug company, Ranbaxy Laboratories Ltd. Harpal Singh is Malvinder Singh's father-in-law. One imbalance that works in India's favour is its lower salaries. A top cardiac surgeon in India makes about $330,000 a year compared with $5 million in the U.S., says Anupam Sibal, director at Apollo Hospital New Delhi.

Cosmetic and Plastic Surgery

This is a surgical specialty that corrects disfigurement caused by burns, tumor, congenital defects, developmental abnormalities, trauma, infection, disease or injuries, improves appearance and self esteem and restores function. Cosmetic and Plastic Surgery is mainly concerned with correcting problems and enhancing appearance of exposed areas of the body and the face. Reconstructive Plastic Surgery is another term that is used in this context mainly referring to surgical procedures that correct severe functional impairments, fix physical abnormalities, and compensate for tissue lost to trauma or surgery.

Some disfigurations corrected include hair restoration (hair implants, hair flaps, and scalp reductions), rhinoplasty (reshaping or re-contouring of the nose), stalling of the aging process (face lift, cosmetic eyelid surgery, brow lift, sub-metal lipectomy for double chin), dermabrasions (sanding of the face), otoplasty for protruding ears, chin and cheek enlargement, lip reductions, various types of breast surgery and reconstruction and liposuction.

The problem of loose upper arm skin usually occurs after weight loss. This problem is more common in people who have lost a lot of weight. If you were over weight, the skin of your arm has to stretch to accommodate the increased volume of your upper arm. After weight loss, the skin usually fails to tighten and sags. Brachioplasty is performed to correct this problem of loose hanging skin of your arms. Brachioplasty is performed as an outpatient procedure in the plastic surgeon's office under local anesthesia with sedation. The entire procedure of Brachioplasty takes about an hour per arm. The surgeon makes zigzag, elliptical or triangular incisions along the inner surface of upper arm. The space contained between the incisions is exactly the area of skin that would be removed. Removal of loose skin tightens the surface of the arm however, it does not remove the fat. That is why it is usually recommended that Brachioplasty be accompanied with liposuction as well to remove extra fat from your arms. Make sure that you make arrangements for some one to accompany you as you will be allowed to go home after a couple of hours following Brachioplasty procedure.

Benefits of Brachioplasty

- Brachioplasty will help you get rid of the extra fat and skin after losing weight. Although this requires you to undergo a Brachioplasty procedure, the results are well worth it. To be able to get the lean and shapely arms that you have always longed for, Brachioplasty is the best option available.
- Brachioplasty is performed under local anesthesia, does not require hospitalization and you can return to work and resume your daily activities within 2 weeks.

What is Body Lift?

Body Lift or Total Body Lift is a Cosmetic and Plastic Surgery procedure performed to reshape your body to it's natural curves and contours. Body Lift is a surgical procedure where the loose and hanging skin of the entire body is tightened and implants are inserted, all in one procedure. Body Lift basically reshapes the breasts, chest, arms, thighs, hips, back, waist, abdomen and knees after losing weight (for example those people who lose lot of weight after undergoing weight loss surgeries like Gastric Bypass, Laparoscopic Gastric Bypass, Gastric Banding), aging and multiple pregnancies. Body Lift can be:

- *Central Body Lift*—This procedure is also called Belt Lipectomy. In Central Body Lift, excess skin and fatty tissue is removed circumferentially from the belly, hips, back, buttocks, and outer thighs.
- *Lower Body Lift*—Lower Body Lift is performed to shape buttocks and thighs by removing excess skin and fat from these areas.

Body Lift can be combined with other Cosmetic and Plastic Surgery procedures like Liposuction, Power Assisted Liposculpture (PAL), Tummy Tuck, Thigh Lift, Arm Lift, Breast Reduction, Breast Augmentation, and Breast Lift. Skin Grafting may also be performed in places of the body where needed. These procedures not only remove excess skin and fat, they also improve the unsightly stretch marks and create an uplifted, shapely, youthful and fuller appearance.

If you have lost large amounts of weight (50-300 lbs.) and have loose, hanging skin on your face, breasts, back, belly and thighs, or if you want to lose weight (especially if you suffer from central obesity) that is resistant to diet and exercise, if you have folds of loose, hanging skin due to aging or multiple pregnancies that might pose a danger of cellulitis or abscess, then you are an ideal candidate for Body Lift. This procedure can either be performed in isolation or in combination with other body contouring and weight loss procedures like Liposuction, Tummy Tuck, etc. If you are severely obese, are a smoker or an alcoholic or do not have a stable mental state to undergo a major surgical procedure and follow post-operative instructions to obtain optimum benefit or if you are allergic to the medication used for general anesthesia, then you are not an ideal candidate for Body Lift.

Body Lift is performed in a hospital setting under general anesthesia and can take about 5-7 or may be 10 hours depending on what other cosmetic surgery procedures are performed along with it. The Body Lift surgery is usually performed to remove excess skin from the belly first, i.e. from the area between the belly button and pubic hair and tightening of abdominal muscles is also performed. Excessive skin is removed, belly button is repositioned, remainder of the skin is approximated and the incision is sutured. The surgeon will then turn you on your side, make incisions in your buttock and back area, remove fat and excess skin to try and normalize the curves and contours of your sides and back. Body Lift also involves Liposuction of the buttocks, thighs and abdomen areas. Lastly, your surgeon will work on the flabby arms (commonly called bat wings) and make them shapely. As mentioned above, Liposuction, Power Assisted Liposculpture (PAL), Tummy Tuck, Thigh Lift, Arm Lift, Breast

Reduction, Breast Augmentation, Breast Lift and Skin Grafting can all be performed at the same time, whatever your need may be.

Body Lift is a comprehensive procedure that can take care of flabby, bulges in different parts of your body. The best results are obtained when Body Lift is performed by skillful and experienced cosmetic surgeons. This procedure is as safe as multiple shorter cosmetic surgeries. The contours of your body will be better defined and if you commit yourself to exercising regularly and eating sensibly, chances are that the results of Body Lift will be good for the rest of your life. Body Lift is a revolutionary surgical procedure that quickly, safely and effectively re-shapes the normal contours of your body. Most people who undergo Body Lift are quite satisfied with the results. The procedure of Body Lift is unified approach to treat and skin laxity as a result of aging, pregnancy and dramatic weight loss. Body Lift is a remarkable procedure which can help you get started on the way to a new, more fulfiling life of normalcy and a level of self-esteem that you may have never imagined.

Alternatives to Body Lift

- *Liposuction* is commonly used in both men and women to remove localized excess fat deposits that are resistant to dieting and exercise.
- *Power Assisted Liposculpture (PAL)*—Power Assisted Liposculpture uses a powerized cannula which moves back and forth through the fat tissue in a rapid motion.
- *Tummy tuck,* also known as Abdominoplasty or Panniculectomy is a procedure where large amount of skin and fat are removed from the middle and lower part of the abdomen.
- *Thigh Lift* is a procedure which is performed to remove loose and excessive (hanging) skin around your thighs and buttocks, thus to tighten them and improve it's appearance and texture.
- *Arm Lift*—Brachioplasty or Arm Lift is a procedure where loose and excess skin are removed from your arm.
- *Breast Reduction* is a surgical procedure designed to remove excessive fat, glandular tissue, and skin from large and pendulous breasts, making them smaller, lighter, and firmer.
- *Breast Augmentation or Breast Implant Surgery* is a surgical procedure in which the size and shape of a woman's breast is enhanced by inserting an artificial breast implant behind each breast.
- *Breast Lift or Mastopexy* is a surgical procedure which is commonly performed in men and in women to reshape sagging or drooping breasts and to give them a firm, youthful contour.
- *Skin grafting* is a surgical procedure by which skin or a skin substitute is used to replace the damaged skin or provide a temporary wound covering.

Body Lift is fondly called the *Face Lift* of your body. The resulting body contour shows a remarkable and significant improvement in the areas of the belly, pubic region, hips, back, and buttocks and will bring you to the range of normal body contour.

What is a Breast Implant?

A breast implant is a soft shell or a rubber sac that is filled with silicone gel or saline (salt-water). The feel of the implant is very natural and close to the feel of the normal breast tissue. They are available in several different sizes to accommodate different patient's needs and surgeon's preference. The surface texture of the implant can be smooth or contoured. There are different approaches used for Breast Augmentation surgery:

(1) *Infra-mammary Breast Augmentation*—This is the most commonly used approach for Breast Augmentation operation. In this approach an incision is made in the crease just below the breast where the breast tissue meets the chest wall.
(2) *Peri-areolar Breast Augmentation*—In this approach a semi-circular incision is made around the lower part of the areola (areola is the dark area of skin surrounding the nipple).
(3) *Trans-axillary or Axillary Breast Augmentation*—In this approach an incision is made in the armpit to insert the breast implant.
(4) *Trans-umblical or Umblical Breast Augmentation*—In this approach, a breast implant is inserted through the umbilicus or belly button with the help of an endoscope.

Breast Augmentation surgery takes about 2-3 hours. Most commonly you can go home the same day or the following day. The sutures are covered with a gauze dressing to promote speedy healing. The outcome of Breast Augmentation is very satisfactory and successful. Your breasts will be enlarged for life. Clothes fit better and it certainly boosts your self-confidence and self esteem. Some cases of leakage or breaking of the breast implant have been reported. In this case, a second Breast Augmentation surgery may be needed. The breast tissue is actually pushed to the surface as the breast implant is inserted behind the breast tissue. Following Breast Augmentation surgery it might become easier to perform breast self-examination to gain familiarity with your breast tissue. Of course, the obvious benefit Breast Augmentation is improved look of your breasts and your overall body image remains undisputed without any doubt. Breast Lift is designed to regain your youthful look and vigor. This procedure of Cosmetic and Plastic Surgery is used world wide by women as well as men to improve the appearance of drooping, sagging breasts. Breast Lift is performed in conjunction with Breast Augmentation to increase their size and give firmness. Breast Lift is a very popular surgery and the number of men and women undergoing Breast Lift has increased tremendously (214%) in the past five years. The beauty of Breast Lift is that it enhances your body image and maintains the normal shape of your breast as closely as possible. The operation for Breast Lift is an excellent option that reverses the changes that occur in your breast due to weight loss, pregnancy, breast feeding and aging. The goal of your plastic surgeon will be to restore the normal contour and firmness of your breasts as closely as possible. You will be extremely pleased with the results of Breast Lift surgery if you completely understand the procedure and make an informed decision but at the same time have realistic expectations.

What is Breast Reduction?

Breast Reduction is a surgical procedure designed to remove excessive fat, glandular tissue, and skin from large and pendulous breasts, making them smaller, lighter, and firmer. During Breast Reduction, the size of the areola is also reduced in proportion to the breast size. Breast Reduction is also performed in men for the correction of Gynecomastia. Breast Reduction surgery is performed to alleviate both your physical and psychological problems due to large breasts. Physical problems include upper back and neck pain and discomfort, deep and sore indentations on the shoulder from bra straps, rashes on the under surface of the breast due to sweat and moisture and difficulty finding clothes or bra that fit you well. Psychological problems include feeling self-conscious due to large breasts. All the above reasons are definite indications for Breast Reduction surgery. Breast Reduction is also performed in men who have large breasts. Although certain health conditions and medications are known to cause male breast enlargements (Gynecomastia), there is no other known cause for this problem in men. If you are a woman who has large, pendulous breasts and are not planning on having any more children, if you have chronic headache, upper back or neck pain, then you are an ideal candidate for Breast Reduction surgery.

Benefits of Breast Reduction

- Breast Reduction surgery not only alleviates your anxiety of being self-conscious about large, sagging breasts but it also relieves physical discomfort like chronic neck and back pain and skin rashes. Of course to say the least, Breast Reduction adds tremendously to your self-confidence and self-esteem as it enhances your body image and allows you to enjoy wearing clothes that you might have avoided to wear in the past. Breast Reduction also allows you freedom to enjoy sports and physical activities that might have been painful or uncomfortable due to bouncing of large and heavy breasts.
- You can feel the breast tissue better during Breast Self-examination as the surrounding excessive fat surrounding the glands and ducts has been diminished

How much can you save by your world-class treatment in India?

The best part about treatment in India is that you enjoy world-class medical advantages at a fraction of the cost in comparison with destinations like US, Europe, Africa and the Middle East. The greatest cost savings is typically found in orthopedic/cardiac procedures (75-90% lower fees outside of the United States). If you have received quotes in the US for $10,000, you can expect the same procedure to cost between $2,500 and $5,000 or less. If one is uninsured or under insured for medical treatment in U.S.A., the better option is to come to India. The significant cost reduction enables you purchase a round trip air ticket, recuperative holidays post-treatment in a exotic beach location in India and return home saving money. India aims to replicate the Thai model, which is still the first Asian destination for International Patients. Here are some examples of your medical price savings.

Nature of Treatment	Approximate Cost in India ($)	Cost in other Major Healthcare Destination ($)	Approximate Waiting Periods in USA / UK (in months)
Open heart Surgery	4,500	> 18,000	9 - 11
Cranio-facial Surgery and skull base	4,300	> 13,000	6 - 8
Neuro-surgery with Hypothermia	6,500	> 21,000	12 - 14
Complex spine surgery with implants	4,300	> 13,000	9 - 11
Simple Spine surgery	2,100	> 6,500	9 - 11
Simple Brain Tumor - Biopsy - Surgery	 1,000 4,300	 > 4,300 > 10,000	6 - 8
Parkinsons - Lesion - DBS	 2,100 17,000	 > 6,500 > 26,000	9 - 11
Hip Replacement	4,300	> 13,000	9 - 11

Where do the cost savings come from?

The answer lies in the economics of health care in the United States and the amount of fraud and waste that is present in the U.S. health care

Bargain Prices

Treatment	*India*	*US*
Coronary Artery Bypass Grafting	$6,600	$60,000
Knee Replacement (single knee)	$6,500	$22,000
Rhinoplasty (nose job)	$2,000	$10,000
Bone Marrow Transplant	$26,000	$2,50,000
Root Canal Treatment	$100	$1000

Procedure	*Cost (US $)*	
	United States	*India*
Liver Transplant	3,00,000	69,000
Cataract Surgery	2,000	1,250

system. 80% of all health care dollars that go through their office cover nothing but paperwork. As a medical tourist in another country, you eliminate these paperwork shufflers. And right there, you can save as much as 80% right off the bat. In the United States, your money is going to the insurance company and then the insurance company money is being used to pay paper shufflers.

Dental procedure	*Cost in US (US$)*		*Cost in India (US$)*
	By General Dentist	By Top End Dentist	By Top End Dentist
Smile designing	-	8,000	1,000
Metal Free Bridge	-	5,500	500
Dental Implants	-	3,500	800
Porcelain Metal Bridge	1,800	3,000	300
Porcelain Metal Crown	600	1,000	80
Tooth impactions	500	2,000	100
Root canal Treatment	600	1,000	100
Tooth whitening	350	800	110
Tooth colored composite fillings	200	500	25
Tooth cleaning	100	300	75

Some cost saving figures in dental treatment at a glance!

Case Study: An 87 year old US citizen who needed a mitral valve replacement turned to Madras Medical Mission Hospital, Chennai, India as no hospital would touch him being a high risk patient. He underwent a triple by-pass surgery years ago that cost him $40,000 in contrast the mitral valve surgery, a more complex and expensive surgery cost only $8,000 here in India. (The patient's damaged mitral valve was replaced with a bio-prosthetic valve whose life is said to be 15 years.) (The India Post Newspaper Publication, USA; Feb. '05)

Uninsured, Uninsurable or Underinsured : Americans increasingly traveling overseas

In the United States, health care is exorbitantly expensive, and each year millions of Americans find themselves unable to pay for the health care they want or need because they are either uninsured, uninsurable or underinsured. Over 47 million Americans have no health insurance at all, and millions more are forced to forgo 'elective procedures' that do not qualify for coverage by insurers. An estimated 120 million Americans live without any form of dental insurance. A recent study describes fifty-percent of bankruptcies in 2001 as being related to medical crises*, and each year millions of Americans are forced to choose between incurring crushing debt or foregoing medical procedures.

Medical Tourism has emerged as a viable health care alternative for many Westerners for a variety of reasons. Furthermore, an increasing number of Western-trained physicians from the developing world have returned to their country of origin to practice. The result is that a "perfect storm" of positive factors have come together to offer real, high quality medical alternatives to Westerners faced with significant costs or waiting times at home. What may accelerate the trend is that some pioneering U.S. corporations, swamped by rising health care costs, are taking a serious look at medical outsourcing. Blue Ridge Paper Products of Canton, N.C., a manufacturing company, may soon offer employees outsourcing as a health care option. The carrot? The patient would get to pocket some of the firm's substantial savings.

Americans looking to save money on medical procedures are increasingly traveling overseas for surgeries not covered by their insurance to avoid costly hospital stays in the United States. The trend is being driven by rising health care costs and frustrated ranks of uninsured American workers, said John Knox, a spokesman for MedSolution, a Vancouver, B.C.-based company that brokers transactions between American patients and foreign hospitals. Surgeries are cheaper in Third World countries where salaries and litigation expenses are lower, Lindland said.

Service providers

There are several service providers; some of them are mentioned elsewhere. One website, www.mediescapes.com that aims to be an extensive resource for International patients needing affordable medical care in India at the same level one could expect from a "first-world" country service but with an third world prices tag!. The three main steps to complete successfully a treatment abroad are:

(a) Your medical insurance (private or governmental) or if any other, and be sure of having sufficient funds.
(b) Your medical travel itinerary.
(c) Your treatment procedure well explained itself.

Many major employers in the U.S. are self-insured, which means they pick up the tab for much of their employees' medical care. That's why three major corporations that collectively cover 240,000 lives asked Dr. Arnold Milstein, national health care "thought leader" at the consultancy Mercer Health and Benefits, to assess the best places to outsource elective surgeries. Procedures in Thailand and Malaysia, he found, cost only 20% to 25% as much as comparable ones in the U.S.; top-notch Indian hospitals sell such services at an even steeper discount. The bottom line: If more private payers sent patients abroad for uncomplicated elective surgeries, the savings could be enormous. "This has the potential of doing to the U.S. health care system what the Japanese auto industry did to American carmakers," says Princeton University health care economist Uwe Reinhardt.

Employees who opt for India would get to take along a family member, says Darrell Douglas, Vice-President of human resources, and the whole experience, including a recuperative stay at a hotel, would be covered. IndUShealth, a medical tourism start-up in Raleigh, N.C., will make all arrangements and coordinate care between U.S. and Indian providers. The sweetener: the company will share with these intrepid employees up to 25% of savings garnered from the outsourcing.

Would people actually travel 10,000 miles for medical care just to make a few bucks? Polls commissioned by Milstein suggest that few consumers would opt for surgery abroad for incentives below $1,000. But raise the ante above $1,000, and the equation changes. Among people who have sick family members, about 45% of the underinsured or uninsured declare they would get on the plane; even 19% of those who have insurance say they're game. Above $5,000, the percentage of takers climbs to 61% and 40%, respectively.

Is the quality of care in foreign hospitals high enough? To cater to an international clientele, many private hospitals abroad are applying for accreditation (many of them successfully) from the Joint Commission International, the global arm of the institution that accredits most U.S. hospitals.

A corresponding boom is taking place among Western agencies that funnel patients to Asia. Eight have popped up in Canada, where national health care can mean a yearlong wait for elective surgery. In the U.S. several firms are aiming at the roughly 61 million people who are uninsured or underinsured. Planet Hospital's founder, "Rudy" Rupak Acharya, says his agency, which in the past seven months has sent some 200 patients abroad, got 11,000 inquiries in March alone. He has just retained Mercer to help him develop an insurance plan for the uninsured that will combine primary and emergency care in the U.S. with surgery abroad.

Patrick Marsek, managing director of the agency MedRetreat, says his company sent 200 people abroad last year and is already processing 320 this year. He is demanding a deposit of $195 from customers because people posing as patients have been looking for information to start up their own agencies.

Why would someone travel to India and not to Thailand?

The cost difference between treatment in India and Thailand is favourable to India. Also India offers what you call a language advantage—a patient would surely prefer a country where English is widely spoken. Also, it is believed that the facilities in India are more suited for International patients.

How can you trust Indian Doctors?

Well, many highly qualified doctors have had some form of training from abroad, especially USA and UK. Indian surgeons and doctors are known for their skill and research throughout the world.

Why is India most suitable?

Indian corporate hospitals excel in cardiology and cardiothoracic surgery, joint replacement, orthopedic surgery, gastroenterology, ophthalmology, transplants and urology to name a few. The various specialties covered are Neurology, Neurosurgery, Oncology, Ophthalmology, Rheumatology, Endocrinology, ENT, Pediatrics, Pediatric Surgery, Pediatric Neurology, Urology, Nephrology, Dermatology, Dentistry, Plastic Surgery, Gynecology, Pulmonology, Psychiatry, General Medicine and General Surgery

The various facilities in India include full body pathology, comprehensive physical and gynecological examinations, dental checkup, eye checkup, diet consultation, audiometry, spirometry, stress and lifestyle management, pap smear, digital Chest X-ray, 12 lead ECG, 2D echo colour doppler, gold standard DXA bone densitometry, body fat analysis, coronary risk markers, cancer risk markers, carotid colour doppler, spiral CT scan and high strength MRI. Each test is carried out by professional M.D. physicians, and is comprehensive yet pain-free.

There is also a gamut of services ranging from General Radiography, Ultra Sonography, Mammography to high end services like Magnetic Resonance Imaging, Digital Subtraction Angiography along with intervention procedures, Nuclear Imaging. The diagnostic facilities offered in India are comprehensive to include Laboratory services, Imaging, Cardiology, Neurology and Pulmonology. The Laboratory services include biochemistry, hematology, microbiology, serology, histopathology, transfusion medicine and RIA.

All medical investigations are conducted on the latest, technologically advanced diagnostic equipment. Stringent quality assurance exercises ensure reliable and high quality test results.

CUTTING-EDGE VACATIONS

In the U.S. insurers negotiate discounts, but the uninsured pay retail rates for medical procedures. Here's how the prices of one surgical tourism agency compare. Its packages include airfare and hospital and hotel rooms, but costs can climb if there are complications.

Procedure	*U.S. Insurer's cost*	*U.S. Retail price*	*India*	*Thailand*	*Singapore*
Angioplasty	$25,704 to $37,128	$57,262 to $82,711	11000	13000	13000
Gastric bypass	$27,717 to $40,035	$47,988 to $69,316	11000	15000	15000
Heart bypass	$54,741 to $79,071	$122,424 to $176,835	10000	12000	20000
Heart-valve replacement (single)	$71,401 to $103,136	$159,326 to $230,138	9500	10500	13000
Hip replacement	$18,281 to $26,407	$43,780 to $63,238	9000	12000	12000
Hysterectomy	$9,591 to $13,854	$20,416 to $29,489	2900	4500	—
Knee replacement	$17,627 to $25,462	$40,640 to $58,702	8500	10000	13000
Mastectomy	$9,774 to $14,118	$23,709 to $34,246	7500	9000	12400
Spinal fusion	$25,302 to $36,547	$62,778 to $90,679	5500	7000	9000

Some Other Services

Tummy tuck

Tummy tuck or abdominoplasty surgery is a major surgical procedure that involves the abdominal area. The abdominal skin is trimmed and excess fat is removed. The stomach muscle is also tightened by stitching them together. The end result is a slimmer waistline. Being a major surgical operation, the recovery period can take anywhere from 6 to 12 months before you can enjoy the full benefits of a tummy tuck. A major surgery like a tummy tuck normally entails spending a few nights at the clinic or hospital to be prepared to fork out a bit more cash for a room. Once you have been discharged from the room or clinic, be prepared to budget for follow-up visits to the tummy tuck specialist. The first few visits will be to remove the dressing and to check on the healing of the scar while monitoring your overall recovery progress. The doctor will also be prescribing you some medication to help you through the rest of your recovery.

Gynecology services and women's hospitals

Many hospitals have women check-up programs designed to detect the earliest signs of disorders of the breast and the organs of reproduction as well as catering to the contraceptive needs of women. A mammogram, an ultrasound of the pelvis and a pap-smear of the cervix are an integral part of any good medical check-up for women. Specialist medical as well as surgical care is available for all types of gynecological problems like menstrual abnormalities, prolapsed, fibroids and other tumors of the uterus and ovaries, tubal recanalization by microsurgery and care of the infertile couple. State-of-the-art gynecological surgery is available with world class equipment and expertise using minimally invasive techniques.

Abnormal Uterine Bleeding

Heavy or irregular bleeding can disrupt your life. Having to be constantly on guard with pads can distract you at work, an evening out with friends and worse still you may feel worn out. You may wonder if this is normal and if so what is causing this. Normal menstrual cycle ranges from 24-35 days length, with an average bleeding for 2-8 days. The menstrual cycle is governed by a hormone "Estrogen" in the first half of the cycle which helps the lining of the uterus to grow. Mid-cycle hormonal surge causes the ovary to usually release an egg, which triggers the 2nd hormone called Progesterone to act on and nature the endometrium. At the end of the cycle, the hormone levels drop when there is no pregnancy and the lining is shed with blood, which is called Menstruation.

Executive Health Check-up

It's designed for busy professionals on the go (okay, so I'm faking it a bit) and involves several hours of all sorts of tests, and a follow-up session a few days later. It starts at 8:30 a.m., after 12 hours of fasting. The reception area looks like hotel lobby, in fact the entire place is spic n' span, with lots of natural light, potted plants, marble floors and views of the gardens.

I quickly check-in and am introduced to Mr. Singh, the hospital traffic co-ordinator. He leads me from appointment to appointment; readjusting my schedule depending on line-ups to make sure wait time is minimal.

The near-painless blood-taking is followed by a glass of glucose and the handing over of a cute and discrete little bag containing my sample containers. Then, it's off for a chest X-ray. The room looks like every other

X-ray room on the planet, sterile and steely. The gowns aren't exactly award-show great, but they cover all the essential bits with more flair than usual. The radiologist cheerfully chats about Toronto doctors he's worked with as he takes snaps of my inner being.

From there, Mr. Singh takes me to my electrocardiogram test in the garden-view diagnostic centre. As she wires me up, the nurse tells me it's International Women's Day and that I should do something special with my friends. She is going to the movies later with her pals. She also administers my pulmonary function test, and cheerleads as I huff and puff, encouraging me to greater windy heights than I thought possible.

Next door is my ultrasound. Another nice gown and clean, professional room. Again the doctor has colleagues in Canada, and we commiserate about the weather as she pokes and prods.

Mr. Singh takes my lunch order and then, in quick succession, I have my bone density tested, a post-glucose blood test, a treadmill test and a meeting with a G.P. The G.P. answers all my questions with patience—so much so that I start making up problems just to see if he'll kick me out, like my G.P. back home does. He doesn't, he just answers in a relaxed and friendly way, which is why I now know that toenails grow slower than fingernails (seems that circulation is poorer in the feet.) Time well spent, I think.

The same level of professional care holds through my next batch of appointments with the gynecologist, cardiologist, ophthalmologist and physiotherapist. Finally, a break for lunch, a nice light sandwich and juice that I eat in the garden.

Then, more appointments. The ear, nose and throat man discovers my deep (because it is several centimetres inside my head), dark (because, contrary to popular belief, there are no light bulbs in there) secret. Apparently I have slighted retracted eardrums. All the flying, probably. He prescribes some medicine, which I get for a few dollars at the hospital pharmacy. Then more tests. I barely spend any time in the waiting room, but what little I do, I end up next to a couple from Arizona who are on the same check-up circuit. They are more experienced, though.

Having been to India before, they also knew to stock up on cheap medicine, prescription glasses (she got two pairs, including prescription sunglasses, for $40 U.S.) and to see a dentist (he is contemplating nine teeth implants for $2,000 U.S.)

End result: Seven hours of tests, half a dozen doctor appointments, a personalized diet plan, all my charts and scans to take back home, a nice lunch and a couple of slightly retracted eardrums. Total cost: $100 (U.S.) Sitaram Bhartia, an excellent non-profit research institute, is a favourite of Indian politicians and bureaucrats, but is less well known to tourists.

Talks and views

Niraj Sharan: In Australia, medical tourism is a new concept. We are tying up with our hospital chains in India.

Stan Correy: And the Indians have done their research on what may attract Australians to medical tourism.

Niraj Sharan: Yes, especially the dental surgery—no doubt there's a lot of opportunities, especially as it's not covered under the insurance policy overseas, and in comparison to costs overseas it's very cheap in India.

Stan Correy: There's been a plethora of Australian media stories in recent weeks about long waiting lists in our public hospitals, higher fees in private hospitals and not enough dentists. So will the Indian corporate hospitals find a lucrative market? "In certain cases, it would make economic sense if you wanted to have a holiday and combine it, say, with having your teeth done." And with the money you save, you can pay for a little holiday afterwards. Dentistry is now a major cost for families, and most of the private insurance programs restrict you to a number of visits or a number of procedures per year.

Stan Correy: Poland and Hungary offer special cheap dental tours to other Europeans. India, Thailand, South Africa and the Caribbean also offer the joys of being an 'orthodontal tourist'.

Ian Crombie: So I got out there, met at the airport, VIP treatment, taken to a private hospital in Chennai, which is the modern name for Madras. I had a suite, which was a room with an en suite bath, choice of menu, daily newspapers, and it was like staying in a resort hotel. I got to meet Dr, Reddy; he is the founder of the Apollo Hospital Group, and he wanted to know how I'd been treated, whether I was satisfied and all that, and he took a great sort of interest. And there were other expats there at the same time, having hip replacements. There was a Kuwaiti having something done to his spine, etc. the anaesthetist was British trained, the cardiologist was British trained, and of course Dr, Vijay himself was British trained. So based on that, I thought, Why the hell not? I mean there is nothing the Apollo Group doesn't do. "The anaesthetist was British trained, the cardiologist was British trained, and of course Dr, Vijay himself was British trained. So based on that, I thought, Why the hell not?" In other words, I want competent people. It turned out

Stan Correy: Ian Crombie didn't feel lonely as he waited for surgery. There were several other non-Indian medical tourists.

Pauline Gately: Trade in services itself is not an area that's well understood, and part of the reason it's not well defined or understood, it's not like trade in other commodities. Part of the reason also that health services and health expenditure has risen is because of course of rising incomes, demographic changes, aging populations. And the development and diffusion and uptake of new drugs and new technologies.

Stan Correy: Countries like Australia have been slower than other parts of the world to build themselves up for the potential business opportunities. As well, there's a general suspicion of Australians going to other countries for medical treatment.

Aadiyta Mattoo: If you were able to buy these services from other countries, it's not difficult to see that the ability to buy a service more cheaply outside your country than in your own country, can make you better-off.

Stan Correy: In the Gulf State of Dubai they've built a luxurious Health Care City. Western health care corporations such as the Mayo Clinic, and Harvard Medical International are falling over themselves to get into this medical city.

Stan Correy: That health conference in Dubai took place last week. Dean of Surgery at the University of Sydney is Professor Andrew Coats. He's recently returned from the Middle East where he visited Dubai Health Care City.

Andrew Coats: I think what we're seeing is very much part of the development of the Middle East; Dubai is a prime example, where we're seeing an area staking a place in the marketplace say for high quality area within the Middle East where people can get First World quality, hotels, resources, infrastructure, and health is a very major aspect of that. They have traditionally gone to the UK or the US, and the people in Dubai believe that if you set-up First World quality health care in Dubai, people will travel from the adjacent Middle East, and I think that's probably a fairly safe bet.

Stan Correy: So in a sense, it's not only what's happening in India or Asia, that kind of centre, or medical city, is also driving the competition in this medical area.

Andrew Coats: Yes. For some countries it will be good quality health care at low cost, in other countries it will be the highest quality health care at a higher cost, and others will offer a geographical advantage, and that's where Dubai might fit in where they can say, We can offer you a US, UK, Australian quality health care, but you don't have to fly eight to twelve hours to get there.

Derek Morgan: This is probably what we're now seeing as the development of a second wave in terms of medical tourism.

Stan Correy: The second global wave of medical tourism is creating new players, new companies, that are not health specialists, but facilitators, brokers between the international patient and the hospital networks.

Derek Morgan: There are two forces I think, that are external to the health care market, which are really contributing to this. The first I mentioned earlier on, is the relative decline of the cost of air travel across the world. And the second is the rise of the internet. "The internet enables increasingly knowledge-rich patients to seek out service providers, to make comparisons for themselves, or for specialist firms to grow up in order to broker patients and specialist services."

Stan Correy: Medical insurance and medical broking are not the same thing. A medical broker is someone who operates as a middleman who, for a fee, will act as a go-between to find the best deal for your personal needs. Medical insurance is self-explanatory, but there are very few medical insurers who will let you take your insurance cover to another country.

Leslie Smith: We then found individuals calling us, asking us for help, saying that they were on an NHS, National Health Service waiting list, couldn't get surgery and were suffering considerable pain levels.

Stan Correy: India is becoming a popular destination for Americans, and there are 47-million poor Americans who have no medical insurance at all, and who might simply die because they can't pay for treatment.

Bob Couch: And you know, you've got to remember we're retired. I mean I'm 81 you know. We're not broke, but these are big sums of money to take out of the bank, because we haven't got the income, we're just living on our savings all the time.

Stan Correy: Before his operation he had to fill in a questionnaire regarding his medical history and the normal documents that patients sign before surgery.

Leslie Smith: I'm particularly concerned always with hundreds and hundreds of patients, you're going to get things go wrong because they're under the surgical knife and anesthesia. So things will go wrong, and I just want to make sure the patients are fairly treated, they can sue properly in the appropriate country, they can be reimbursed, they can be brought home.

Stan Correy: How do you come under as a financial company?

Leslie Smith: No, we're still under the insurance regulator here for our insurance advice. But so far, the industry of facilitating patients to other hospitals around the world, without giving medical advice, there's no regulator for that as far as I'm aware in Europe at this time. I think there will be in the future.

Stan Correy: Acting as a broker for international patients is in its early days, and Leslie Smith admits that there are large regulatory issues involved. Many countries don't have the protective legal systems westerners are used to.

Derek Morgan: You've identified a difficult issue within this whole sort of boutique market that's now developing. What is the legal status? we don't really know. We're not entirely sure. Complications do arise in any potential operation that is undertaken. You can't guarantee that health care and the sequelae to operations are always going to run smoothly, there will always be issues about problems that arise. And how one deals with those on a patient who, let's say, has made a contract with a company or a broker in London to travel to Johannesburg for surgery, to travel on to another country for recuperative holiday and such like, and something goes wrong in the operation itself, trying to resolve these legal issues really is going to become a quite fundamental issue over the next 10 or 15 years. And of course it's going to differ from jurisdiction to jurisdiction. It may even differ from where the patient comes from.

Stan Correy: You can have a hip replacement in India, or heart surgery in Dubai, or dental work in Malaysia, but you may find it hard to get insurance, or a legal comeback if you're badly treated.

Leslie Smith: The interesting thing about Singapore and in Thailand, is the involvement of state government, where they're investing millions of dollars in state-of-the-art hospitals, recognizing that the kind of health tourism from Australasia or Japan is hard currency, which is dollars. "They have all the skills there, they have huge number of nurses and they can do this just as good as the westerners, if not better."

Stan Correy: So let's hitch a ride on one of those big white aeroplanes, full of medical tourists from UK, Canada and the US, refugees from overstretched and expensive health care systems. Waiting with open arms and beds are a whole chain of new Indian health care corporations. The Escorts Group, Fortis Health care, Max Health care, Wockhardt, and the largest, the Apollo Group, which is the most aggressive in promoting its business abroad. They're also lobbying the Indian government to make India more attractive for medical tourism.

Sangita Reddy: I think in any other sector some things can wait, it's not as critical. But health care is life. And also we come from a culture of people expecting the government to provide health care, as we transition from a country where the private sector is playing such an important role. It's important for the private sector and the public to work together and try and give more efficient solutions, reach people quicker, extend our reach, and there are many examples of win-win solutions when we work together.

Stan Correy: Indian corporate hospitals say business is good and they offer world class treatment. But there are critics who see medical tourism as a sick concept. In India, NGOs say the reason we're hearing so much about medical tourism is that too much money is being spent on building expensive hospitals, and that the vast majority of ordinary Indians can't afford them.

Ravi Duggall: Without regulated health care market insurance will find it very difficult to operate because the younger people are not insuring themselves. So you have a very small, about 2%, of the population which seeks this kind of voluntary insurance, and the private sector has stayed away, the study that they did, the private insurance companies said they've gone into life insurance or other general insurance, but they have stayed away from health because they realise that the people who are insuring themselves are high risk people. So that would have been a good base for many of these elite hospitals to fill up their vacant occupancies. But that has somehow not worked. So the other option is now looking to developed countries to cater to their over-supply of patients which they can't handle.

Stan Correy: Apollo and other Indian hospital corporations have recently asked the Indian government to relax foreign investment guidelines to allow international health insurance companies to set-up in India. But insurance companies demand better government regulation of health care. In India, the only accreditation these relatively new groups have isn't by any health authority. Apollo, for example, is accredited by Crisil, an Indian financial and credit rating company which isn't really the same thing.

Ashok Ananthram: If you look at the Apollo Group, we are touching 60,000 cardiac surgeries to date. At a success rate of well past 95%, 98%. Now JCI, etc. is a tangible proof of the fact that the systems, your processes, your entire hygiene, perhaps the quality of blood, etc. is at international levels. I think we need to get international accreditation to be counted amongst the world's best.

Stan Correy: And after you had the operation, what was the experience like then?

Ian Crombie: I spent a couple of weeks in Chennai. In the Taj Hotel, where I came across Warnie and Gilchrist and all the other lot about to play the second Test Match down there, and we had a great time. And during that time that I was in the hotel, every day they sent over a nurse to make sure the dressing, the stitches were OK. They also sent a physio across every day to make sure I was doing my exercises. I mean, you couldn't have asked for better care.

Stan Correy: In the Bloomberg's article, it says you paid a total of 5,000 pounds for the trip.

Ian Crombie: By the time I would have paid for my air fare, plus my hotel stay, yes, it would have come out at about 5,000 pounds.

Stan Correy: Outsourcing of IT has already given the Indian economy a huge boost, and it's no secret that India has turned around from being one of the poor countries of the world to an emerging economic power. There's talk of Indian medical care being worth billions of dollars.

Guy Ellena: I don't believe that they've established management of hospitals in such a strong way, that they can guarantee consistent quality of health care, a consistent quality of services around health care. They have fantastic doctors, no doubt, I mean OK a lot of them being trained either in India, but also trained in the US, in the UK, in Australia, and different countries. If something was to happen, or people started to be dissatisfied, because if big numbers were really to flock into India I think the system would be very much stressed.

Stan Correy: He's concerned that the Indian health care corporations may be over-hyping the market for medical tourists.

Guy Ellena: The private sector is not going to address the needs of the entire population, because they have private hospitals, they need to generate profits, if not OK they would close the doors. Clearly they need to sell their services to a population that can pay.

Stan Correy: Ellena's more critical perspective on the profits to be made from medical tourism comes from first-hand experience.

Guy Ellena: I'm traveling all around the world. We are financing hospitals in Latin America, in Central Europe, in Russia, in East Asia, Africa, all over the world. They all believe that they have a comparative advantage. There have been, up to 9/11, it's true, a trend where wealthy patients from the Middle East felt reluctant, or a difficulty, to be treated in the US because of getting a visa, or they didn't feel comfortable to go, and they have moved back to other places where is easier. Europe, and/or to some extent the subcontinent or Thailand. But still these are very, very small numbers.

Stan Correy: Once a trend and hype bubble gets rolling in the global economy, it's hard to stop. Everyone wants to be a health care hub. The surgery itself, it seems, is first class in the best places. And it's much cheaper than what you pay in the UK, the USA and Australia. But it's not only all about providing better health care. It's about business and commerce and trade.

Debra Lipson: Our members, along with thousands of unrepresented workers, are now being confronted with proposals to literally export themselves to have certain "expensive" medical procedures provided in India. When you're there, you give up your legal rights that you have here. You can't sue if there's malpractice. Who would send their 7-year-old child or their 80-year-old grandmother to a foreign country for surgery and you couldn't do anything if something goes wrong? Exacerbating this crisis by attempting to outsource health care is not only shameless; it does nothing to solve the nation's skyrocketing health care costs.

So America is also aware of its shortcomings and wants to improve its health care. If it does it may have impact the medical tourism plans of countries across the globe.

Some more details: BUMRUNGRAD HOSPITAL (BANGKOK, THAILAND

Before we discuss the Organization, functions and activities of the hospital, let us briefly review in brief the important administrative machinery in Thailand.

Since its inception, this hospital has achieved a high status based upon its quality operations.

Milestones

- Opened 200-bed facility: September 17, 1980.
- Listed on the Stock Exchange of Thailand: 1989.
- Expanded facility commissioned: January 1, 1997.
- Joint Commission International Accreditation: February 2002; reaccredited: April 2005.
- Joint Commission International: October 2006.
- Disease or Condition-Specific Care Certifications: October 2006.

Mission

The hospital has a loudable objective of serving patients. The hospital has its mission to provide world class health care with care and compassion.

Ownership

Bumrungrad Hospital (BH) is a Government Hospital run as a public company traded on the Stock Exchange of Thailand. The majority shareholders are Bangkok Insurance Public Company Limited and the Sophonpanich family, one of Thailand's most respected business families. The company form of organization provides flexibility and autonomy to the hospital and the day-to-day interference of the government is avoided. The hospital is running efficiently in a company form. There is a new set-up that our Indian hospitals at territory level should be run in company or corporation form to avoid day-to-day political interference and promote efficiency.

Patients are considered the VIPs and they are the main focus of hospital authorities. The mission is put in practice and is not merely a decorative piece.

The hospital is progressing fast. It expands its area of operation frequently. For example, in 1997, it promoted the following additional facilities:

Facility (Opened 1997)

- Largest private hospital in South East Asia
- One million square feet
- 12 stories plus basement parking
- Fully licensed medical heliport
- US Hospital (NFPA) building/fire standards
- Hospital 2000 information system
- Hospital wide wi-fi network coverage

Patient Volumes and Revenues

- The result of efficient running of hospital can be seen in the increase of patients and revenue.
- Over 1.2 million patients treated per year (outpatient and inpatient).
- Over 430,000 are international patients from over 190 different countries.
- US $220 million turnover in 2006.

The success and failure of any organization depends upon the quality of personnel especially at its top level. The hospital is very careful in the selection of medical experts to meet the needs of the patients. It has been rightly said that human rather than capital is the key to development. The hospital is staffed with the following human resources:

- American-led international management team.
- Over 3,000 employees.
- Over 900 physicians and dentists, most with international training/certification.

The hospital has inpatient capacities and outpatient facilities of high quality.

- 554 Inpatient Beds
  - 500 Medical/Surgical/OB/Pediatrics
  - 26 Adult Intensive Care
  - 14 Cardiac Care (CCU)
  - 9 Pediatric Intensive Care
  - 5 Level III Neonatal Intensive Care
- 57 Deluxe rooms, 21 VIP Suites and 2 Royal Suites.

Outpatient Facilities

- 135 examination suites
- Capacity 3,500 OPD patients per day
- Ambulance and mobile critical care fleet
- Outpatient Surgery Centre
- 24-hour emergency care including emergency cardiac catheterization.

Outpatient Centres

- Allergy Centre
- Eye and ENT Centre
- Plastic Surgery Centre
- Aviation Medicine Centre
- Eye Laser Refraction Centre
- Pulmonary Physiology Centre
- Behavioural Health Centre
- Fertility Centre
- Radiology Centre
- Breast Screening Centre
- Health Screening Centre
- Rehabilitation Centre
- Children Centre
- Heart Centre
- Skin Centre
- Dental Centre
- Horizon Regional Cancer Centre
- Skin Laser Centre
- Diabetes Centre
- Medical Centre
- Sleep Disorder Centre
- Dialysis Centre
- Neurology Centre
- Stroke Centre
- Digestive Disease Centre
- Orthopedic Centre
- Surgical Centre

- Early Intervention Centre
- Pathology Centre
- Urology Centre
- Emergency Centre
- Physiotherapy Centre
- Women's Centre
- Endoscopic Centre

Special Facilities

- 2 Cardiac Catheterization Laboratories
- 2 Cardiac Operating Theaters
- 19 Operating Theaters
- Interventional Radiology
- MRI, CT and Lithotripsy
- Neonatal Critical Care Transport
- Nuclear Medicine
- Radiation Therapy (Linear Accelerator)
- PACS Radiology
- VitalLife Wellness Centre
- 64-slice CT Scanner
- Surgical Navigation System

International Representative Offices

Australia, Bangladesh, Cambodia, Canada, Ethiopia, Hong Kong, Indonesia, Macau, Mongolia, Myanmar, Nepal, Netherlands, Nigeria, Oman, Seychelles, Sri Lanka, Sweden, Taiwan, Vietnam, Uganda, Ukraine.

Special Interracial Services

- International Patient Centre: interpreters, international/airport concierge service, embassy assistance, VIP airport transfers, e-mail correspondence, international insurance coordination and international medical coordinators, vise extension counter, Diet helm Travel Thailand counter, airline ticket counter, prayer room.
- Bumrungrad Hospitality Residence: 74 fully serviced apartments connected to the hospital
- Bumrungrad Hospitality Suites: 51 fully serviced apartments with pool and fitness facilities.

Quality and Certification

- The first private hospital awarded Thailand Hospital Accreditation
- Asia's first hospital accredited by the US-based Joint

Commission International (JCI); the first hospital in Asia to be reaccredited.

- First hospital outside the US to receive two JCI Disease or Condition-Specific Care Certifications (Primary stroke Program and Acute Myocardial Infection with ST Segment Elevation (STEMI) Program.
- Awarded the Best Small Cap Company by Asia Money's 2003 Survey.
- Internationally Certified Laboratory

Social Responsibility

Established in 1990, Bumrungrad Hospital Foundation is dedicated to helping the underprivileged in Thailand access free health care services. The Foundation has provided over 100,000 Thais with free medical services ranging from check-up programs to heart surgery for children.

HEALTH SCREENING CENTRE

Keeping your health in check

The hospital has developed an innovative centre which can prevent major risks. It is rarely available in any hospital. We, in India, should follow this and set-up health screening centre.

Prevention is the best medicine and annual health screenings are key to your well being. Often the early stages of diseases present no symptoms, or the symptoms may be so mild that they go unnoticed. The earlier a problem is detected, the more effectively it can be treated.

Preparing for your Visit

General Instructions

- Do not eat or drink anything except plain water for at least 9 hours prior to check up in case of Upper GI X-ray, please keep fasting.
- Please bring along your ID card or passport and arrive 10 minutes before the scheduled appointment time.
- Stool and urine samples will be collected on the day of examination.
- If you have a pre-existing medical condition, please bring along any test results or reports you have for the doctor to review.

If you schedule a stress test

- Please bring your jogging shoes.
- If you need to eat before the stress test, then eat a light snack only and avoid fatty foods, caffeine, and alcohol.

- If you are under treatment or taking medication for any medical or physical condition, please notify the nurse in advance.
- If you are suffering any chest pain or breathing difficulty, please notify the nurse in advance.

Instruction for abdominal ultrasound

Drink plenty of water before the ultrasound exam. The test requires a full bladder for best results. Do not void prior to the ultrasound examination.

Payment

Pre-payment is required for all check up programs.

Location

The Health Screening Centre is located on the 11th floor of Bumrungrad International Clinic.

Hours of operation

07:00-15:00 hrs everyday.

Appointments

Please make your appointment at least 3 days in advance.
To make or change an appointment:
Tel: 66(0)2667 1555 Fax:+66 (0) 2667 295
Online appointment:www.bumrungrad.com

BONES AND JOINT CENTRE

Some of life's greatest pleasures are simple things—a walk along the beach, a round of golf with friends or a good night's sleep. But the simple pleasures we often take for granted remain out of reach for people living with painful, debilitating bone and torturous joint problems.

Longer life expectancies have made joint pain—especially in the knees and hips—a growing problem in Thailand and around the world.

Serious bone—related conditions, whether caused by aging, injury, or diseased like arthritis and osteoarthritis, can quickly wreak havoc on one's ability to do normal daily activities and enjoy a decent quality of life.

In the past, treating serious bone and joint conditions often required traumatic and complex major surgery, with up to a full year of recovery time, and frequently left significant scarring.

What a difference a few years has made! Advances in medical technology and techniques have revolutionized technology and techniques have revolutionized the treatment of bone and joint problems. Joint replacement is a prime example of these exciting changes. To learn more, Better Health spoke to Dr. Sitthiporn Orpain, an orthopedic surgeon specializing in joint replacement.

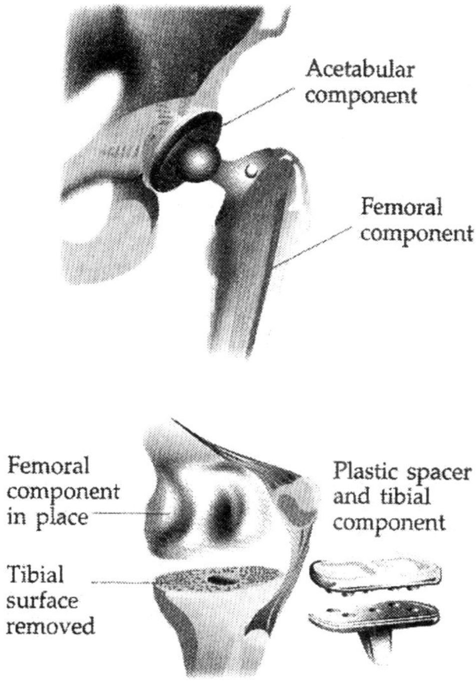

Pictured : Hip (top) and knee replacement components.

The sources of joint pain

Joints are where two bones are joined by connective tissue called cartilage. Cartilage acts as a protective cushion to allow the joint to support body weight and move comfortably. But when the cartilage is damaged by disease, infection, wear-and-tear or injury, the result is often painful inflammation, stiffness and reduced mobility.

"While there are many causes of joint pain," explained Dr. Sitthiporn, "Osteoarthritis and other degenerative joint diseases are among the most common. These conditions cause a break-down in the cartilage that affects the normal workings of the joint. As the cartilage wears away, the two bones rub against each other, causing great pain.

Aging is a key risk factor for developing osteoarthritis, especially after the age of 50. Obesity, a family history of osteoarthritis and being in overall poor health also increase one's risk.

"The first symptoms people usually notice are pain, stiffness, and reduced flexibility of a joint," Dr. Sitthiporn noted. "The area around the joint may become swollen as an unusual fluid builds up, and that can worsen the pain each time weight is exerted on the joint," Osteorathritis is a progressive disease whose symptoms and severity worsen over time, so early detection is very important to successful treatment.

Rheumatioid arthritis also leads to serious joint damage. This condition causes chronic inflammation of the joint that results in pain, stiffness, and swelling. "The repeated inflammation causes damage to the bone and cartilage," Dr. Sitthiporn added. "While joint pain and stiffness caused by osteoarthritis usually affect one knee or one hip, the pain and stiffness from rheumatoid arthritis tends to affect both hips or both knees at the same time."

Diagnosis and Treatment

To diagnose the cause of joint pain, your doctor will usually begin with a through physical examination and ask about your medical and family histories. Specialized tests, such as a biopsy, X-rays, MRI scans, and arthroscopy help confirm the diagnosis and determine the severity of the condition. Blood tests are sometimes used to check for the presence of rheumatoid arthritis of infection.

Patients diagnosed with mild to moderate osteoarthritis can usually be treated without surgery. Doctors may recommend a combination of options including—

- Weight reduction for overweight or obese patients.
- Rest or activity modification.
- Medication to relieve pain and inflammation.
- Physiotherapy.
- Using a brace or walking aid.

The Joint Replacement Revolution

More serious cases may require the complete replacement of the damaged joint. As Dr. Sitthiporn explained, "For many people, joint problems become so severe to the point where the patient suffers a serious decline in quality of life. In many of these cases, a good option is to replace the damaged knee or hip with an artificial joint."

Ten years ago, the idea of replacing a real hip or knee joint with an artificial one may have seemed quite radical. Today, joint replacement is among the most successful treatments for serious joint conditions; it has already brought great relief to thousands of long-suffering patients. Here's detailed look at the knee and hip replacement procedures.

Knee Replacement

The knee joint is formed where the lower part of the thighbone (femur) connects with the upper part of the shinbone (tibia) and the kneecap (patella). Shock-absorbing cartilage covers the surfaces of these bones.

During a typical knee replacement surgery, the damaged areas of the thighbone, shinbone and kneecap are first removed. The surgeon then smoothes and reshapes the ends of the remaining bones to ensure an optimal fit of the artificial knee components.

Major knee surgery used to require long hospital stays and up to a year of recovery time. That's no longer the case, as Dr. Sitthiporn explained: "knee replacement usually requires 4-7 days in the hospital. The recovery period depends on a patient's general health, age, and other factors, but many patients resume their normal activities within three months."

Once the knee has sufficiently healed, patients are often advised to incorporate a comprehensive exercise programme into their daily routine. Low-impact activities like swimming and walking are highly recommended, as they can help improve blood circulation, endurance, flexibility and muscle strength, without putting too much pressure on the knees.

Hip Replacement

The hip is a large "ball-and-socket" joint that bears much of the body's weight and movements. The ball of the joint at the top of the thighbone (femoral head) moves within the hollow socket (acetabulum) of the pelvis. A layer of cartilage allows the ball to glide smoothly inside the socket.

During the total hip replacement procedure, the surgeon removes the ball part of the joint and replaces it with a prosthetic ball. The ball is attached to a stem that fits into the hollowed-out space in the thighbone. Damaged cartilage and bone are removed from the socket, and a cup-like component is inserted in its place.

Hip replacement surgery has rapidly become a leading choice for treating severe hip problems, with shorter hospital stays and faster recovery times compared to traditional hip surgery.

Younger patients with less-serious hip problems are also benefiting from major advances in technology and techniques through a procedure called hip resurfacing. According to Dr. Sitthiporn, "Hip resurfacing is a less-invasive, bone-conserving surgical technique that has already allowed thousands of people in their 40s and 50s to resume active lives and delay or eliminate the need for total hip replacement.

Unlike the prosthesis used in total hip replacement, the resurfacing prosthesis allows the head to be preserved and reshaped. The resurfaced bone is then capped with a metal prosthesis. As with total hip replacement, the socket is fitted with a prosthesis.

Is joint replacement right for me?

As people pursue active lifestyles well into their 60s, 70s and 80s, joints need to stay strong and healthy. But the added years means more wear-and-tear on knees and hips, and increased risk of serious disease and injury.

Joint replacement surgery has established an impressive record for safety and successful post-treatment results, eliminating pain and restoring mobility in patients who don't respond to other treatments. All medical procedures, including joint replacement and resurfacing, involve some level of risk and may not be suitable for every patient. Your doctor will explain the treatment options and recommend the best course of treatment for your individual situation.

"It's important for patients to have realistic expectations about joint replacement surgery," said Dr. Sitthiporn. "While most patients are able to resume most normal activities without pain, it won't enable them to run a marathon! Not all patients are good candidates; for example, people who are obese may have to be excluded."

Exercise and Healthy Joints

The right exercise is essential for keeping bones and joints healthy. Even for people being treated for joint problems, regular exercise can still help reduce joint pain and stiffness. Be sure to consult your doctor before starting any exercise program.

It's best to choose non-weight bearing, low-impact exercises like walking or swimming as they are safer for joints compared to more vigorous high-impact exercises such as jogging.

Stretch: Warm up by gently stretching the muscles in the front of the thigh (quardriceps), the side of the thigh, and the back of the thigh (hamstrings); stretching reduces pressure on the knees and hips that occurs during exercise.

Strengthen: Strengthening exercise increase muscles strength, a key to supporting bones and joints.

Swimming is an ideal exercise for those with arthritis as it can increase mobility and build muscle strength. An unlike exercise on dry land, the water helps reduce the amount of stress on the body's hips, knees and spine.

You don't have to be a fitness fanatic or "gym rat" to reap the benefits of regular exercise. Look for opportunities in your daily routine to add some exercise and increase your level of activity. Take the stairs instead of the elevator, or try a nightly after-dinner walk with your family. Your bones and joints will be glad you made the effort.

Minimally-invasive: Less trauma, faster recovery

Dramatic advancements have been made in recent years in the effectiveness and durability of prosthetic replacement joints thanks to better design, materials and production methods. At the same time, similar advances have come in the way of new and improved surgical techniques that require smaller incisions and causes less trauma to surrounding areas.

"The minimal-incision surgery technique minimizes trauma to muscles, tissue and tendons and results in less bleeding during surgery," explained Dr. Sitthiporn, "Patients typically experience less pain after surgery, so they can be up and walking around sooner, and their hospital stay is usually shorter as well."

IMAGE GUIDED NAVIGATION SYSTEM—POINTS THE WAY TO HIGH-TECH SURGERY SUCCESS

Joint replacement surgery has quickly become one of the most popular and successful treatment options for patients with serious joint and bone conditions. A successful joint replacement operation depends on several factors, most notably the precise and accurate alignment of the joint component. Accurate alignment during surgery is critical to a patient's future mobility, and its helps maximize the longevity of the prosthetic components. A new generation of image-guided navigation systems like the one in use at Bumrungrad is giving surgeon a powerful tool to perform many successful procedures including joint replacement.

Real time 3-D positioning

Image-guide navigation systems for surgery operate in a similar way to the latest navigation systems for cars and ships that help pinpoint the driver or captain's precise location and guide them on their journey. The system provides surgeons with clear and detailed images and positioning calculations, in 'real-time' on a computer screen, giving the surgeon a clear view of the area where the operation is being performed.

Computer navigation gives the surgeon visual information on the precise positioning during a surgical procedure, including joint replacement surgery which is performed using smaller incisions. As a result, the minimally invasive procedure can be highly reliable and accurate.

During a joint replacement procedure, the surgeon first places temporary markers on and around the joint bones at the positions that have been located using the system's infrared camera. Next, the system tracks the position of each marker while the surgeon guides the joint through a variety of motions. The computer processes the data and generates a highly detailed 3-dimensional image of the joint.

A complement of the minimally-invasive surgery

This new technology is a perfect complement to minimally-invasive surgical procedures, that give patients an easier and faster recovery. Traditional surgery usually involves large incision that cut through muscles tissue and cause a lot of bleeding during surgery. On the other hand, minimally-invasive surgery uses small punctures in the skin to perform the surgery. Lesser trauma to the surrounding tissue means less post-operative pain, quicker restoration of mobility, and shorter hospital stays. Patients can now look forward to a much faster return to their normal lifestyle.

FIRST IN ASIA: SWISSLOG PHARMACY ROBOT—NOW SERVING BUMRUNGRAD PATIENTS

The pharmacy of the future has arrived in Asia. Bumrungrad International recently introduced the region's first 'Pharmacy Robot'—a fully-automated drug management system being used by many leading medical centres around the world.

The accuracy of the system is one of its unique strengths. The traditional system of preparing and dispensing medications in hospitals is inherently complex; there can be more than 100 steps from the time a prescription is written to the time a patient receives the medication. Technology reduces errors by reducing complexity, avoiding over-reliance on memory, simplifying critical processes, and increasing efficiency. The system will allow highly-trained pharmacists and technicians to spend less time on routine tasks, and more time on patient care.

Automated packaging and dispensing systems for filling patient orders are becoming common in US hospitals as a result of increased public knowledge about medication errors. Bar coding helps reduce medication errors during dispensing and administration. A unit-dose drug is created when a single drug is taken from its bulk container and put into a labeled package. Bar coding of unit doses allows nurses to easily verify that the right dose of the right drug is being given to the right patient at the right time.

The automated robot system will help Bumrungrad care for the more than 1 million patients from 190 different countries who come to the hospital each year. "The automated drug management system is part of the hospital's continuing commitment to patient safety," explained Dr. Karoon Mekanontchai, Bumrungrad's Medical Director. "The system should increase patients' confidence in the hospital's quality."

HEPATITIS PREVENTION

The hepatitis B virus has been around for generations, but it receives relatively little attention from the media or from the public at large. Most people are unaware that they're infected, and the serious, sometimes deadly consequences can take decades to appear. But make no mistake, hepatitis B has quietly become a major health threat to millions of people in Thailand, and millions more throughout Asia and around the world.

The ABCs of Hepatitis

The word hepatitis means inflammation of the liver, which is usually caused by a viral infection. There are many types of hepatitis (A, B, C, D, AND d). While hepatitis A is the most prevalent, it goes away on its own and does not lead to long-term liver damage. Hepatitis B has far more serious consequences, including liver scarring, cirrhosis of the liver, and liver cancer. It can also be fatal.

It's estimated that more than 350 million people around the world have been infected with the hepatitis B virus, and nearly 75% of them are Asian. Thailand has one of the highest rates of infection; nine million Thais have the HBV virus.

To gain a better understanding of this serious threat, Better Health spoke with Dr. Virasak Wongpaitoon, M.D., a gastroenterologist and hepatologist with many years' experience treating patients infected with hepatitis.

How does infection occur?

The hepatitis B virus is transmitted through three main routes; unprotected sexual contact, exposure to blood or bodily fluids such as semen or vaginal secretions of a person who carries the virus, and 'vertical' transmission from mother-to-child during childbirth. Most patients diagnosed with chronic hepatitis B as adults became infected during infancy or childhood. In addition to the risk of mother-to-child infection during childbirth, Dr. Virasak noted that children are at higher risk due to normal activities and surrounding. "There is a high incidence of hepatitis B infection in places with lots of children," he explained. "At school or on the playground, children play together, and it's common that they scrape or cut themselves and expose an open wound. Because children's immune systems are still developing, they're more vulnerable to infection. "Many children's immune systems are strong enough to completely kill the virus. In others, most of the virus is killed-off, but they still carry the virus and can infect others. In serious cases, the HBV virus proves too strong for the immune system, and symptoms of chronic hepatitis B will eventually become apparent during adulthood (usually between the ages of 20 and 40).

Dr. Virasak stressed one of the most dangerous aspects of the HBV virus; Most people don't realize they've been infected. "Infection typically produces no symptoms at all, or only mild symptoms such as a fever or aches and pains that go away within a few days", he explained. "There is a high prevalence of hepatitis B in Thai people because there are few symptoms at the time of infection. As a result, patients don't seek medical treatment, the disease continues to progress, and they can spread the virus to others."

The dangers of Hepatitis B

- More than 9 million Thais—and nearly 300 million people across Asia—carry the hepatitis B virus (HBV).
- Most people don't know they're infected, and they can spread the virus to many others.
- Infants and children are at the greatest risk of infection.
- Chronic hepatitis B can lead to serious, potentially fatal liver problems including cirrhosis, liver cancer and liver failure.

Infant and Childhood Dangers

In the majority of infections that occur during adulthood (termed 'acute'), the body's strong immune system is able to produce antibodies that completely kill off the HBV virus within a few months after infections. These antibodies provide lifetime protection against becoming re-infected. Patients who are unable to kill-off the virus within six months face the future health threats of 'chronic' hepatitis such as cirrhosis and liver cancer. And as HBV carriers they can pass the infection on to others.

When infection occurs during infancy or childhood, the hepatitis B virus is much more threatening. With few or no symptoms at the time of infection, it's often years before an infected child has a blood test for hepatitis B. That's more than enough time during the critical years before the immune system has fully developed for the HBV virus to multiply and progress to the point of inflicting serious liver damage—usually without any noticeable signs or symptoms of the disease.

Vaccination and Prevention

Despite its serious nature, hepatitis B can be easily prevented through vaccination, regular medical check-ups, and avoiding the risk factors for transmitting the virus.

The vaccine against hepatitis B has proven highly effective in offering a lifetime of protection against the virus. These days, most newborns receive the vaccine soon after birth.

Avoiding the major risk factors for transmission of the virus is critical to reducing the rate of HBV infection. In addition to practicing safer sex, "if you haven't been tested for the virus." Dr. Virasak advised, "or if you haven't been vaccinated, talk to your doctor. And don't share personal items such as razor blades and toothbrushes."

If You Think You Are Infected...

For patients who worry that they may be infected with the HBV virus, a simple blood test is used to check for the presence of the virus in the bloodstream. If the virus is detected, additional test may be recommended to check for the presence of antibodies, and your doctor may also prescribe a liver function test and ultrasound examination to determine the extent of any damage to the liver.

Recently-infected patients (i.e. those with acute hepatitis B) require a lot of rest until any symptoms go away. Among patients diagnose with chronic hepatitis B, those who show no symptoms and have normal liver function usually don't require medication. Some patients with chronic hepatitis B may need medication that can effectively reduce or completely eliminate the HBV virus. Your doctor will set-up a schedule for regular check-ups and monitoring of the disease's progression to ensure earlier detection of potential problems including cirrhosis, scarring and cancer.

To lessen the risk of future health problems, Dr. Virasak recommends that all patients with HBV "should consult their doctor before taking any medication, abstain from drinking alcohol, get regular medical check-ups, and lead a healthy lifestyle. That means reducing stress, practicing good nutrition and exercise habits, and avoiding the risk factor that can spread the virus to others."

STEM CELL TREATMENT

Stem cell transplantation has received worldwide media attention and has shown great potential for treating many serious illnesses. To provide more insight and understanding on this very complex topic,

Bumrungrad's website (www.bumrungrad.com) now includes a section that provides information and Bumrugrad's position on stem cell treatment issues.

Clinical studies have already shown stem cell treatments to be effective for treating certain blood-related disorders, and experienced Bumrungrad physicians offer treatments in those proven areas.

To learn more about developments in stem cell treatment, simply visit www.bumrungrad.com/stemcell. You'll find a special briefing on Stem Cell Treatment that answers the most frequently-asked questions on this important and fast-developing topic.

HYPERBORIC OXYGEN THERAPY UNIT

Bumrungrad International's new Hyperbaric Oxygen Therapy (HBOT) Unit is now open, offering therapeutic benefits to inpatients and outpatients who suffer from certain illness and conditions. The HBOT (high pressure) treatment is a non-invasive and painless course of treatment originally developed to treat scuba and deep-sea divers with the dangerous condition called decompression sickness. However, it is now being used to treat several other conditions. For example, HBOT can reduce the effects of toxic substances, alleviate gas-bubble obstructions, promote wound healing, increase oxygen delivery to injured tissue, and improve infection control.

"Breathing 100 percent pure oxygen, under higher-than-normal atmospheric pressure, increases the amount of oxygen in the blood," noted Dr. Karoon Mekanonthchai, Bumrungrad International's Medical Director. "This can help and fight-off infection, reduce swelling and aid the growth of new blood vessels—benefits that cannot be achieved by breathing oxygen in a regular room."

MEN'S HEALTH

If you are a man over 40 and you answered "yes" to more than two questions, it's time to take action. Our men's health experts can help you with problems that threaten your life, or just diminish your lifestyle:

- Andropause
- Back and knees
- Diabetes
- Erectile dysfunction
- Infertility
- Fitness and weight
- Hair loss
- Heart disease
- Prostate problems
- Stroke

Andropause is the result of a decline in male hormone (testoterone) levels which can occur with aging.

The decline in hormones, coupled with unhealthy diet, stress, and lack of exercise, can cause health problems. You don't have to accept these problems as investiable and unmanageable. You can do something to remain in control of your health and lifestyle.

Men Centre at Bumrungrad International is a team of doctors who study, understand, and treat the health issues faced by men as they age. You start with an initial evaluation with a Men Centre doctor. He will give you advice and may recommend appropriate treatment by a specialist on the Men Centre team. The team includes experts in cardiology, urology, orthopaedics, hormones, psychiatry, nutrition, anti-aging medicine—whatever you need to get back to looking, feeling, and living better.

Our experts enjoy access to the hospital's stat-of-the-art technology. For example, laser treatment of the prostate to relieve painful urination; 3-D imaging of bones and joints; and sophisticated blood testing that profiles hormone and micronutrient levels.

ANDROPAUSE AND ERECTILE DYSFUNCTION (ED)

For men over 40, getting older doesn't have to mean living with declining health. Thanks to extensive research and new treatment advances, male andropause can be diagnosed and treated successfully.

There's a ring of truth to the old saying that "Life begins at 40," Entering the middle part of life is supposed to be a positive experience, and a time to feel more settled, established and comfortable.

But for a great number of men, life beyond the age of 40 can feel more like the end of good health, with unexplained fatigue, insomnia, depressed feelings and a general lack of enthusiasm for living—not unlike the difficulties many women encounter during menopause. For some middle-aged men, the physical and mental toll of everyday living means a profound decline in quality of life.

Given the similarities to the symptoms of female menopause, this condition has been referred to as "male menopause", or "mid-life crisis." Some used to believe it was just a normal part of the male aging process. Others questioned whether it was all just a state of mind.

So what exactly is it that these men are experiencing? And what is the best way to deal with it? For answers, Better Health turned to Dr. Pansak Sugkraruek, an endocrinologist and fertility expert with vast experience treating men for what is now called andropause.

What is Andropause?

Years ago many doctors believed that male 'menopause' symptoms were merely an unavoidable part of the aging process; consequently, relatively little research effort was made to understand what exactly was causing the condition. Thanks to intensive research in recent years, science now has a clear understanding that andropause results from declining levels of several male hormones.

"People used to equate these symptoms in men with those that occur during female menopause, and so the term 'male menopause' was coined," says Dr. Pansak. "Extensive research in recent years has shown that the term doesn't properly describe the male condition. While the symptoms are similar in both men and women, the causes are very different.

For women, menopause begins when the ovaries stop functioning and no longer produce hormones. "In men, hormone production continues," Dr. Pansak explains, "but certain bodily conditions impair a man's hormone production to such an extent that this hormone deficiency begins to have a noticeable effect on some important body function."

"The correct term to describe this process is testosterone deficiency syndrome or androgen deficiency of the aging male," says, Dr. Pansak. "In simple terms, this is andropause."

Andropause and Hormone Deficiency

The impact of hormone deficiency in men is usually gradual and often goes unnoticed at least initially. "As the condition progress it can lead to a significant impact in both physical and psychological terms on a man's quality of life," Dr. Pansak explains. "Andropause affects a man's self-esteem and how he relates to others. Men with hormone deficiency often feel frustrated, irritable, subdued and pessimistic. Their muscles contract while body fat increases. They often experience insomnia, emotional turbulence, less sharp thinking, a decreased sex drive and erectile dysfunction. Serious cases can eventually lead to clinical depression."

Andropause affects more than just testosterone. "All hormones experience a decline," Dr. Pansak continues. "One of the first to decline is melatonin, the so-called 'hormone of the night.' Melatonin is normally secreted after sundown and helps a person feel sleepy as bedtime approaches, allowing him to fall into deep healthy sleep around midnight. In a healthy man, the pituitary gland produces a variety of hormones during deep sleep. The first of these is the growth hormone which preserves one's youthfulness and counters the aging process."

"The thyroid gland then produces a hormone that converts food into energy," explains Dr. Pansak. "A healthy thyroid hormone function gives a man energy to enthusiastically engage in activities. The adrenal gland produces the antioxidant hormone DHEA that slows the aging process."

The male sexual hormone testosterone is the last hormone produced. "This hormone helps one think decisively, reasonably and positively as a healthy man should," says Dr. Pansak. "It also supports bone and muscle strength and regulates body fat and body contour. That's why men with normal hormone levels usually don't have 'beer belly.' Their bodies are strong and their mood is good."

The Dangers of Male Hormone Deficiency

If left untreated, male hormone deficiency poses a number of potentially serious health risks, including fragile bones, weak muscles, erectile dysfunction, hypertension, heart disease and stroke.

"With decreased hormone levels, body at increase and accumulated around the waistline," notes Dr. Pansak. "The beer belly is one sign of male hormone deficiency. The criterion is a waistline in excess of 94 centimeters for westerners and 90 centimeters for easterners."

Beer Belly Dangers

While most of us are aware of the health risks that come with being overweight, the specific dangers for men with excessive fat accumulation around the waist are less well understood, but no less serious

"Think about it: When a man has a 'spare tire' around his waist, he's unlikely to have the energy or the desire to stay active," Dr. Pansak explains. "This lack of activity means he's not using enough energy to burn his daily calorie intake, and that leads to even more fat buildup. This increased fat clogs blood vessels and leads to hypertensions. It can also cause dyslipidemia, the condition of having too much 'bad' cholesterol and not enough 'good' cholesterol. This can significantly raise a man's risk for stroke, a potentially deadly condition."

This unhealthy state can also affect a man's sexual health. "Clogged blood vessels affect the supply of blood to the genitals," says Dr. Pansak. "This can cause erectile dysfunction. Excess fat accumulates in the genital muscles, further worsening the symptoms. This is a prime example of how the body's many systems are interconnected."

Dr. Pansak stresses the importance of consulting a doctor at the first sign of difficulty in achieving a normal erection. "Your doctor may recommend a hormone level test to check for possible deficiencies," he explains. "Your doctor can recommend a treatment strategy for sexual impotency as well as other steps to address one's overall health situation."

Treating Hormone Deficiency

Hormone Supplement Therapy

The old saying "Getting old is natural, feeling old is optional" certainly applies to male hormone deficiency. Today's modern lifestyles are far different from earlier generations. People tend to spend more time working and less time sleeping, and most of us endure greater stress from everyday living. Our fast-paced world leads to eating on-the-run and sleeping just a few hours a night, while leaving less time for exercise and relaxation. These factors all contribute to premature hormone deficiency.

Dr. Pansak shares his experience: "I see more and more men in their 30s who come to me because of loss of sexual desire and erectile dysfunction, hair loss or obesity. Dealing with their problems requires a holistic approach, to diagnose and treat the full range of health issues to produce a successful treatment outcome."

"Sexual impotency is an important indicator of male health problems, so we have to check blood sugar and body fat levels, hormone levels, the health of the prostate gland, and understand a patient's lifestyle and family history to see what changes may be needed," says Dr. Pansak. "Hormone supplement therapy is often recommended as part of the treatment plan. After a period of taking hormone supplements, patients usually experience noticeable improvements to their health and wellness, which are often accompanied by weight loss and improved sexual function. A patient's mood and overall happiness usually also improves."

Hormone supplement therapy has an impressive record of safety for effectively treating men suffering from andropause. All medical treatments and procedures involve some level of risk and may not be suitable for everyone. Your doctor will explain the risks involved and recommend the course of treatment that's right for your individual situation.

Lifestyle Modification

Dr. Pansak emphasizes the hormone-related differences between men and women. "The female body stops producing female hormones during menopause", he explains. "Replacement therapy is usually recommended to mitigate the negative effects. On the contrary, the male body never stops producing male hormones. The levels of hormones decline, but they can be restored. Doctors will advise their patients on specific lifestyle changes that can help increase hormone production. For some patients—usually older men with greater hormone deficiency—doctors will also prescribe male hormone supplements to be taken on a regular basis".

There are simple guidelines that all men can follow to improve their overall health and limit the effects of hormone deficiency. Dr. Pansak recommends:

- Going to bed early enough to ensure that you fall into deep sleep by midnight;
- Exercising most days for 45 minutes per workout (or 300 total minutes each week) as opposed to the 30 minutes per workout guideline for the general population;
- Eating a healthier diet; and
- Adopting a positive attitude in order to avoid depression and insomnia.

According to Dr. Pansak, unhealthy living is often the biggest single factor in causing male hormone deficiency. So making healthy lifestyle changes under the supervision of a medical specialist can prove highly effective in returning to better health. Middle age really can be the beginning of a happier, healthier life. As the famous comedian George Burns said, "You can't help getting older, but you don't have to get old".

Erectile dysfunction (ED)

Q: *What are the most common myths and misconceptions about ED?*

A: One common misconception is that emotional and psychological

Do you have hormone deficiency? Find out by taking this quiz.

Are you experiencing these symptoms?

Sexual health:	Yes	No
1. Decreased sex drive	☐	☐
2. Difficulty achieving and/or maintaining an erection	☐	☐
General health:		
3. Decreased strength and stamina	☐	☐
4. Fatigue or lack of energy	☐	☐
5. Depression	☐	☐
6. 'Shrinking' or having a hunched back	☐	☐
7. Difficulty concentrating at work	☐	☐
8. Feeling unhappy or pessimistic about life	☐	☐
9. Decreased athletic capabilities	☐	☐
10. Falling asleep or nodding off during the day	☐	☐

If you answered YES to questions 1 or 2, or if you answered YES to at least 3 of the general health questions, you may be experiencing male hormone deficiency. Consult your doctor for a physical examination and a hormone level test.

Source: www.andropause.com

problems are the main causes. In truth, it's just opposite; research has shown that physical causes account for over 80% of ED cases.

Another popular myth is that ED is an unavoidable part of the aging process. Yes, a man's hormone levels diminish with age, and he may need more stimulation to achieve a healthy erection. But age alone does not cause ED.

Q: *What are the most common causes of ED? What are the key risk factors?*

A: Difficulty achieving an erection can be caused by any number of factors, either physical, psychological, or a combination of the two. A number of medical conditions are known to cause ED, including some arterosclerosis, heart and vascular diseases, diabetes, prostate conditions including enlargement and cancer, disease affecting the nerves and brain (e.g. multiple sclerosis, Parkinson's disease, Alzeimer's disease), and vascular conditions that affect blood vessels and circulation.

Unhealthy living-excessive stress, obesity and poor nutrition lack of exercise tobacco use, excessive alcohol consumption and drug use, among other-s can lead to ED. It's also a potential side effect resulting from a number of prescription medications, medical procedures and surgeries.

Age also plays a role; studies show ED affects about one out of 20 men aged 40, but about one out of four men aged 65.

ED can also be a symptom of a potential undiagnosed medical condition; which is one of many reasons why it is important for men to talk to their doctor about ED.

Q: *What treatment options are most effective?*

A: There has been tremendous progress in the number and effectiveness of treatments of ED. The best treatments include medications (taken orally), penile implants, and penile pumps. Doctors often recommend lifestyle modifications such as exercise, smoking cessation, and stress reduction, all of which help improve erectile function and overall health.

Q: *What advice should be given to men who may be suffering from ED but are reluctant to seek help?*

A: Men should know that it's normal feel anxious about talking to your doctor about ED. Men have always been less likely than women to make regular doctor visits, and there's a stigma in almost every society that men should be able to handle their problems by themselves, and that feeling vulnerable or seeking help is a sign of weakness.

Doctors have been successfully treating men with ED for many years. With even more effective treatment option available now, whatever anxiety men may feel about seeking help always pales in comparison to the anxiety and potentially serious medical problems that can result from not seeking help.

PET/CT

Every year, cancer claims the lives of millions of people. It continues to be a leading cause of death among Thais. But it doesn't have to be that way. Many types of cancer are treatable and curable if detected early.

Recent advances in technology are helping detect cancerous cells earlier and with greater precision and accuracy, making it possible to save potentially millions of lives. One of the most exciting innovations in cancer detection is PET/CT (Position Emission Tomograph/Computed Tomograph) technology. In the few short years since its introduction, PET/CT has become one of the most highly effective tools for early detection of cancerous cells.

PET/CT provides an anatomical map of the body with 64 slices per revolution in only 0.33 seconds. It produces high resolution 2-dimensional and 3-dimensional images capable of revealing even tiny traces of cancerous tissue—as small as 3 millimeters in size. Its effectiveness helps doctors to plan medical treatments and scheduled suitable to each patient individually.

Dr. Narongsak Kiatikajornthada, Hematology and Oncology specialist at Bumrungrad International Hospital, explains how PET/CT technology is used to pinpoint the exact location and size of tumors and to quickly determine the exact stage of cancer. "The procedure begins with an injection of FDG, an analog of glucose that is tagged to the radionuclide F 18," Dr. Naraongsak says. "Tumors trap more FDG than other organs, so PET/CT can identify gamma rays in the rapidly growing tumors. This helps doctors to detect and diagnose cancer faster and easier."

The scanner pinpoints the exact location of tumors that may have gone unnoticed by other CT or MRI diagnostic tools. Besides cancer, PET/CT can also detect some brain diseases such as Alzheimer's disease and epilepsy.

With early detection being among the most important factors for successful cancer treatment, Bumrungrad patients are already reaping significant benefits through more successful and less traumatic treatment regimens.

NEW INTERNATIONAL CLINIC

Following its July 31 grand opening, the brand new 53,000-square meter Bumrungrad International Clinic is now delivering an unrivaled patient experience in a warm, comfortable and friendly environment.

The 22-storey building was designed to be the ideal place for patients and doctors to meet for consultation and medical services. The clinic is equipped with world-class medical technology and equipment and offers a full range of facilities, including spacious lobby and seating areas, an international food centre, retail shops, and a lounge for Bumrungrad patients and Healthy Living Club Members.

The Bumrungrad International Clinic delivers on its promise of a one-stop, one-location service with ease and convenience from start to finish. New technology delivers more streamlined patient registration and online medical records availability. More convenience is offered with diagnostic imaging services available right inside patient consultation rooms, and expanded laboratory automation to provide faster and more accurate test results. Patients can even pay their bills and pick-up prescribed medicine on the same floor.

With the opening of the new outpatient building. Bumrungrad International is Thailand's largest private hospital, with 250 outpatient consultation rooms and the capacity to welcome upto 6,000 patients each day.

The Bumrungrad International Clinic incorporates many medical services and specialist centres, including:

- Medical Coordination Centre
- Health Screening Centre
- Respiratory Efficiency Testing
- Rehabilitation Centre
- Surgical Clinic
- Men Centre
- Endocrinology Services
- Nutrition therapy
- Diagnostic radiology
- Heart Centre
- Dialysis.
- Specialists in infectious disease, lung disease, internal medicine, allergies, orthopedics and rheumatism, hematology, urology, neurology, neurosurgery and breast surgery.

Bumrungrad International now serves more than 12 million Thai and International patients each year from 190 countries all over the world and is acknowledged as a pioneer in Medical Tourism. More recently, The Wall Street Journal Asia named Bumrungrad one of the best companies in Thailand.

WELLNESS PROGRAMMES; VITALLIFE

Anti-Aging Programs

A thoughtful anti-aging program will lead to optimal health.

It is a way to manage health risks so you can be sure that you are as healthy as can be.

The VitaLlife approach is an integrated and personalized plan that combines nutritional, hormonal, and physical therapies to slow the aging process and improve your functionality.

Make it your way to a longer and healthier life.

I. EXECUTIVE ANTI-AGING

Consultations

- Physician: Anti-Aging Medicine
- Physician: Functional Medicine
- Physician: Sports Medicine
- Registered: Dietician

Laboratory Evaluations

- *Antioxidants*

  Vitamin C (Ascorbate), Vitamin A (Retinol), Vitamin E (Alpha-Tocopherol), Gamma-Tocopherol, Beta-Carotene, Alpha-Carotene, Coenzyme Q 10 (Ubiquinone), Lycopene

- *Vitamins and Minerals*

  Folate (Vitamin B9), Vitamin B12, Chromium Copper, Ferritin, Magnesium, Selenium, Zinc

- *Hormones*

  LH, FSH, Estradiol, Testosterone*, Progesterone**, TSH, Free T3, Free T4, DHEA-S

- *General*

  Complete Blood Count (CBC)

- *Inflammatory Markers*

  ESR, CRP

- *Cardiac Profile*

  Cholesterol, Triglycerides, HDL, LDL (calc)

- *Insulin Resistance*

  Fasting Plasma Glucose (FPG), Insulin

- *Liver and Kidney Function*

  AST, ALT, Alkaline phosphatase, Creatinine

- *Gout*

  Uric Acid

- *Tumor Markers*

  CEA, AFP, PSA

- *Other Laboratory Evaluations*

  Urine Analysis (UA), Stool Analysis

Investigations

- Bio-Physical Assessment
- Chest X-Ray
- EKG
- Bone Scan (hip and spine)
- Ultrasound of the Whole Abdomen
- Ultrasound of the Prostate (trans-rectal)*
- Mammogram with ultrasound breast**
- Pap Smear**

THB 35,000 (Female)
THB 34,000 (Male)
* Male only
** Female only

2. COMPREHENSIVE ANTI-AGING

Consultations

- Physician: Anti-Aging Medicine
- Physician: Functional Medicine
- Physician: Sports Medicine
- Registered: Dietician

Laboratory Evaluations

- *Antioxidants*

Vitamin C (Ascorbate), Vitamin A (Retinol), Vitamin E (Alpha-Tocopherol), Gamma-Tocopherol, Beta-Carotene, Alpha-Carotene, Coenzyme Q 10 (Ubiquinone), Lycopene

- *Vitamins and Minerals*

Folate (Vitamin B9), Vitamin B12, Chromium Copper, Ferritin, Magnesium, Selenium, Zinc

- *Hormones*

LH, FSH, Estradiol, Testosterone*, Progesterone*, TSH, Free T3, Free T4, DHEA-S, IGF-1

- *General*

Complete Blood Count (CBC)

- *Inflammatory Markers*

ESR, CRP

- *Cardiac Profile*

Cholesterol, Triglycerides, HDL, LDL (calc)

- *Insulin Resistance*
  Fasting Plasma Glucose (FPG), Insulin

- *Liver and Kidney Function*
  AST, ALT, Total Bilirubin, Alkaline Phosphatase, Albumin, BUN, Creatinine

- *Gout*
  Uric Acid

- *Iron Study*
  Serum Iron, Ferritin

- *Tumor Markers*
  CEA, AFP, PSA*

- *Special Laboratory Evaluations*
  Oxidative Damage Markers
  MDA (Malonyldiadehyde)
  Carbonyl Proteins
  Allantoins
  80HdG (8-Hydroxy deoxyguanosine)
  Gluathione
  Essential and Metabolic Fatty Acids
  Omega 3, Omega 6, Omega 9,
  Saturated Fatty Acids
  Even Carbon Atom Fatty Acids
  Urinary Organic Acids
  Functional Deficit of Vitamins
  Metabolite Indicators of Energy Production
  Gut Dysbiosis Markers
  Sulfate Detoxification
  Neurotransmitters

- *Other Laboratory Evaluations*
  Urine Analysis (UA), Stool Analysis.

Investigations

- Bio-Physical Assessment
- Chest X-Ray
- EKG
- DEXA Scan (whole body)

Body Fat Analysis

Bone Mineral Density

- Ultrasound of the Whole Abdomen
- Ultrasound of the Prostate (Trans-rectal)*

- Mammogram with ultrasound breast**
- Pap Smear**

THB 69,000 (Female)
THB 68,000 (Male)
* Male only
** Female only
A healthy body is one in biochemical balance with nature.

A personalized VitalLife supplement program will replenish your body's reserves, strengthen your immune system, and make up for deficiencies that come from poor diet or a hectic daily schedule.

We custom design and compound nutritional supplements to ensure your body has the right balance of vitamins, minerals, and antioxidants to achieve peak physical and mental performance.

I. ANTIOXIDANTS

Consultations

- Physician: Functional Medicine

Laboratory Evaluations

- *Antioxidants*

Vitamin C (Ascorbate), Vitamin A (Retinol), Vitamin E (Alpha-Tocopherol), Gamma-Tocopherol, Beta-Carotene, Alpha-Carotene, Coenzyme Q10 (Ubiquinone), Lycopene

THB 5,800

2. MICRONUTRIENTS

Consultations

- Physician: Functional Medicine

Laboratory Evaluations

- *Antioxidants*

Vitamin C (Ascorbate), Vitamin A (Retinol), Vitamin E (Alpha-Tocopherol), Gamma-Tocopherol, Beta-Carotene, Alpha-Carotene, Coenzyme Q10 (Ubiquinone), Lycopene.

- *Vitamins and Minerals*

Folate (Vitamin B9), Vitamin B12, Chromium Copper, Ferritin, Magnesium, Selenium, Zinc

THB 9,200

3. ANTIOXIDANTS-LIFESTYLE

Consultations

- Physician: Functional Medicine
- Physician: Sports Medicine
- Registered Dietician

Laboratory Evaluations

- *Antioxidants*

Vitamin C (Ascorbate), Vitamin A (Retinol), Vitamin E (Alpha-Tocopherol), Gamma-Tocopherol, Beta-Carotene, Alpha-Carotene, Coenzyme Q10 (Ubiquinone), Lycopene.

Investigation

- *Bio-Physical Age Assessment*

THB 10,300

4. MICRONUTRIENTS-LIFESTYLE

Consultations

- Physician: Functional Medicine
- Physician: Sports Medicine
- Registered Dietician

Laboratory Evaluations

- *Antioxidants*

Vitamin C (Ascorbate), Vitamin A (Retinol), Vitamin E (Alpha-Tocopherol), Gamma-Tocopherol, Beta-Carotene, Alpha-Carotene, Coenzyme Q10 (Ubiquinone), Lycopene.

- *Vitamins and Minerals*

Folate (Vitamin B9), Vitamin B12, Chromium, Copper, Ferritin, Magnesium, Selenium, Zinc.

Investigation

- *Bio-Physical Age Assessment*

THB 13,700

5. EXECUTIVE WELLNESS

Consultations

- Physician: Functional Medicine
- Physician: Sports Medicine
- Registered Dietician

Laboratory Evaluations

- *Antioxidants*

Vitamin C (Ascorbate), Vitamin A (Retinol), Vitamin E (Alpha-Tocopherol), Gamma-Tocopherol, Beta-Carotene, Alpha-Carotene, Coenzyme Q10 (Ubiquinone), Lycopene.

- *Vitamins and Minerals*

Folate (Vitamin B9), Vitamin B12, Chromium, Copper, Ferritin, Magnesium, Selenium, Zinc.

- *General*

Complete Body Count (CBC), Fasting Plasma Glucose (FPG).

- *Inflammatory Markers*

ESR, CRP

- *Cardiac Profile*

Cholesterol, Triglycerides, HDL, LDL (calc)

- *Liver and Kidney Function*

AST, ALT, Alkaline Phosphatase, Creatinine

- *Gout*

Uric Acid

- *Tumor Markers*

CEA, AFP

- *Other Laboratory Evaluations*

Urine Analysis (UA), Stool Analysis.

Investigation

- Bio-Physical Age Assessment
- Chest X-Ray, EKG, Ultrasound of the Whole Abdomen

THB 19,500

6. COMPREHENSIVE WELLNESS

Consultations

- Physician: Functional Medicine
- Physician: Sports Medicine
- Registered Dietician

Laboratory Evaluations

- *Antioxidants*

  Vitamin C (Ascorbate), Vitamin A (Retinol), Vitamin E (Alpha-Tocopherol), Gamma-Tocopherol, Beta-Carotene, Alpha-Carotene, Coenzyme Q10 (Ubiquinone), Lycopene.

- *Vitamins and Minerals*

  Folate (Vitamin B9), Vitamin B12, Chromium, Copper, Ferritin, Magnesium, Selenium, Zinc.

- *General*

  Complete Body Count (CBC).

- *Inflammatory Markers*

  ESR, CRP

- *Cardiac Profile*

  Cholesterol, Triglycerides, HDL, LDL (calc)

- *Insulin Resistance*

  Fasting Plasma Glucose (FPG), Insulin

- *Liver and Kidney Function*

  AST, ALT, Total Bilirubin, Alkaline Phosphatase, Albumin, BUN, Creatinine

- *Gout*

  Uric Acid

- *Iron Study*

  Serum iron, Ferritin

- *Tumor Markers*

  CEA, AFP

- *Special Laboratory Evaluations*

  Oxidative Damage Markers

  MDA, Carbonyl Proteins, Allantoins, 80HdG, Glutathione

  Essential and Metabolic Fatty Acids

  Omega 3, Omega 6, Omega 9, Saturated Fatty Acids, Even Carbon Atom Fatty Acids

  Urinary Organic Acids

  Functional Deficit of Vitamins, Indicators of Energy Production, Gut Dysbiosis Markers, Sulfate Detoxification, Neurotransmitters

- *Other Laboratory Evaluations*
  Urine Analysis (UA), Stool Analysis

Investigation

- Bio-Physical Age Assessment
- Chest X-Ray, EKG, DEXA Scan (whole body), Ultrasound of the Whole Abdomen

THB 54,000

Weight-Loss Programs

The VitalLife weight loss program is designed to help you lose pounds but not feel hungry... to keep your energy levels up without stimulants!

Our system begins with a thorough diagnosis of your weight status and the reasons for it. Then we will prescribe nutritional supplements just right for you. Enjoy the VitalLife food supplements, and after you have reached your goals, we will give you a maintenance plan to keep you looking and feeling your best.

I. WEIGHT LOSS INITIAL SCREENING

Consultations

- Physician

Laboratory Evaluations

- Complete Blood Count (CBC)
- Serum Iron
- Thyroid Function

TSH, Free T4, Free T3

- Insulin Resistance

FPG, Insulin

- Cardiac Profile

Cholesterol, Triglycerides, HDL, LDL (Calc)

- Liver Function

AST, ALT, Alkaline Phosphatase

- Kidney Function

BUN, Creatinine

- Electrolytes

Sodium, Potassium, Chloride, Bicarbonate

- Uric Acid, Calcium
- Urinary Microalbumin/Creatinine Ratio

Investigations

- EKG
- Dexa Scan

Body fat analysis

Bone mineral density

THB 10,000

2. HIPRO RAPID WEIGHT LOSS

HiPro—4 Month Program
1 month Hi-Pro Rapid Weight Loss
3 months Maintenance

Consultations

•Physician	5 sessions
•Exercise Physician	6 sessions
•Registered Dietician	7 sessions
Investigations	
• Blood Tests	2
• Urine Tests	2
• DEXA Scan	1
Supplements	
• Nutraceuticals	4 months supply
• VitalLife Functional Food	1 months supply
(Protein Shakes)	
THB 58,000	
HiPro—5 Months Program	
2 months	Hi-Pro Rapid Weight Loss
3 months	Maintenance
Consultations	
• Physician	7 sessions
• Exercise Physician	6 sessions
• Registered Dietician	7 sessions
Investigations	
• Blood Tests	4
• Urine Tests	4
• DEXA Scan	2
• EKG	1
Supplements	
• Nutraceuticals	5 months supply
• VitalLife Functional Food	2 months supply
(Protein Shakes)	
THB 88,000	
HiPro—6 Month Program	
3 months	Hi-Pro Rapid Weight Loss
3 months	Maintenance
Consultations	
• Physician	9 sessions
• Exercise Physician	6 sessions
• Registered Dietician	7 sessions
Investigations	
• Blood Tests	7
• Urine Tests	6
• DEXA Scan	2
• EKG	2

Supplements

• Nutraceuticals	6 months supply
• VitalLife Functional Food (Protein Shakes)	3 months supply

THB 118,000

3. FOUR MONTHS WEIGHT LOSS PROGRAM

Consultations

• Physician	1 session
• Exercise Physician	5 sessions
• Registered Dietician	5 sessions

Investigations

• Blood Tests	1
• DEXA Scan	1

Supplements

• Nutraceuticals	4 months supply

THB 42,000

4. TAILORED WEIGHT LOSS PROGRAMS FOR SPECIAL NEEDS

For individuals who are not residents of Bangkok and need to return home after the screening test.

Consultation with
• Physician via e-mail or telephone
Supplements
• As prescribed
Price based on actual

Vitality Programs

Hormone replacement therapy results in a more active and VitalLife.

It counters the effects of andropause in men and menopause in women. A hormone replacement program increases sexual desire and fulfilment, generates a higher level of motivation, and helps you be more focused and affirmative in your daily decision-making.

We start with a comprehensive screening to know your levels of wellness, prescribe an appropriate program designed specifically for you.... then monitor your state of wellness on a regular basis so that you maintain maximum vitality.

Signs and Symptoms of Hormone Deficiency

Male

- Fatigue, loss of energy
- Loss of memory or concentration
- Loss of sex drive or libido
- Loss of morning erections or sexual performance
- Backache, joint pains or stiffness
- Loss of fitness

- Depression, lacking motivation
- Irritability, anger or bad temper
- Anxiety or nervousness
- Feeling over-stressed

Female

- Hot flashes and sweats
- Lethargy, loss of energy
- Depression, moodiness
- Tension, irritability, anxiety
- Loss of memory or concentration
- Headaches
- Droopy breasts
- Loss of sex drive or libido
- Vaginal dryness, urinary symptoms
- Hair and skin changes

1. VITALITY

Consultations

- Physician : Anti-Aging Medicine

Laboratory Evaluations

- Hormones

LH, FSH, Estradiol, Testosterone*, Progesterone**, DHEA-S

- General

Complete Blood Count (CBC)

- Liver Function

AST, ALT

- Tumor Marker

PSA*

- Other Laboratory Evaluation

Urine Analysis (UA)

Investigations

- EKG
- Bone scan (hip and spine)
- Ultrasound of the Prostate (trans-rectal)*
- Mammogram with ultrasound breast**
- Pap Smear**

THB 13,000 (Female)

THB 12,000 (Male)

2. VITALITY-LIFESTYLE

Consultations

- Physician : Anti-Aging Medicine
- Physician : Sports Medicine
- Registered Dietician

Laboratory Evaluations

- Hormones

LH, FSH, Estradiol, Testosterone*, Progesterone**, DHEA-S
• General
Complete Blood Count (CBC)
• Liver Function
AST, ALT
• Tumor Marker
PSA*
• Other Laboratory Evaluation
Urine Analysis (UA)
Investigations
• EKG
• Bio-Physical Age Assessment
• Bone scan (hip and spine)
• Ultrasound of the Prostate (trans-rectal)*
• Mammogram with ultrasound breast**
• Pap Smear**
THB 17,000 (Female)
THB 16,000 (Male)

3. EXECUTIVE VITALITY
Consultations
• Physician : Anti-Aging Medicine
• Physician : Sports Medicine
• Registered Dietician
Laboratory Evaluations
• Hormones
LH, FSH, Estradiol, Testosterone*, Progesterone**, TSH, Free T3, Free T4, DHEA-S, IGF-1
• General
Complete Blood Count (CBC), Fasting Plasma Glucose (FPG)
• Cardiac Profile
Cholesterol, Triglycerides, HDL, LDL (calc)
• Liver and Kidney Function
AST, ALT, Alkaline Phosphatase, Creatinine
• Gout
Uric Acid
• Tumor Marker
CEA, AFP, PSA*
• Other Laboratory Evaluations
Urine Analysis (UA), Stool Analysis
Investigations
• Bio-Physical Age Assessment
• Chest X-Ray
• EKG
• Bone scan (hip and spine)
• Ultrasound of the Whole Abdomen

- Ultrasound of the Prostate (trans-rectal)*
- Mammogram with ultrasound breast**
- Pap Smear**

THB 24,000 (Female)
THB 23,000 (Male)

4. HORMONE SCREENING PANEL

Consultations
- Physician : Anti-Aging Medicine

Laboratory Evaluations
- Hormones

LH, FSH, Estradiol, Testosterone*, Progesterone**, TSH, Free T3, Free T4, DHEA-S, IGF-1

THB 9,000
*Male only
**Female only

HEALTHY LIVING CLUB

Bumrungrad International hospital offers the Healthy Living Club program to provide affordable international-standard health care with additional privileges.

Care benefits

Register for a Main Membership Card and pay only 6,300 baht for 3 years and receive a privilege coupon for the Executive Health Check-up program valued at 6,300 baht. You are then eligible for a Supplementary Card for any member of your family for only 3,000 baht for 3 years and receive an additional privilege coupon worth 3,000 baht towards an Executive or Comprehensive Check-up.

Value benefits

For inpatients	:	30% discount for an inpatient room*
For outpatients	:	15% discount for medicine and medical supplies**, Laboratory Test***, X-ray

Remarks: Discounts exclude doctors' consultation fees and special medical equipment.

* Except meals, nursing services and other services
** Except special medicine such as Chemotherapy
*** Except special lab

Members are eligible for outpatient discounts upon registration. Inpatient discounts may be received starting 7 days after registration.

Convenience benefits

- Free access to Wi-Fi internet

- Access to the Napa Lounge in the Bumrungrad Clinic building
- Receive Better Health magazine, delivered to your home free
- Pre-booking privileges for our public health seminars
- Other additional privilege programs are offered to members only.

*Other benefits**

Get special discount privileges from retailers at Bumrungrad, such as Booskorn Flower Shop, New City, Baby and Children, Get The Books, Ayame Japanese restaurant and Portofino Italian Restaurant. Also get special giveaway privileges when purchasing food and beverages at Au Bon Pain and McDonald's.

CONCLUSION

The hospital is providing preventive, promotive and curative services efficiently and promptly. The reasons for this are:

(a) Patient centreed approach.
(b) Excellent staff.
(c) A combination of preventive and curative approach.
(d) Subsidized services to weaker sections.
(e) High Tech specialized centres.
(f) Special arrangements to foreigners.

Index